FOURTH EDITION

Becoming a Helper

Marianne Schneider Corey
Private Practice/Consultant

Gerald Corey
California State University, Fullerton
Diplomate in Counseling Psychology,
American Board of Professional Psychology

BROOKS/COLE
™
THOMSON LEARNING

Australia • Canada • Mexico • Singapore • Spain • United Kingdom • United States

BROOKS/COLE

THOMSON LEARNING ™

Sponsoring Editor: *Julie Martinez*
Editorial Assistant: *Catherine Broz*
Assistant Editor: *Shelley Gesicki*
Marketing: *Caroline Concilla/Megan Hansen/ Tami Strang*
Production Editor: *Tessa Avila*
Production Service: *The Cooper Company*

Manuscript Editor: *Kay Mikel*
Cover Design: *Lisa Henry*
Cover Image: *José Ortega*
Indexer: *Mimi Lawson*
Print Buyer: *Vena Dyer*
Typesetting: *Scratchgravel*
Printing and Binding: *WebCom, Ltd.*

For more information about this or any other Brooks/Cole product, contact:
BROOKS/COLE
511 Forest Lodge Road
Pacific Grove, CA 93950 USA
www.brookscole.com
1-800-423-0563 (Thomson Learning Academic Resource Center)

Printed in Canada

10   9   8   7   6   5   4   3   2   1

Library of Congress Cataloging-in-Publication Data

Corey, Marianne Schneider.
  Becoming a helper / Marianne Schneider Corey, Gerald Corey.—4th ed.
    p. cm.
  Includes bibliographical references (p.) and index.
  ISBN 0-534-35614-1
    1. Human services—Vocational guidance—United States. 2. Social service—Vocational guidance—United States. I. Corey, Gerald. Becoming a helper. II. Title.

HV10.5 .C67   2001
361.3'2'02373—dc21

                                                                    2001052548

To you, our readers.

May you make a significant difference

in the lives of others.

Photography by Dawn Harman

MARIANNE SCHNEIDER COREY is a licensed marriage and family therapist in California and is a National Certified Counselor. She received her master's degree in marriage, family, and child counseling from Chapman College. She is a Fellow of the Association for Specialists in Group Work (ASGW) and was the recipient of ASGW's Eminent Career Award in 2001. She also holds memberships in the American Counseling Association; the Association for Spiritual, Ethical, and Religious Values in Counseling; the Association for Counselor Education and Supervision (both national and regional); the Western Psychological Association; and the Association for Specialists in Group Work.

Marianne has been actively involved in leading groups for different populations, providing training and supervision workshops in group process, facilitating a self-exploration group for graduate students in counseling, and co-facilitating training groups for group counselors and weeklong residential workshops in personal growth. She sees groups as the most effective format in which to work with clients and finds it the most rewarding for her personally. With her husband, Jerry, Marianne has conducted training workshops, continuing-education seminars, and personal-growth groups in Germany, Ireland, Belgium, Mexico, and China, as well as regularly doing these workshops in the United States. In her free time Marianne enjoys traveling, reading, visiting with friends, and hiking.

Marianne has co-authored several articles in group work, as well as the following books (published by Brooks/Cole/Thomson Learning):

- *Issues and Ethics in the Helping Professions,* Sixth Edition (2003, with Gerald Corey and Patrick Callanan)
- *Groups: Process and Practice*, Sixth Edition (2002, with Gerald Corey)
- *I Never Knew I Had a Choice,* Seventh Edition (2002, with Gerald Corey)
- *Group Techniques,* Second Edition (1992, with Gerald Corey, Patrick Callanan, and J. Michael Russell)
- *Becoming a Helper,* Fourth Edition (2003, with Gerald Corey)

Marianne has made several videos (with accompanying student workbooks) for Brooks/Cole: *Ethics in Action* CD-ROM (Student Version); *Ethics in Action* (Institutional Version); and *The Evolution of a Group.*

Marianne and Jerry have been married since 1964. They have two adult daughters, Heidi and Cindy. Marianne grew up in Germany and keeps in close contact with her family there.

About the Authors

GERALD COREY is Professor Emeritus of Human Services at California State University at Fullerton. He received his doctorate in counseling from the University of Southern California. He is a Diplomate in Counseling Psychology, American Board of Professional Psychology; a licensed psychologist; a National Certified Counselor; a Fellow of the American Psychological Association (Counseling Psychology); and a Fellow of the Association for Specialists in Group Work.

Jerry received the Outstanding Professor of the Year Award from California State University at Fullerton in 1991, and was the recipient of the Association for Specialists in Group Work's Eminent Career Award in 2001. He teaches both undergraduate and graduate courses in group counseling, as well as courses in experiential groups, the theory and practice of counseling, and ethics in counseling practice. With his colleagues he has conducted workshops in the United States, Canada, Germany, Ireland, Belgium, Scotland, Mexico, and China, with a special focus on training in group counseling. He often presents workshops for professional organizations, special intensive courses at various universities, and residential training and supervision workshops for group leaders. In his leisure time, Jerry likes to travel, hike and bicycle in the mountains, and drive his 1931 Model A Ford.

In addition to five books Jerry Corey co-authored with Marianne Schneider Corey, other recent publications, all with Brooks/Cole/Thomson Learning, include:

- *Theory and Practice of Counseling and Psychotherapy*, Sixth Edition (and *Manual*) (2001)
- *Case Approach to Counseling and Psychotherapy*, Fifth Edition (2001)
- *The Art of Integrative Counseling* (2001)
- *Theory and Practice of Group Counseling*, Fifth Edition (and *Manual*) (2000)

Jerry is co-author, with his daughters Cindy Corey and Heidi Jo Corey, of an orientation-to-college book entitled *Living and Learning* (1997), published by Wadsworth. He is also co-author (with Barbara Herlihy) of *Boundary Issues in Counseling: Multiple Roles and Responsibilities* (1997) and *ACA Ethical Standards Casebook*, Fifth Edition (1996), both published by the American Counseling Association.

He has also made three videos on various aspects of counseling practice: (1) *Student Video and Workbook for the Art of Integrative Counseling* (2001, with Robert Haynes); (2) *The Evolution of a Group: Student Video and Workbook* (2000, with Marianne Schneider Corey and Robert Haynes); and (3) *Ethics in Action* CD-ROM (Student Version) (2003, with Marianne Schneider Corey and Robert Haynes). All of these student videos and workbooks are available through Brooks/Cole.

Contents

CHAPTER **3**

Helper, Know Thyself   65

CHAPTER **4**

Understanding Life Transitions   87

CHAPTER **5**

Stages in the Helping Process   108

CHAPTER **6**

Common Concerns of Beginning Helpers   *139*

CHAPTER **7**

Values and the Helping Relationship   *165*

CHAPTER **8**

Cultural Diversity in the Helping Professions   *189*

CHAPTER **9**

Ethical and Legal Issues Facing Helpers 214

CHAPTER **10**

Managing Boundary Issues 252

CHAPTER **11**

Working in the Community 278

CHAPTER **12**

Understanding Special Populations   *300*

CHAPTER **13**

Working With Groups and Families   *322*

CHAPTER **14**

Stress and Burnout   *343*

CHAPTER **15**

Take Care of Yourself   *364*

Preface

Many books deal with the skills, theories, and techniques of helping. Yet few books concentrate on the problems involved in becoming an effective helper or focus on the personal difficulties in working with others. In writing this book, we had in mind both students who are planning a career in human services, counseling, psychology, couples and family therapy, social work, or related professions and helpers who have just begun their careers. We intend this book to be used as a supplement to textbooks dealing with helping skills and with counseling theory and practice. Earlier editions of *Becoming a Helper* have proved useful for introductory classes in human services, social work, and counseling as well as classes in practicum, fieldwork, and internship.

We focus on the struggles, anxieties, and uncertainties of helpers. In addition, we explore in depth the demands and strains of the helping professions and their effects on the provider. We begin with a discussion of the motivations for seeking a career in the helping professions. We encourage our readers to examine their personal motives and needs for helping, and we challenge them to be honest in assessing what they will get from their work. We challenge students to take a proactive stance in their educational program. Being active applies to selecting field placements and internships as well as getting the most from supervision. Therefore, we offer some practical strategies for ensuring quality experiences in fieldwork and profiting from supervision.

We discuss the importance of helpers knowing themselves and encourage readers to explore their family-of-origin experiences, focusing on how earlier relationships continue to influence the quality of later ones. We look at how helpers deal with their own life transitions and discuss the implications of this process when working with the clients' life crises.

We provide an overview of the stages of the helping process, with a brief discussion of the skills and knowledge required to be a successful agent at each of these stages. The focus of this discussion is not on skill development but on the personal characteristics that enable helpers to be effective. Because helpers ask clients to examine their behavior to understand themselves more fully, we ask helpers to be equally committed to an awareness of their own lives. Without a high level of self-awareness, a helper may obstruct clients' progress, especially when these clients are struggling with issues the helper has avoided facing.

Beginning and seasoned helpers encounter common problems in their work related to dealing with resistance, transference and countertransference, and clients who are challenging. Forming a sense of ethical awareness and learning to resolve professional dilemmas is a task facing all helpers. We raise a number of challenges surrounding current ethical issues as a way to sensitize readers to the intricacies of ethical decision making and managing boundaries.

We explore the belief systems of helpers and discuss the positive and negative effects that a variety of beliefs and assumptions can have on one's practice. Values are an integral part of the client-helper relationship, and we devote considerable attention to an analysis of how values influence helping. We develop the thesis that the job of helpers is not to impose values but to help clients define their own value system. Special consideration is given to understanding and working with culturally diverse populations.

We also deal with understanding one's role as a helper in the community; we discuss the group process and the value of working with groups and families in human services work. Other topics covered in the book are stress and burnout and ways to stay alive and vital, both as a person and as a professional.

Although this book should be useful to any student planning to enter the helping professions, our backgrounds are in the field of counseling, and this orientation comes through in our approach. Therefore, those who want to work in the counseling aspects of the human services are likely to find this book especially meaningful. We have tried to write a personal book that will stimulate both thought and action. At the end of each chapter we encourage readers to commit to some specific action that will move them closer to their goals.

New in This Edition

Whenever possible, new references have been added to bring discussions up to date; in this fourth edition, more than 160 references have been added. Three new chapters have been added and several chapters have been reorganized and largely rewritten. A new feature, InfoTrac College Edition Resources, has been provided at the end of each chapter. Students will be able to access additional information on chapter topics on the Internet using this resource. Exercises from the *Ethics in Action* CD-ROM have been incorporated in the chapter activities for Chapters 7, 8, 9, and 10.

Chapter 3, Helper, Know Thyself, is new to this edition and includes an expanded discussion on how your family of origin influences you and your approach to helping. Chapter, 10, Managing Boundary Issues, is also new and reflects the ongoing debate among helpers regarding relationships with clients and former clients, accepting gifts from clients, and sexual attraction in the helping relationship. The third new chapter is Chapter 12, Understanding Special Populations. This chapter addresses the problems helpers face with clients who are HIV-positive or who have AIDS, clients with disabilities, and clients who are elderly.

In addition, the chapters on values and ethics in the helping professions have been reorganized and expanded to include discussions about religion and spirituality, value conflicts between helper and client, the importance of seeking consultation when dealing with difficult clients, the ethics of working in a managed care environment, and a thoughtful look at helping clients make end-of-life decisions. Throughout the book we have kept the focus on how helpers may be affected by the problems they face and the choices they make in service to their clients.

Supplements

Instructor's Resource Manual

This edition has available an *Instructor's Resource Manual.* It contains suggestions for teaching the course, course objectives, key terms, class activities to stimulate interest, transparency masters, and a bank of test items, discussion questions, and online test items. Included are many multiple-choice, true-false, matching, and short essay questions from which the instructor can choose.

Codes of Ethics for the Helping Professions

Each of the major mental health professional organizations has its own code of ethics. The codes listed at the end of Chapter 9 are available as a package, which can be purchased at a nominal cost as an accompanying supplement to this textbook. We recommend that you familiarize yourself with the basic standards for ethical practice of the various mental health professions. Codes of ethics for specific organizations also can be accessed through the Internet or by contacting the professional organizations directly.

Ethics in Action CD-ROM *(Student Version)*

A new integrated learning package designed to enhance the fourth edition of *Becoming a Helper,* entitled *Ethics in Action* CD-ROM (Student Version), can be bundled with this textbook. This new CD-ROM is designed to bring to life, through video role-play segments, the ethical issues and dilemmas that helpers often encounter. The program provides ample opportunity for discussion, self-exploration, and problem solving through self-inventories and exercises designed for interactive learning geared directly to the vignettes shown.

    Ethics in Action CD-ROM is divided into three parts: Ethical Decision Making, Values and the Helping Relationship, and Boundary Issues and Multiple Relationships. This interactive self-study program challenges students to deal with the complexity of ethical issues and encourages reflection on their perspectives on each of the issues presented. By viewing the video and completing the exercises, students will be in a better position to get involved in class discussions. The more students become involved in this learning package, the more their understanding of ethical practice will be enhanced.

    Ethics in Action CD-ROM (Student Version) is available from Brooks/Cole and can be purchased at a discount when packaged with *Becoming a Helper.*

Acknowledgments

A number of reviewers provided insightful comments and reacted to the fourth edition, and we would like to thank them. They include Mary Jo Blazek, University of Maine at Augusta; Jamie Bludworth, doctoral student, Arizona State University; Phil Durrant, Niagara College, Ontario, Canada; Susan Ericksen, Utah State

University; Allen Ivey, University of Massachusetts; Bette Katsekas, University of Southern Maine; and Howard Rosenthal, St. Louis Community College.

We want to thank George Williams of The Citadel for his review of *Becoming a Helper*, and as well we thank the following students in his class who provided thoughtful comments and suggestions: Leslie Dunlap, Suzan Familia, Sara Ray, Kelley Richardson, Tusha Richardson, and Amy Subryd. We also thank Conrad Fuentes and Galo Arboleda of California State University at Fullerton, who had their students write reactions to our book, and Susan Ericksen's students at Utah State University.

The following individuals provided us with prerevision reviews, which were most valuable in helping us shape this edition: Patricia Cianciolo, Northern Michigan University; James Colangelo, Long Island University; Rob Lawson, Western Washington University; Judy Miranti, Our Lady of the Holy Cross; Richard Watts, Baylor University at Waco; and Guy Wylie, Western Nebraska Community College.

The members of the Brooks/Cole team continue to offer support for all our projects. It is a delight to work with a dedicated staff of professionals who go out of their way to give their best. These people include Julie Martinez, the editor of counseling and human services; Cat Broz, who coordinated the reviewing process; Tessa Avila, the production manager on the project; Cecile Joyner of the Cooper Company, the production editor; and Kay Mikel, the manuscript editor of this edition, whose fine editorial assistance kept this book reader friendly. We appreciate Mimi Lawson's work in compiling the index.

Marianne Schneider Corey
Gerald Corey

CHAPTER *1*

Are the Helping Professions for You?

Focus Questions

Aim of the Chapter

Examining Your Motives for Becoming a Helper

Our Own Beginnings as Helpers

A Helping Career Is Not for Everyone

Portrait of the "Ideal Helper"

*Selecting a Professional Program
and Career Path*

*Self-Assessment: An Inventory of Your
Attitudes and Beliefs About Helping*

By Way of Review

What Will You Do Now?

InfoTrac College Edition Resources

Focus Questions

1. What has attracted you to the helping professions? Who in your life has been instrumental in your decision to consider this role for yourself?

2. What is your main motivation for wanting to be a helper? What personal needs of yours are likely to be met through your work as a helper?

3. Think of a time when you very much needed help from a significant person in your life or from a counselor. What did you most want from this person? What did he or she do that was either a help or a hindrance to you?

4. Think about the attributes of an effective helper. What are a few traits or characteristics that you would identify as being the most important?

5. At this time in your life, how prepared (from a personal standpoint) do you feel you are to enter one of the helping professions? If you were applying to a graduate program or for a job in the field, you might be asked these questions: "What qualities, traits, attitudes, values, and convictions are central to the person who you are?" "How might these personal characteristics be either assets or liabilities for you as you pursue a career in the helping professions?"

6. If you could pursue a career in one of the helping professions at this time, what would your ideal vision be? What kind of work particularly appeals to you? With what clients would you most like to work? What kind of human service work would bring you the greatest meaning and satisfaction?

Aim of the Chapter

As you consider a career in one of the helping professions, you are probably asking yourself these questions:

- Are the helping professions for me?
- Do I know enough to help others?
- Will I be able to secure a job?
- Will I be able to apply what I am learning in my education to my job?
- Will this career be satisfying in the long run?

This book is intended to help you answer these and other questions about your career. The focus of the book is on *you* and on what you need personally and professionally to be the best helper possible. We also emphasize the realities you are certain to face when you enter the professional world. You will be best able to cope with the demands of the helping professions if you get an idea now of what lies ahead.

We begin this chapter by inviting you to examine your reasons for wanting to become a helper. We challenge you to clarify your personal and professional motivations, and we share our own experiences as beginning helpers to demonstrate that learning to become a helper is a process, with its ups and downs. This chapter also introduces you to the attributes of an effective helper. Although we do not believe there is one perfect pattern of characteristics that identifies "ideal" helpers, we do present some attributes as a catalyst to encourage you to think about the characteristics you possess that could either help or hinder you in your work with others. Because most students express concerns about what professional program will best help them attain their career objectives, we explore the differences among various educational routes. We also examine some of the major factors to consider in selecting a career in the helping professions. Although you may think you know the career path you want to pursue, we encourage you to keep your options open while you are reading this book and taking this course. You will probably work in several different positions within a career area, and many human service professionals change careers at different points in their lives. For instance, they may begin by providing direct services to clients in a community agency but later on shift to administering programs.

Finally, keep in mind as you read this book that we use the terms *helper* and *human services professional* interchangeably to refer to a wide range of practitioners, including social workers, counselors, clinical and counseling psychologists, couples and family therapists, pastoral counselors, mental health nurses, community mental health workers, and rehabilitation counselors.

Examining Your Motives for Becoming a Helper

In choosing a career in the helping professions, you would do well to begin by examining your motivations for pursuing this path. It is imperative that you be honest with yourself about the reasons you are considering entering this field. For many of us, becoming a helper satisfies some of our personal needs, such as the need to make a difference in the lives of others. As you reflect on the needs and motives we discuss in this section, ask yourself this question: "How do my personal needs either enhance or detract from my ability to be an effective helper?"

Typical Needs and Motivations of Helpers

We have observed a variety of motivations in our own students and trainees in the helping professions. We encourage you to recognize your motivations and needs, to accept them, and to become aware of how they influence the quality of your interactions with others. Let's examine some of the reasons you may have for becoming a helper.

The need to make an impact.   Perhaps you are hoping that you will exert a significant influence on the lives of those you serve. You may have a need to know that you are making a positive difference in people's daily existence. Although you recognize that you will not be able to change the world, you are likely to derive satisfaction from empowering individuals. When clients are not interested in changing or do not want your help, however, you may become frustrated. If your worth as a person is tethered to the need to make a difference, you are likely to become disillusioned and disappointed rather quickly. Your professional work is one source for finding meaning in your life, but be sure to explore other avenues as well.

The need to return a favor.   The desire to emulate a role model often plays a part in the decision to be a helper. Someone special, perhaps a teacher or a therapist, may have entered your life in a very influential way, or the influential person may be a grandmother, an uncle, or a parent. Many therapists whom we know have acknowledged that they were greatly influenced by their experience in personal therapy to seek the education needed to become therapists themselves.

The need to care for others.   You may have been a helper from a very early age. Were you the one in your family who attended to the problems and concerns of other family members? Do your peers and friends find it easy to come to you to unload their burdens? If you are a "natural helper," you may have sought out training to capitalize on your talent. One of the pitfalls of being a caregiver to significant people in your life is that very often no one attends to your needs. As a result, you may not have learned to ask for what *you* need. You can easily become personally and professionally burned out, or emotionally exhausted, if you do not learn to ask for help when you need it. Skovholt (2001) writes about the importance of sustaining the personal self: "Individuals in the caring professions are experts at one-way caring. Others are attracted to them because of their expertise and caring attitude" (p. 147). He cautions helping professionals to become aware of the dangers of one-way caring in their professional lives. If helpers hope to function effectively in a professional role, it is essential that they learn and practice the art of self-care.

One professional we contacted reported that, of the 33 people in the training program at his institute, half identified themselves as "rescuers" in alcoholic families. In his view, they were recruited at birth and trained daily to stabilize the family. Many of our own students are adult children of alcoholics who adopted the role of peacemaker in their families. Although this pattern is not necessarily problematic, it is important that such helpers become aware of their dynamics and learn how they operate in both personal and their professional lives.

If the pattern described here fits you, you may profit from reevaluating your early decision to focus on taking care of others to the exclusion of taking care of yourself. If you burden yourself with the full responsibility of always being available for everyone who might need your help, you are likely to find that you will soon have little left to give. It is crucial to have a healthy balance between taking care of others and taking care of yourself. You also need to be able to let others care for you.

The need for self-help.   An interest in helping others often stems from an interest in dealing with the impact of your own struggles. For example, you may have experienced the difficulties of growing up in an abusive family, and you may still be vulnerable due to your early wounding. In your professional work you are likely to encounter a number of individuals who have struggled with similar concerns. Some women who were involved in abusive marriages eventually become counselors who specialize in working with battered women. Some men who were abused as children develop particular professional interests in counseling abused children and youth.

One of our colleagues told us that a guest speaker in his class shared her view that helpers should not be working with victims if they are unwilling to work with perpetrators. Her point was that helpers' objectivity is impaired if they are unwilling to explore all the different aspects of the abusive scenario. Be aware of your own personal issues.

Healers are most often able to heal others out of their own experience with psychological struggle. It is the wounded healer, more so than the well-adjusted helper, who can be authentically present for others searching to find themselves. If you have struggled successfully with a problem, you are able to identify and empathize with clients who come to you with similar concerns.

Sometimes highly disturbed individuals may themselves be studying to become helpers. If you are not on the road to resolving your own pressing problems, it is unlikely that you will be effective in helping others find solutions to their problems. Furthermore, engaging in intense work with others can intensify your own pain. Before you attempt to deal with the lives of others, examine your own life situation. For example, a female counselor who works with women who are victims of spousal abuse may try to work out her own unfinished business and conflicts by giving plenty of advice and pushing these women in certain directions. Because of her unresolved personal problems, she may show hostility to the abusing husband, especially if she becomes overinvolved with family dynamics. She might also make the assumption that what "worked" for her will fit for everyone else also. This topic is addressed more fully in Chapter 3.

The need to be needed.   Very few helpers are immune to the need to be needed. The problem arises when you deny that you want to feel needed. It may be psychologically rewarding to you to have clients say that they are getting better because of your influence. These clients are likely to express their appreciation for the hope that you have given them. You may value being able to take care of other people's wants, and you may get a great deal of satisfaction from doing so. To us, satisfying this need is perhaps one of the greatest rewards of being helpers. We hope that you will not be apologetic about having this need and will not deny that you like being needed and appreciated. If this need is consistently in the forefront, however, it can overshadow the needs of your clients. Some helpers foster dependency by encouraging their clients to call them often.

If you depend exclusively on your clients to feel like a useful human being, your self-worth is on shaky ground. The reality is that many clients will not express appreciation for your efforts, nor will some of them make changes in their lives. Furthermore, agencies often provide feedback only when your performance does not meet the expected standards. No matter what you accomplish, the institution may expect more of you. Eventually, you may feel that whatever you do will not be enough. Wanting to feel appreciated for what you are doing for others can be perfectly all right. The danger exists when you *must* receive appreciation and recognition to feel worthwhile.

The need for money.   Some helpers have come to enjoy the financial rewards of their work, but if you need to make a great deal of money, we suggest that you look elsewhere than the helping professions. In most cases, beginning helpers are not likely to get rich. Many professionals feel that they are not adequately compensated financially for their contributions.

You certainly do not need to feel guilty for wanting to earn a good living. If you were to donate most of your services and had to struggle to make ends meet, you might soon find yourself resenting all that you were giving to your clients. However, financial motives can work against establishment of therapeutic relationships. If you make how much you are earning from each client your primary concern, you are likely to keep clients coming to you when it is no longer in their best interest.

The need for prestige and status.   You may have hopes of acquiring a certain level of prestige, if not a certain income level. Yet if you work in an agency, many of the consumers of the services you offer will be economically disadvantaged. You will be working with people on probation, those with various addictions, and people who are mandated to see you, which means that frequently you may not be given the prestige and the status you deserve. For this reason, it is important that you evaluate status within yourself rather than measuring it by what others give you.

Conversely, you may work in a setting where you can enjoy the status that goes along with being respected by clients and colleagues. If you have worked hard and become good at what you do, allow yourself to accept the prestige you have earned. You can be proud yet still be humble. If you become arrogant as a result of your status, however, you may be perceived as unapproachable, and clients may be put off by your attitude. You also may become prone to accepting far more credit for your clients' changes than you deserve. Some clients will put you on a pedestal, and you may come to like this position too much. Remember, those on a pedestal have only one place to go—down. If you want your self-esteem to rest on a solid foundation, it is essential that you look within yourself to meet your status needs rather than looking to others to provide you with affirmations that you are indeed a worthwhile person.

The need to provide answers.   Many of our students seem to have a strong need to give others advice and to provide the "right answers." For example, some of our students say they feel inadequate if their friends come to them with a problem and they are not able to give them concrete advice. Yet their friends may really need to be listened to and cared for rather than to be told "what they should do." Although you may find satisfaction in influencing others, it is important to realize that your answers may not be best for them. Your purpose is to provide direction and to assist clients in discovering their own course of action. If you find that your need for providing advice and answers sometimes gets in the way of effectively relating to others, we encourage you to bring this up in your sessions with your supervisor.

The need for control.   Related to the need to provide others with advice and answers is the need to control others. Most of us have some need for self-control and many also have the need to control others at times. Some have a great need to control what others are thinking, feeling, and doing. You might ask yourself these questions: Are you convinced that some people should think more liberally (or more conservatively)? When people are angry, depressed, or anxious, do you sometimes tell them that they should not feel that way and do your best to change their state of mind? Do you at times have a strong need to change the way people who are close to you behave, even if what they are doing does not directly affect you? Although some helpers have a need to control under the guise of being helpful, it can be a productive exercise to reflect on what the outcomes might be if you gave more and more control to those you encountered. Is your purpose to control the lives of others, or is it to teach others how to regain effective control of their own lives?

The need for variety and flexibility.   Working in the helping professions, you will come into contact with many culturally diverse groups and individuals. You may also experience many different approaches to helping. You may work with individuals, couples, groups, families, organizations, or whole communities. Flexible hours and being able to work in different settings are benefits without a price tag. You may have been drawn to the helping professions because of the wide variety of ways you can derive meaning from your work.

How Your Needs and Motivations Operate

We often say that in the ideal situation your own needs are met at the same time that you are meeting your clients' needs. Most of the needs and motives we have discussed can work either for or against a client's welfare. If you are unaware of your needs, however, there is a much greater likelihood that your own needs will determine the nature of your interventions. If you are attempting to work through unconscious personal conflicts by focusing on the problems of others, for example, there is more chance that you will use your clients to meet your own needs. In addition, you may be in trouble if some of these needs assume such a high priority that you become obsessed with satisfying them. For instance, if your need for control is so high that you consistently attempt to determine the path that others take, you could easily interfere with your clients' development of independence and freedom.

Helpers who meet their own needs at the expense of their clients are depriving their clients of the quality of care to which they are entitled. If you feel a strong need to provide answers to every problem a client presents, for example, you are meeting your own need rather than working in the best interest of your client. As you reflect on the needs we have discussed, think about how they might either enhance or interfere with your ability to help others. If you have not yet worked with clients, recall your actions in situations with friends or family members who were struggling with some problem. How did you relate to them as they were searching for the best course of action? Do your best to identify how any of these needs can become problematic if you deny them, become obsessed with them, or meet them at the expense of others.

It is unlikely that any single motive drives you; rather, needs and motivations are intertwined and can change over time. Even though your original motives and needs change, your desire to be a helper may remain unchanged. Because personal growth is an ongoing process, we encourage you to periodically reexamine your motives for being a helper. It can be a valuable tool toward self-awareness.

Our Own Beginnings as Helpers

This is a personal book in two ways. It is personal in that we encourage you to find ways to apply the book to yourself. In addition, we have written the book in a personal manner, sharing our own views and experiences whenever we think it is appropriate and useful. As a concrete illustration of how personal motives and experiences can affect career choice, we discuss some of our own motivations for becoming helping professionals and remaining in the field.

Beginning a helping career is not always easy and can involve anxiety and uncertainty. Although at this point we feel more confident than when we were beginning our careers, we have not forgotten our own struggles. We, too, had to cope with many of the fears and self-doubts discussed in the previous pages. By sharing our own difficulties with you, we hope to encourage you not to give up too soon. At this point in our professional lives, we continue to take time to reflect on both what we are giving and what we are getting through our varied work projects.

Marianne Corey's Early Experience

I was a helper long before I studied counseling in school. From childhood on I responded to the needs of my brothers and sisters. At age 8, I was made almost totally responsible for my newborn brother. I not only took care of him but also attended to other members of an extended family.

My family owned a restaurant in a German village. The restaurant, which was in our home, was the meeting place for many of the local men. These men came mostly to socialize rather than to eat and drink. For hours they would sit and talk, and I was taught that I had better listen attentively. Furthermore, I learned that I should not repeat the personal conversations and gossip to other townspeople. At this early age I learned three very important skills: attentive listening, empathic understanding, and confidentiality. It became apparent to me that a variety of people found it easy to talk to me and tell me about their personal problems.

In my growing-up years I felt liked and respected by most people. I remember feeling compassion, especially for those who had a difficult or unusual life situation. For example, I recall seeing a woman who had a psychotic episode standing naked by an upstairs window. She threw her clothes and furniture out of the window as onlookers baited her. I felt sad and thought that she must be very unhappy. I also had special feelings for two persons in my village who were considered "town drunks." I was curious about why they wanted to drink.

I have always been interested in looking beyond the façade that people present to others. I became convinced that people could be more than they appeared if they were willing to make an effort to change. My belief was not typical. In my immediate cultural environment the normative message was that "this is fate, and there is nothing you can do about it."

In my own life I overcame many obstacles and exceeded my dreams. As a result, I am often successful in challenging and encouraging my clients not to give up too soon when limits are imposed on them. Through my work I derive a great sense of satisfaction when I have been instrumental in the lives of individuals who are willing to take risks, to tolerate uncertainty, to dare to be different, and to live a fuller life because of their choices. When clients show appreciation for what I have done for them, I enjoy hearing it. However, I always let them know that their progress stems only partially from my efforts; the rest comes from their hard work.

In my life now I find it easy to give to my friends, family, and community as well as to clients. It seems natural to me to give both personally and professionally. It continues to be a struggle for me to find a good balance between giving to others and taking for myself. Although I am considered a good giver, I realize that I am a slow learner when it comes to making my needs known and asking for what I want.

It is interesting for me to compare my cultural conditioning and early role in my family with my development as a professional caregiver. Although I seemed to assume the role of caring for my brothers and sisters "naturally," I did not feel quite as natural when I began formal helping. In my first practical experiences as part of my undergraduate program in behavioral sciences, I had my share of self-doubt.

In one of my earlier internships I was placed in a college counseling center. I remember how petrified I was one day when a student came in and asked for an appointment and my supervisor asked me to counsel this client. The feedback that I received later from my supervisor on how confident I had appeared was very incongruent with what I had felt. Here are some of the thoughts that ran through my head as I was walking to my office with this client: "I'm not ready for this. What am I going to do? What if he doesn't talk? What if I don't know how to help him? I wish I could get out of this!" In my self-absorption I never once considered any of my client's feelings. For instance, how might he be approaching this session? What fears might he be having?

I was much more aware of myself than of my clients. I took far too much responsibility, put much pressure on myself to "do it right," and worried a lot about what harm I might do. I did not allow my clients to assume their rightful share of the responsibility for making changes. I often worked much harder than they did, and sometimes it seemed that I wanted more for my clients than they wanted for themselves. I think I had a tendency to exaggerate my capacity for causing harm because of my fears and insecurities as a helper. When I shared with my supervisor my concern about feeling so responsible for the outcomes of our sessions and about hurting my clients, she responded "You are assuming more power than you have over your clients or than they will give you."

Another time I told my supervisor that I had doubts about being in my profession, that I was overwhelmed by all the pain I saw around me, and that I was concerned that I was not helping anybody. I remember being very emotional and feeling extremely discouraged. My supervisor's smile surprised me. "I would be very concerned about you as a helper," he said, "if you never asked yourself these kinds of questions and were not willing to confront yourself with these feelings." In retrospect, I think he was telling me that he was encouraged for me because I was acknowledging my struggles and was not pretending to be the all-competent counselor who was without fears.

As a beginning counselor I was acutely aware of my own anxieties. Now I am much better able to be present with my clients and to enter their world. Although I am not anxiety-free, I am not watching myself practicing therapy. Furthermore, although I take responsibility for the counseling process, I do not see myself as totally responsible for what goes on in a session, and I am usually not willing to work harder than my clients.

At one time I wanted to abandon the idea of becoming a counselor and instead considered teaching German. I was very aware of comparing myself with professionals who had years of experience, and I thought I should be as effective as they were. I eventually realized that my expectations were extremely unrealistic, because I was demanding that I immediately be as skilled as these very experienced people. I had been giving myself no room for learning and for tolerating my rudimentary beginnings.

One of my professional activities now is working with beginning helpers. I find that they are often in the same predicament I was when I began working with others. These students seem focused on how much I know and how easy interventions seem to come to me. By contrast, they feel discouraged with their lack of knowledge and with how much they have to struggle to find "the right thing to say." They usually sigh with relief when I tell them about some of my beginnings and admit that I do not see myself as an expert but as someone who has a certain amount of expertise in counseling. I want most to convey to them that learning never stops and that beginnings are difficult and, at times, discouraging.

Jerry Corey's Early Experience

When I was in college studying to become a teacher, I hoped to create a different learning climate for students than I was experiencing as a learner. I wanted to help others, and it was important for me to make a difference. I recognize now that the need to make a significant difference has been a theme for the more than 30 years I have been in the helping professions. As a child and as an adolescent, I did not feel that my presence made that much difference. In many ways, during my early years, I felt that I did not fit anywhere and that I was unrecognized and useless. I was surrounded by a large, extended immigrant Italian family who often spoke in their native language, which I did not understand. There was a good deal of pain attached to feeling ignored, and one of my early decisions was not to let myself be ignored. This took the form of making myself a nuisance, which of course resulted in negative attention. But I assumed that this type of recognition was better than being ignored! In college I experienced some success and found some positive routes to being recognized. Later, when I began my teaching career, I began to see that I could make a difference, at least within the confines of my classroom. In addition to helping students enjoy learning, I also got personal satisfaction from knowing that I was a useful person, which was quite different from my perception of myself during my youth. In fact, I think that I depended (and still do) to a large extent on my professional accomplishments for my sense of identity.

At the beginning of my career as a counseling psychologist, I did not feel confident, and I often wondered whether I was suited for the field. I recall as being particularly difficult the times that I co-led a group with my supervisor. I felt incompetent and inexperienced next to my co-leader, who was an experienced therapist. Much of the time I didn't know what to say or do. It seemed that there was little place for me to intervene, because my co-leader was so effective. I had many doubts about my ability to say anything meaningful to the members. It just seemed that my supervisor was so insightful and so skillful that I would never attain such a level of professionalism. The effect of working with an experienced group leader was to heighten my own sense of insecurity and inadequacy.

Another thing that I found difficult was practicing individual counseling in a university center. When I began as a practicing counselor, I frequently asked myself what I could do for my clients. I remember progress being very slow, and it seemed that I needed an inordinate amount of immediate and positive feedback. When after several weeks a client was still talking about feeling anxious or depressed, I immediately felt my own incompetence as a helper. I frequently found myself thinking: "How would my supervisor say this? What would he do?" I even caught myself copying his gestures, phrases, and mannerisms. Many times I felt that I did not have what it took to be an effective counselor, and I wondered if I had pursued the wrong path.

I often had no idea of what, if anything, my clients were getting from our sessions. Indications of whether clients were getting better, staying the same, or getting worse were typically very subtle. What I did not know at the time was that clients need to struggle as a part of finding their own answers. My expectation was that they should feel better quickly, for then I would know that I was surely helping them. I also did not appreciate that clients often begin to feel worse as they give up their defenses and open themselves to their pain. When I saw clients expressing their fear and uncertainty about their future, it brought out my own lack of certainty that I could help them. Because I was concerned about saying "the wrong thing," I often listened but did not give too many of my own reactions in return.

Even though it is uncomfortable for me to admit this, I was more inclined to accept clients who were bright, verbal, attractive, and willing to talk about their problems than clients who seemed depressed or unmotivated to change. Those whom I considered "good and cooperative clients" I encouraged to come back. As long as they were talking and working, and preferably letting me know that they were getting somewhere with our sessions, I was quick to schedule other appointments. Those clients who seemed to make very few changes were the ones who increased my own anxiety. Rather than seeing their own part in their progress or lack of it, I typically blamed myself for not knowing enough and not being able to solve their problems. I took full responsibility for what they did during the session. It never occurred to me that the fact that they did not return for another session might have said something about them and their unwillingness to change. I had limited tolerance for uncertainty and for their struggle in finding their own direction. My self-doubts grew when they did not show up for following appointments. I was sure that this was a sign that they were dissatisfied with what they were getting from me.

I particularly remember encouraging depressed clients to make an appointment with one of the other counselors on the staff. I learned in my own supervision that working with depressed clients was difficult for me because of my reluctance to deal with my own fears of depression. If I allowed myself to really enter the world of these depressed clients, I might get in touch with some of my anxiety. This experience taught me the important lesson that I could not take clients in any direction that I had not been willing to explore in my own life.

Although I no longer engage in counseling people individually, I do teach counselors and write textbooks on counseling practice. Had I not challenged my fears and self-doubts, I am quite certain that I would not be a counselor educator and an author today.

A Helping Career Is Not for Everyone

As is clear from our accounts, both of us had self-doubts. We certainly do not see it as a disgrace if you wonder whether a helping profession is right for you. If you keep the question of whether you want to pursue a helping career open, you are bound to have periods of self-doubt. At times you may feel excited about the prospects of your career choice, and at other times you may feel hopeless and discouraged. Be tolerant of these ambivalent feelings. Don't make the decision whether to pursue a helping career by yourself, based on your initial experiences. We encourage you to be open to the pattern of consistent feedback you receive from faculty members, supervisors, and your peers. In some situations you may hear that you are not suited for a particular field. If people have concerns about your entering that helping profession, be willing to listen and to consider what they have to say. Such feedback is certainly hard to accept. Your first inclination may be to decide that the person does not like you, yet the advice may be in your best interest. If you hear such a recommendation, ask for specific reasons for this evaluation and find out what alternatives the person can suggest to you.

You will ultimately have to make the decision of whether the helping profession is for you, but before you decide, consult with supervisors, colleagues, friends, and others who know you best. Give yourself credit for being able to change. If you are willing to remain open and apply the effort needed to change, you may find that your limitations can also be your assets.

The inclination to give up too soon is often greatest when you first have to apply what you have learned in your courses. A most difficult time will be when you step out of the lab and into the real world. The chances are that you will find that what worked in the lab will not work so well in real-life helping situations. In the lab you may have worked with fellow students who role-played clients who were cooperative. Now you are facing some clients who, no matter how hard you try, are not responding to you. Realize that it will take time and experience to learn how to apply your knowledge of theories and techniques to actual situations. At first your attempts at helping may seem artificial and rehearsed. You will probably be more aware of this artificiality than your clients. Again, allow yourself the time to gain a greater sense of ease in applying what you have learned and in functioning in your role as a helper.

Portrait of the "Ideal Helper"

Although it is useful to imagine the characteristics of the "ideal helper," even the most effective helpers do not meet all of these criteria. If you try to match the ideal picture we are about to paint, you will be needlessly setting yourself up for failure and frustration. But it is surely possible to become a more effective helper if you are aware of those areas that need strengthening. You can hone your existing skills and acquire new ones. You can integrate knowledge that will enhance your abilities. You can make personal changes that will enable you to be more present and powerful as you intervene in the lives of your clients. With these possibilities in mind, consider this picture of a helper who is making a significant difference:

- You are committed to an honest assessment of your own strengths and weaknesses. You recognize that who you are as a person is the most important instrument you possess as a helper.
- You are open to learning and have a basic curiosity. You realize what you do not know, and you are willing to take steps to fill the gaps in your knowledge.
- You have the interpersonal skills needed to establish good contact with other people, and you can apply these skills in the helping relationship.

- You genuinely care for the people you help, and this caring is expressed by doing what is in their best interest. You are able to deal with a wide range of your clients' thoughts, feelings, and behaviors.
- You realize that it takes hard work to bring about change, and you are willing to stick with clients as they go through this difficult process. You are able to enter the world of your clients and see the world through their eyes rather than imposing your own vision of reality on them.
- You realize that clients often limit themselves through a restricted imagination of possibilities for their future. You are able to inspire clients to dream and to take the steps necessary to fulfill their dreams in reality. You realize that you are unable to inspire clients to do in their lives what you are unable or unwilling to do in your own life.
- You are willing to draw on a number of resources to enable clients to move toward their goals. You are flexible in applying strategies for change, and you are willing to adapt your techniques to the unique situation of each client.
- In working with clients whose ethnic or cultural background is different from yours, you show your respect for them by not fitting them into a neat mold.
- You take care of yourself physically, mentally, psychologically, socially, and spiritually. You do in your own life what you ask of your clients. If you are confronted with problems, you deal with them.
- You question life and engage in critical self-examination of your beliefs and values. You are aware of your needs and motivations, and you make choices that are congruent with your life goals. Your philosophy of life is your own creation, not one that has been imposed on you.
- You are capable of establishing meaningful relationships with at least a few significant people.
- Although you have a healthy sense of self-love and pride, you are not arrogant.

This is not a complete list, and no one fits the portrait of the "ideal helper" perfectly. Our intent in presenting this list is not to overwhelm you but to provide you with some characteristics that are worthy of reflection. You might be telling yourself that you lack many of these characteristics. An unskilled helper can become a skilled one, and all of us can become more effective in touching the lives of the clients we encounter. We hope you will assess your personal characteristics that could work either for or against you in your role as a professional helper. In addressing the question "Are the helping professions for me?" you are encouraged to use this book as a catalyst for honest self-reflection.

Many training programs offer some self-exploration experiences in which students can become more aware of how their personal attributes manifest themselves in relationships. In your practicum and internship seminars, there are typically opportunities to focus on ways in which your personal style influences your ability to establish helping relationships with clients. If your program does not offer formal personal-growth experiences, seek these resources in the community. Much of the rest of this book will deal with the interplay between you as a person and your work as a professional helper. Our underlying assumption is that the best way to prepare for a dynamic career is to come to a fuller appreciation of the richness of your being and to be able to use your own life experiences in your evolution in the helping professions.

Selecting a Professional Program and Career Path

Students planning to enter one of the helping professions sometimes fall into the trap of idealizing the profession. In their minds, they may build up the glory of helping others, seeing only the positives. They may envision themselves as being able to help virtually everyone who comes to them, and even reaching those who do not seek their counsel. Although having ideals and goals to strive for is part of being a helper who makes a difference, it is easy to paint an unrealistic picture of what your career as a helper will be like. You need to engage in ongoing reality testing to maintain a balanced outlook. You can test your vision by talking to various practitioners in many different settings. Ask them to tell you what they do in a typical week. Inquire about their motivations for choosing and remaining in the helping professions. Ask especially about the rewards, challenges, and demands of their work.

When you begin fieldwork, you will be able to test many of your ideas and expectations against the real world of work. This is a good time to reflect on your motives and needs for considering helping as a career. Observations in various field settings and practical experience working with different client populations will provide a more accurate picture of how your career is likely to satisfy your needs for becoming a helper in the first place.

At this point, you may not even be certain you want to pursue a career in the helping professions. If you are enrolled in a 2-year community college program in human services, you may be wondering whether it would be best for you to get a job when you complete your program. A wide range of human services jobs are available, including skills training, social service assistants, work with the mentally handicapped, outreach workers in the community, work with parolees or in prison settings, work in the area of substance abuse, and a host of community agency settings. Human services programs at the bachelor's degree level often train students for entry into a wide range of jobs, some of which include youth corrections, crisis shelters, career counseling, youth programs, residential treatment centers, mental health units, senior citizens centers, nursing homes, and agencies for people with disabilities. It is generally true that the higher your educational level the more career options are open to you. However, you may want to get a job for a time to gain experience once you complete a community college program or a 4-year program. Later you may see the need to return to school for a graduate degree in one of the helping professions.

Whether you are an undergraduate or a graduate student, you have probably experienced some anxiety in selecting the right program. We encourage students to be open to new ideas. There are no absolute guidelines or perfect choices. Gather program material from several universities and talk with professors and students. Talking with professionals about their work experience can also broaden your perspective. Ask about the specific educational and practical background that they most value. In selecting a program, ask yourself these questions: "Will the program give me what I need to do the work I want to do? Does the orientation of the program fit with my values? Am I compatible with the program?"

If you are taking an introductory course on the helping professions as an elective and are undecided about pursuing a career in the field, you can take selected courses and fieldwork classes to explore your interest in continuing. We have met students who remained in a course of study even though they had discovered that they were not enthusiastic about the field. They were hesitant to change because doing so could be interpreted as a failure. Others are reluctant to change majors because they would face added requirements for graduation. It seems to us that such students are likely to fail in the long run if they do not pursue their real interests.

If you find yourself in a program that you really do not like, consider getting out. But be sure you evaluate the overall direction of the program rather than a specific course or requirement that you do not like. One of our graduates complained that some of the classes she had to take were unrelated to her career interests. Specifically, she could not understand why research-oriented and grant-writing courses were required. However, she discovered that these courses were valuable in helping her land a job. In hindsight, she found value in a part of her education that she at one time had thought was meaningless.

Deciding Which Professional Route to Take

Students often ask which professional specialty we think is best for them. You can take many routes as a helper in the human services: social worker, psychiatric technician, couples and family therapist, mental health counselor, psychologist, or school counselor. Each of these professional specialties has a different focus, yet all have in common working with people.

We tell students that they will have to choose a specialty through a process of reading and thinking about the alternatives. Much depends on what you want to do, how much time you are willing to invest in a program, where you want to live, and what your other interests are. Realize that there is no "perfect profession" and that each profession has advantages and drawbacks.

At the undergraduate level, human services programs train practitioners for community agency work. Human service workers generally carry out specific roles and functions under the supervision of clinical social workers, psychologists, and licensed counselors. At the master's degree level, students can choose among various types of programs, some of which include school counseling, mental health counseling, rehabilitation counseling, counseling psychology, clinical psychology, couples and family therapy, and clinical social work. At the doctoral level, there are generally four approved programs for those wanting to become practitioners: social work, counselor education, counseling psychology, and clinical psychology. Each specialization has its own perspective and emphasizes different roles and functions for practitioners.

Regardless of which of the helping professions interests you the most, you are likely to discover that you will occupy many different positions within an area of specialization. For instance, if you pursue a clinical social work program, you may eventually hold a variety of jobs. You are likely to provide direct service to clients, including casework, counseling, assessment, and community work. You may also assume a role in formulating social policy, doing advocacy work, and writing grants to fund social programs. At some point your professional services may be more indirect, such as supervising interns, working as a consultant, or designing or managing human services programs.

Be open to the vast range of possibilities before you. Do not fall into the trap of convincing yourself that once you accept a position you are locked into that specific job forever. Too often we find that students are overly anxious about making the "right decision," as though there were only one or two positions they would ever occupy. Instead, allow yourself to consider your professional life in a developmental way and explore new possibilities as you gain additional work experience.

Advantages and Disadvantages of Various Specializations

As you read about the various specialty areas of practice described in this section, think about the characteristics that resonate most with your own expectations. Each specialty has much to recommend it, but you will probably find yourself drawn more to one than to the others. The personal characteristics and experience of the counselor often combine favorably with a particular specialization. The professional organization for each specialty is described, and this is a good place to inquire for further information. We have provided contact information for these organizations to facilitate further inquiries.

Social Work

This specialization attends not only to the inner workings of a person but also to an understanding of the person in the environment. A master's program in social work (MSW) prepares students broadly for casework, counseling, community intervention, social policy and planning, research and development, and administration and management. The course work tends to be broader than that in counseling, and it focuses on developing skills to intervene and bring about social change on levels beyond the individual. Although clinical social workers are engaged in assessment and treatment of individuals, couples, families, and groups, they tend to view environmental factors as contributing strongly to an individual's or a family's problems. In addition to academic courses, a supervised internship is part of the social worker's preparation for either direct or indirect social services. Several instructors who teach in the human services program at our university, all of whom are social workers, provided these comments about the course of study required for an MSW:

- In my own education, I found that my social work program was broad-based, so less time was devoted to learning specific therapeutic techniques. I was frustrated with this as a student because I was eager to become a therapist. Now I am quite grateful for the background in policy and research.
- The MSW gives tremendous career flexibility because of the range of practice, including clinical practice, administration, community organization, planning, and policy areas.
- Because of the range within social work, you can actually change careers without a major retooling. You can go from direct practice to research to teaching to policy and planning.
- A social worker has many options open for securing a position. The MSW degree provides maximum options in regard to specialties. You can specialize in clinical, child, family, group, community, or administration. The MSW is an old, well-established profession with solid support nationwide. You can move from agency to agency, location to location, and state to state more easily than with certain other professional licenses.

National Association of Social Workers (NASW).   NASW membership is open to all professional social workers, and there is a student membership category. The NASW Press, which produces *Social Work* and the *NASW News* as membership benefits, is a major service in professional development. NASW also provides a number of pamphlets on relevant topics. For further information about NASW or to obtain the NASW *Code of Ethics* (1999), contact:

National Association of Social Workers
750 First Street, N. E., Suite 700
Washington, DC 20002-4241
Telephone: (202) 408-8600 or (800) 638-8799
Fax: (202) 336-8311
Web site: http://www.socialworkers.org

Couples and Family Counseling

The specialization of couples and family therapy is primarily concerned with relationship counseling. It deals with assessing and treating clients from a family-systems perspective. Students in a master's program in couples and family therapy take a variety of courses in assessment and treatment, as well as theory courses. They also do extensive supervised fieldwork with children and adults, couples, and families. Several instructors in our program, who have training and a license in couples and family therapy, offered these perspectives on this professional specialty:

- Having a professional license will open many doors, but the type of license is less important than one's academic courses, life experiences, and internship practice. Most programs in couples and family therapy emphasize clinical applications and involve a great deal of experiential work.

- Couples and family therapy continues to be a developing field. People who do well in this field are innovative, self-directed, and understand themselves, and they are in basic agreement with the tenets of the systems approach.
- The greatest joy for me is to see children and adolescents I helped 20 years ago come back and see me as a group. At such times, the feeling of having made a contribution is overwhelming. There is a sense of having a place in the lives of families and in the history of our civilization.
- One of the drawbacks of this specialty is that many insurance and managed care companies do not pay for couples and family counseling, even though it is a useful service.

American Association for Marriage and Family Therapy (AAMFT).   The AAMFT has a student membership category. Members receive the *Journal of Marital and Family Therapy,* which is published four times a year, and a subscription to six issues yearly of *Family Therapy News.* For membership applications, the *AAMFT Code of Ethics* (2001), or for further information, contact:

American Association for Marriage and Family Therapy
1133 15th Street, N. W., Suite 300
Washington, DC 20005-2710
Telephone: (202) 452-0109
Fax: (202) 223-2329
Web site: http://www.aamft.org

National Council on Family Relations (NCFR).   The NCFR provides a forum for family researchers, educators, and practitioners to share in the development and dissemination of knowledge about families and family relationships, establishes professional standards, and works to promote family well-being. For further information or to request the NCFR's *Ethical Principles and Guidelines* (1997), contact:

National Council on Family Relations
3989 Central Avenue, N. E., Suite 550
Minneapolis, MN 55421

Clinical and Counseling Psychology

Although clinical and counseling psychology are different specializations, there are no rigid boundaries separating their professional functions so we will discuss them together. Although you can be licensed as a social worker, counselor, and couples and family therapist with a master's degree, this is not the case if you wish to refer to yourself as a psychologist. Both counseling and clinical psychology require a doctorate for licensure. Clinical psychologists focus on assessment, diagnosis, and treatment procedures of mildly to severely disturbed persons. They interview clients and write case studies. Counseling psychologists assist relatively healthy people in solving developmental problems and functioning more effectively. They help clients find and use information to make better personal, educational, and occupational choices. Professional psychologists in both specialties often offer psychotherapy to individuals, couples, families, and groups; they may teach or conduct research. Both specializations focus on evaluation of treatments and programs and help clients develop action plans.

American Psychological Association (APA).   The APA has a Student Affiliates category rather than student membership. Journals and subscriptions are extra. Each year in mid-August or late August the APA holds a national convention. Membership includes a monthly subscription to a journal, *American Psychologist,* and a magazine, *Monitor on Psychology,* 11 times a year. For further information or to request the *Ethical Principles of Psychologists and Code of Conduct* (APA, 1992), contact:

American Psychological Association
750 First Street, N. E.
Washington, DC 20002-4242
Telephone: (202) 336-5500 or (800) 374-2721
Fax: (202) 336-5568
Web site: http://www.apa.org

American Counseling Association (ACA).   Student memberships are available to both undergraduate and graduate students enrolled at least half-time or more at the college level. ACA membership provides many benefits, including a subscription to the *Journal of Counseling and Development* and also a monthly newspaper entitled *Counseling Today,* eligibility for professional liability insurance programs, legal defense services, and professional development through workshops and conventions. The ACA puts out a resource catalog that provides information on the various aspects of the counseling profession, as well as giving detailed information about membership, journals, books, home-study programs, videotapes, audiotapes, and liability insurance. For further information or to request the *Code of Ethics and Standards of Practice* (ACA, 1995), contact:

American Counseling Association
5999 Stevenson Avenue
Alexandria, VA 22304 -3300
Telephone: (703) 823-9800 or (800) 347-6647
Fax: (703) 823-0252
Web site: http://www.counseling.org

School Counseling

Neukrug (1999) traces the historical development of school counseling from its beginnings as a response to the needs of vocational guidance to its growing viability as a profession today. Over the past two decades accreditation guidelines for school counseling have been established, which have moved school counseling forward in terms of accountability as a helping profession. Now all states require a master's degree in school counseling, and professional organizations advocate and lobby for legislative initiatives and the establishment of credentialing.

School counselors perform a wide variety of roles and functions in elementary, middle, and secondary schools, including individual counseling, group guidance, group counseling, consultation, and coordination. In addition to working with students, many school counselors consult with teachers, administration, and at times, parents. School counselors work with students on a variety of educational issues, but many of them provide some personal and social counseling as well. From a multicultural perspective, school counselors have the challenge of striving to lessen language barriers, advocating for minority students, sensitizing the school community to cultural diversity issues, assuring that educational materials are relevant for students' culture, and establishing a comprehensive developmental counseling and guidance program (Neukrug, 1999).

American School Counselors Association (ASCA). The ASCA is the major professional organization devoted to school counseling. ASCA has a student membership category with current dues at $45 per year. Members receive the journal *Professional School Counselor* and a newsletter. This group sponsors an annual conference in June. The professional ethics code of the ASCA is *Ethical Standards for School Counselors* (1998). For additional information, contact:

American School Counselor Association
801 North Fairfax, Suite 310
Alexandria, VA 22314
Telephone: (703) 683-2722 or (800) 306-4722
Fax: (703) 683-1619
Web site: www.schoolcounselor.org

National Board for Certified Counselors (NBCC). The National Board for Certified Counselors (NBCC) is a national voluntary certification program. There are no governmental requirements that counselors be certified, but to become a National Certified Counselor (NCC) an individual must complete a master's degree in counseling, have 2 years of post-master's experience, and pass the National Counselor Examination. NBCC also offers specialty certification in the areas of mental health, career, school, gerontology, and addictions counseling. To become certified in a specialty, counselors must first become certified counselors. For further information or to request the NBCC's *Code of Ethics* (1997), contact:

National Board for Certified Counselors
3 Terrace Way, Suite D
Greensboro, NC 27403-3660
Telephone: (336) 547-0607
Fax: (336) 547-0017
Web site: http://www.nbcc.org

Nonlicensed Human Service Workers

It is clear that there are not enough professionally licensed practitioners willing to meet the demand for psychological assistance in many segments of the community. Nonlicensed human service professionals may have a graduate degree, an undergraduate degree, an associate of arts degree, a certificate of competence in some aspect of human services, or some formal training from experts in the field. These nonlicensed workers have a variety of job titles, a few of which include community support worker, human service worker, social work assistant, and community outreach worker. Another example of nonlicensed workers are lay volunteers from the community who receive training and supervision in therapeutic intervention with a wide range of clients. These volunteers work on hot lines, co-lead groups, and engage in other supportive activities. These helpers alleviate the shortage of personnel, and some nonlicensed practitioners may actually be more effective in reaching certain client populations in the community because they have experienced similar problems and learned to deal with them successfully.

A large part of the success of community mental health programs will depend on these nontraditional workers' receiving the training and supervision they need to develop skills for effective intervention. In some instances, nonlicensed human service workers may aid licensed practitioners who lack experience or training in working with various racial, ethnic, and socioeconomic groups. The helping professions are enriched by the contributions of nonlicensed workers.

National Organization for Human Service Education (NOHSE).   NOHSE is made up of members from diverse disciplines—mental health, child care, social services, gerontology, recreation, corrections, and developmental disabilities. Membership is open to human service educators, students, fieldwork supervisors, and direct-care professionals. Student membership is $28 per year, which includes a subscription to the newsletter (the *Link*); the yearly journal, *Human Services Education*; and a discount price for the yearly conference (held in October). For further information about membership in the National Organization for Human Service Education or to request *Ethical Standards of Human Service Professionals* (NOHSE, 2000), contact:

Chrisanne Christensen
Sul Ross State University
Rio Grande College
Rt. 3, Box 1200
Eagle Pass, TX 78852
Telephone: (830) 758-5112
Fax: (830) 758-5001
Web site: http:www.nohse.com

Becoming a Licensed Professional

Obtaining a master's degree or a doctoral degree in counseling, counselor education, social work, psychology, or couples and family counseling may be the beginning of your educational journey as a mental health professional, not the final destination. If you hope to establish even a part-time private practice, or to work in some positions in mental health agencies, you may need to secure a license to practice. The main licenses available in most states include licensed professional counselor, licensed clinical social worker, licensed psychologist, and licensed marital and family therapist. To qualify for a license, an applicant generally must first secure a master's degree (or a doctoral degree for certain licenses) in the professional area of specialization. Beyond the degree a minimum number of hours of supervised clinical work (generally 3,000 hours) is required, and the applicant must pass both a written and an oral examination. Licensure statutes determine and govern professional practice, specifying what the holder of the license can do. A person with a professional license is assumed to have minimal competence in the general practice of clinical work.

Licensure assures the public that practitioners have completed minimum educational programs, have had a certain number of hours of supervised training, and have gone through some type of evaluation and screening. Licenses do not, and probably cannot, ensure that practitioners will competently do what their licenses permit them to do. The main advantages of licensure are protection of the public from grossly unqualified and untrained practitioners and formal representation to the public that practitioners are part of an established profession.

Licenses and credentials usually do not specify the clients or types of problems practitioners are competent to work with, nor do they specify the techniques that counselors are competent to use. Most licensing regulations do specify that licensees are to engage only in those therapeutic tasks for which they have adequate training, but it is up to the licensee to put this rule into practice. If you are interested in securing more information about the licensure process, research the specific licenses available in your state and the requirements for making application for these licenses.

Factors to Consider in Choosing Your Career Path

Making career choices is an ongoing process rather than an isolated event. People generally go through a series of stages when choosing a career path. Information from practitioners and professors can help you define a professional direction. But you cannot rely solely on the advice of others when making your career decisions. In today's world, it is wise to consider the advantages of becoming a generalist. Your chances of gaining employment in a managed care system are greater if you are able to work with a range of client populations in a variety of problem areas. Although you may develop expertise in a specific area, flexibility is often necessary to meet the changing demands in the marketplace.

Ultimately you must decide for yourself which path is likely to best tap your talents and bring you the most fulfillment. In your career decision-making process, consider your self-concept, interests, abilities, values, occupational attitudes, socioeconomic level, parental influence, ethnic identity, gender, and physical, mental, emotional, and social handicaps. We will discuss five of these factors in more detail—self-concept, motivation and achievement, interests, abilities, and values. Apply these areas to yourself as you consider the range of career possibilities you might want to pursue.

Self-concept.   Some writers in career development contend that a vocational choice is an attempt to fulfill one's self-concept. People with a poor self-concept, for example, are not likely to envision themselves in a meaningful or important job. They are likely to keep their aspirations low; as a result, their achievements will probably be low. They may select and remain in a job that they do not enjoy or derive satisfaction from because they are convinced that such a job is all they are worthy of. In this regard, choosing a vocation can be thought of as a public declaration of the kind of person you see yourself as being.

Motivation and achievement.   Setting goals is at the core of the process of deciding on a vocation. If you have goals but do not have the energy and persistence to pursue them, your goals will not materialize. Your need to achieve, along with your achievements to date, is related to your motivation to translate goals into action plans. In thinking about your career choices, identify those areas where your drive is the greatest. Also, reflect on specific personal achievements. What have you accomplished that you feel particularly proud of? What are you doing now that moves you in the direction of achieving what is important to you? What are some of the things you dream about doing in the future? Thinking about your goals, needs, motivations, and achievements is a good way to get a clearer focus on your career direction.

Interests.   Interest measurement is used extensively in career planning. Once you have determined your areas of vocational interest, you can identify possible positions for which these interests are appropriate. You can then focus your attention on those jobs for which you have the abilities required for satisfactory job performance. Working as a volunteer in a community agency is an excellent way to test your interests and abilities. Going to the career center for information, testing, and vocational counseling can also be helpful. Although interests are a significant element, you must also consider whether you have the ability to perform well on the job.

Abilities.   Ability or aptitude is a significant factor in the career decision-making process, and it is probably used more often than any other factor. *Ability* refers to your competence in an activity; *aptitude* is your ability to learn. Scholastic aptitude is particularly significant if you need to enter a graduate program that will be a gateway to a position you seek in the helping professions. Consider the activities you have engaged in where you think you do especially well. Ask yourself what kind of activities you would find rewarding. To get a clearer sense of your aptitude, review your academic strengths and weaknesses. How open are you to academic learning? How quickly do you grasp concepts, and to what degree are you able to apply and use what you know? How far are you willing to go in your schooling?

Values.   Once you have determined how your interests and abilities match with possible career choices, explore your values. It is important to assess, identify, and clarify your values so that you will be able to match them with your career.

Your *work values* pertain to what you hope to accomplish in an occupation. Work values are an important aspect of your total value system. Recognizing those things that bring meaning to your life is crucial if you hope to find a career that has personal value for you. A few examples of work values include helping others, influencing people, finding meaning, prestige, status, competition, friendships, creativity, stability, recognition, adventure, physical challenge, change and variety, opportunity for travel, moral fulfillment, and independence. Because certain work values are related to certain occupations, they can be the basis of a good match between you and a position. Take time to complete the following self-inventory as a way of clarifying some of your values pertaining to work.

Decide how important each of the following values is to you in your work. Write the appropriate number next to each: 4 = most important to me; 3 = important, but not a top priority; 2 = slightly important; and 1 = of little or no importance.

_____ 1. *High income:* opportunity for high pay or other financial gain.
_____ 2. *Power:* opportunity to influence, lead, and direct others.
_____ 3. *Prestige:* opportunity for respect and admiration from others.
_____ 4. *Job security:* security from unemployment and economic changes.
_____ 5. *Variety:* chances to do many different things in a job.
_____ 6. *Achievement:* opportunities to accomplish goals.
_____ 7. *Responsibility:* chance to be in charge of myself and others; being able to show trustworthiness.
_____ 8. *Independence:* freedom from rigid hours or controls.
_____ 9. *Family relationships:* time to be with family in addition to the job.
_____ 10. *Interests:* work that matches my field of interest.
_____ 11. *Opportunity to serve people:* being able to make a difference in the lives of others; helping others help themselves.
_____ 12. *Adventure:* a high level of excitement on the job.
_____ 13. *Creativity:* opportunities to come up with new ideas and do things in creative ways.
_____ 14. *Inner harmony:* peace and contentment through work.
_____ 15. *Teamwork:* opportunities to cooperate with others toward common goals.
_____ 16. *Intellectual challenge:* demands at work for a high level of problem solving and creative thinking.
_____ 17. *Competition:* the need to compete against others.
_____ 18. *Advancement:* opportunities for promotion.
_____ 19. *Continued learning:* chances to update learning and knowledge.
_____ 20. *Structure and routine:* a predictable routine on the job that requires a certain pattern of responses.

Go over the list again and identify your top three values—the ones you deem to be essential in a job you would accept. What does your list tell you? What other values do you consider to be extremely important in work? To clarify some of these values, ask yourself these questions: "Do I like working with a wide range of people? Am I able to ask for help from others when faced with problematic situations? Do I place a value on doing in my own life what I encourage others to do for themselves? How do I feel about offering help to others with their problems? Am I interested in organizing, coordinating, and leading others in work projects? Do I value working on projects I have designed, or do I tend to look to others to come up with ideas for projects with which I can become involved?" Your values and interests are intertwined; knowing them can help you identify areas of work where you will find the most personal satisfaction.

Self-Assessment: An Inventory of Your Attitudes and Beliefs About Helping

Self-assessment is an ongoing process for all helping professionals. Completing this inventory will help you clarify your beliefs and values. The inventory is designed to introduce you to issues and topics presented in this book and to stimulate your thoughts and interest. You may want to complete the inventory in more than one sitting, giving each question your full concentration.

This is not a traditional multiple-choice test in which you must select the "one right answer." Rather, it is a survey of your basic beliefs, attitudes, and values on specific topics related to the helping process. For each question, write in the letter of the response that most clearly reflects your viewpoint at this time. In many cases the answers are not mutually exclusive, and you may choose more than one response if you wish. In addition, a blank line is included for each item so you can provide a response more suited to your thinking or qualify a chosen response.

Notice that there are two spaces before each item. Use the space on the left for your answer at the beginning of the course. At the end of the course, take this inventory again, placing your answer in the space on the right. Cover your initial answers so you won't be influenced by how you originally responded. Then you can see how your attitudes have changed as a result of your experience in this course.

___ ___ 1. The personal characteristics of helpers are
    a. not really that relevant to the helping process.
    b. the most important variable in determining the quality of the helping process.
    c. shaped and molded by those who teach mental health workers.
    d. not as important as the skills and knowledge helpers possess.
    e. _____

___ ___ 2. Which of the following do you consider to be the most important personal characteristic of a good helper?
    a. Willingness to serve as a model for clients
    b. Courage
    c. Openness and honesty
    d. A sense of being "centered" as a person
    e. _____

___ ___ 3. I believe helpers' self-disclosure to their clients
    a. is essential for establishing a relationship.
    b. is inappropriate and merely burdens the client.

    c. should be done rarely and only when helpers feel it would be of benefit to clients.

    d. is useful to reveal how helpers feel toward their clients in the context of the professional relationship.

    e. _____

__ __ 4. If I were working with a client who could no longer continue because of his or her inability to pay my fees, I would most likely

    a. be willing to see this person at no fee, but in return expect him or her to do some type of volunteer work in the community.

    b. give my client the names of several referrals.

    c. suggest some form of bartering of goods or services for therapy services.

    d. adjust my fee to whatever the client could afford.

    e. _____

__ __ 5. Which of the following factors is most important in determining whether the helping process will result in change?

    a. The kind of person the helper is

    b. The skills and techniques the helper uses

    c. The motivation of the client to change

    d. The theoretical orientation of the helper

    e. _____

__ __ 6. Which of the following do you consider to be the most important attribute of an effective mental health practitioner?

    a. Knowledge of the theory of counseling and behavior

    b. Skill in using techniques appropriately

    c. Genuineness and openness

    d. Ability to specify a treatment plan and evaluate the results

    e. _____

__ __ 7. With respect to a fieldwork placement,

    a. I do not feel at all ready to participate in fieldwork.

    b. I would treat it like a job.

    c. I expect to limit myself to working with the kind of clients that I think I want to eventually work with in a job position.

    d. I want to work with clients that I think would be a challenge for me.

    e. _____

__ __ 8. To be an effective helper, I believe I

    a. must have an in-depth knowledge of my client's cultural background.

    b. must be free of any personal conflicts in the area in which the client is working.

    c. need to have experienced the same problem as the client.

    d. must be aware of my own needs and motivations for wanting to enter the helping field.

    e. _____

__ __ 9. With regard to the client-helper relationship, I think

    a. the helper should remain objective and anonymous.

     b. the helper should be a friend to the client.

     c. a personal relationship, but not friendship, is essential.

     d. a personal and warm relationship is not essential.

     e. _____

___ ___ 10. I should be open and honest with my clients

     a. when I like and value them.

     b. when I have negative feelings toward them.

     c. rarely, if ever, so that I will avoid negatively influencing the client-helper relationship.

     d. only when it intuitively feels like the right thing to do.

     e. _____

___ ___ 11. If I were faced with an ethical dilemma, the first step I would take would be to

     a. talk to my supervisor or seek consultation.

     b. attempt to solve the problem myself.

     c. identify the nature of the problem or problems.

     d. talk to my client and strive to involve him or her in working through this dilemma.

     e. _____

___ ___ 12. If I were not getting the kind of supervision I thought I needed and want, my inclination would be to

     a. make the best of the situation and not cause any trouble.

     b. demand that my supervisor provide adequate supervision.

     c. learn assertiveness skills and consistently ask for what I need by way of supervision.

     d. suggest that my peers and I form our own peer-supervision group to talk about the concerns we are facing.

     e. _____

___ ___ 13. If I were an intern and was convinced that my supervisor was encouraging trainees to take on clients with problems beyond their level of education and competence, I would

     a. first discuss the matter with the supervisor.

     b. ask my supervisor to give me extra help and perhaps work with me directly.

     c. ignore the situation for fear of negative consequences.

     d. refuse to engage in delivering any services that I thought were beyond my level of competence.

     e. _____

___ ___ 14. Practitioners who work with culturally diverse groups without having multicultural knowledge and skills

     a. are certainly not going to be able to provide effective services.

     b. are probably guilty of unethical behavior.

     c. will need to acquire the knowledge and skills by taking a course, reading, or engaging in continuing education.

     d. are making themselves vulnerable to a malpractice suit.

     e. _____

___ ___ 15. If I were working with a difficult and resistant client, my approach would likely be to
  a. discuss my reactions to my client's behavior with him or her.
  b. keep my reactions to myself and figure ways that I might get the upper hand with my client.
  c. discuss strategies for reaching difficult clients with a supervisor or colleague.
  d. strive to honor and respect the resistances my client displays and encourage my client to explore his or her attitudes and behaviors.
  e. _____

___ ___ 16. I won't feel ready to offer professional help to others until
  a. I have completed the program I am now in.
  b. I have developed a specialization that will make me an expert in a particular area.
  c. I feel very confident and know that I will be effective.
  d. I have become a self-aware person and developed the ability to continually reexamine my own life and relationships.
  e. _____

___ ___ 17. If a client evidenced strong feelings of attraction or dislike for me, I think I would
  a. immediately want to discuss this matter in my supervision.
  b. not have a clue as to how to respond.
  c. quickly refer my client to another professional.
  d. engage in self-disclosure, letting my client know how I was affected by what he or she said to me.
  e. _____

___ ___ 18. Practitioners who counsel clients whose sex, race, age, social class, or sexual orientation is different from their own
  a. will constantly be tested by these clients, which will make trust almost impossible.
  b. need to understand the meaning of the differences between their clients and themselves.
  c. are likely to be very effective if they are willing to acquire a range of knowledge and skills that will enable them to become culturally competent helpers.
  d. are probably not going to be effective with such clients because of these differences.
  e. _____

___ ___ 19. When I consider being involved in the helping professions, I value most the
  a. money I expect to earn.
  b. status and recognition that will be associated with the job.
  c. knowledge that I will be intimately involved with people who are searching for a better life.
  d. personal growth I expect to experience through my work.
  e. _____

____ ____ 20. With respect to making value judgments in the helping relationship, I
believe helpers should
   a. feel free to make value judgments about their clients' behavior.
   b. actively teach their own values when they think clients need a dif-
      ferent set of values.
   c. remain neutral and keep their values out of the helping process.
   d. encourage clients to question their own values and decide on the
      quality of their own behavior.
   e. _____

____ ____ 21. Helpers should
   a. teach desirable behavior and values by modeling them for clients.
   b. encourage clients to look within themselves to discover values
      that are meaningful to them.
   c. reinforce the dominant values of society.
   d. very delicately, if at all, challenge clients' value systems.
   e. _____

____ ____ 22. I would refer a client to another professional if
   a. I were convinced that I was no longer able to be effective with this
      client for any reason.
   b. I didn't have much experience working with the kind of problem
      the client presented.
   c. any sort of conflict of values existed between my client and me.
   d. the client seemed resistant and was not willing to be open to my
      suggestions.
   e. _____

____ ____ 23. Regarding confidentiality, I believe
   a. there is little hope that trust will be established unless clients can
      be guaranteed absolute confidentiality.
   b. it is ethical to break confidence when there is reason to believe
      that a client will do harm to someone else or will harm himself or
      herself.
   c. it is essential for me to discuss in detail the purpose and limits of
      confidentiality at the first session with a client.
   d. it is ethical to inform the authorities when a client is breaking the
      law.
   e. _____

____ ____ 24. A sexual relationship between a *former* client and a therapist is
   a. ethical if the therapist can prove that the relationship will not
      harm the former client.
   b. considered ethical 2 years after the termination of the professional
      relationship.
   c. ethical only when client and therapist discuss the issue and agree
      to the relationship.
   d. never ethical, regardless of the time that has elapsed.
   e. _____

_____ _____ 25. If a client were to offer me a gift, I would
    a. possibly accept it, but only after fully discussing the matter with my client.
    b. never accept it under any circumstances.
    c. accept the gift only if this was the termination of our professional relationship.
    d. accept the gift if gift-giving were a part of the client's culture and if refusing the gift would be insulting to my client.
    e. _____

_____ _____ 26. With respect to the role of spiritual and religious values in the helping process, I would be inclined to
    a. do my best to keep my own values out of the professional relationship for fear that I would unduly influence my client.
    b. recommend to my client that he or she think about how spirituality or religion could bring new meaning to his or her life.
    c. avoid introducing such topics in a session unless my client initiated this discussion.
    d. routinely conduct an assessment of my client's spiritual and religious beliefs during the intake session.
    e. _____

_____ _____ 27. Regarding the issue of who should select goals in the helping process, I believe
    a. it is the helper's responsibility to select goals.
    b. it is the client's responsibility to select goals.
    c. the responsibility for selecting goals should be a collaborative venture by both client and helper.
    d. the question of who selects the goals depends on what kind of client is being seen.
    e. _____

_____ _____ 28. Concerning the helper's responsibility to the community, I believe
    a. the helper should educate the community concerning the nature of psychological services.
    b. the central role of a helper is that of a change agent.
    c. it is appropriate to function as an advocate for underrepresented groups in the community.
    d. helpers should become involved in helping clients use the resources available in the community.
    e. _____

_____ _____ 29. When it comes to working in institutions or a system, I believe
    a. I must learn how to survive with dignity within a system.
    b. I must learn how to subvert the system so that I can do what I deeply believe in.
    c. the institution will stifle most of my enthusiasm and block any real change.

    d. I cannot blame the institution if I am unable to succeed in my programs.

    e. _____

___ ___ 30. If my philosophy were in conflict with that of the institution I worked for, I would

    a. seriously consider whether I could ethically remain in that position.

    b. attempt to change the policies of the institution by any means possible.

    c. agree to whatever was expected of me in that system so that I would not lose my job.

    d. quietly do what I wanted to do, even if I had to be devious about it.

    e. _____

By Way of Review

Near the end of each chapter we list some of the chapter's highlights. These key points serve as a review of the messages we have attempted to get across. We encourage you to spend a few minutes after you finish each chapter to write down central issues and points that have the most meaning for you.

- A helping career is not for everyone. We hope you will keep open the question of whether it is right for you.

- In deciding whether to pursue one of the helping professions, do not give up too soon. Be prepared for doubts and setbacks.

- Although the "ideal helper" does not exist in reality, a number of behaviors and attitudes characterize effective helpers. Even though you might not reach the ideal, you can progress, especially with the willingness to question what you are doing.

- It is essential that helpers examine their motivations for going into the field. Helpers meet their own needs through their work, and they must recognize these needs. It is possible for both client and helper to benefit from the helping relationship.

- Some of the needs for going into the helping professions include the need to be needed, the need for prestige and status, and the need to make a difference. These needs can work both for you and against you in becoming an effective helper.

- In selecting an educational program, follow your interests. Be willing to experiment by taking classes and by getting experience as a volunteer worker.

• In choosing a career path, consider factors such as self-concept, interests, abilities, values, occupational attitudes, socioeconomic level, parental influence, ethnic identity, gender, and personal limitations in the physical, mental, emotional, and social realms.

• Be willing to seek information about careers in mental health from others, such as professionals in the field and faculty members, but realize that ultimately you will decide which career path is best for you.

• Do not consider the selection of a career as a one-time event. Instead, allow yourself to entertain many job possibilities over your lifetime.

• Realize that you must have a beginning to your career. Be patient, and allow yourself time to feel comfortable in the role of helper. You don't have to be the perfect person or the perfect helper.

What Will You Do Now?

After each chapter review we provide concrete suggestions you can put into action. These suggested activities grow out of the major points developed in the chapter. Once you have read the chapter, we hope you will find some way to develop an action program. If you commit yourself to doing even one of these activities for each chapter, you will become more actively involved in the process of reading and reflecting.

1. If you are an undergraduate and if you think you would like to pursue a graduate program, select at least one graduate school to visit and talk with faculty members and students. If you are in a graduate program, contact several community agencies or attend a professional conference to determine what kinds of positions will be available to you. If you have an interest in obtaining a professional license, contact the appropriate board early in your program to obtain information on the requirements. (The American Counseling Association publishes an updated list of the counselor licensure board addresses and telephone numbers annually, as well as a list of state departments of education for all states.)

2. Ask a helper whom you know about his or her motivations for becoming a helper and for remaining in the profession. What does this person get out of helping clients?

3. Conduct an interview with a mental health professional who works in a position similar to the one you hope to obtain. Before the interview, develop a list of questions that you are interested in exploring. Write up the salient points of your interview, and share the results in your class.

4. The career-guidance center in your college or university probably offers several computer-based programs to help students decide on a career. One

popular program is known as the System of Interactive Guidance and Information (SIGI). This program assesses and categorizes your work values. Taking it will aid you in identifying specific occupations that you might want to explore.

5. Create your own activity or project (for this chapter or any of the chapters to follow). Find some ways to get involved by taking action. Think of ways you can apply what you read in each chapter to yourself. Decide on something specific, a step you can take now, that will help you get actively engaged in a positive endeavor. After reading this chapter, for example, you could decide to reflect on your own needs and motives for considering a career in the helping professions. Review some significant turning points in your life that might have contributed to your desire to become a helper.

6. If you are in a training program, now is an ideal time to begin getting involved in professional organizations. Become an active student member in at least one of the organizations described in this chapter. By joining an organization, you can take advantage of its workshops and conferences. Membership also puts you in touch with other professional with similar interests, gives you ideas for updating your skills, and helps you make excellent contacts.

7. We strongly encourage you to keep a journal as an adjunct to reading this book and taking this course. Write in your journal in a free-flowing and unedited style. Be honest, and use journal writing as an opportunity to get to know yourself better, to clarify your thinking on issues raised in each chapter, and to explore your thoughts and feelings about working in the helping professions. At the end of each chapter, we will provide a few suggestions of topics for you to reflect on and include in your journal writing. For this chapter, consider these areas:

- Write about your main motives for wanting to become a helper. How do you expect your needs to be satisfied through your work?
- Write about factors that have influenced your conception of what it means to be a helper. Who are your role models? What kind of helping did you receive?
- Spend some time thinking about the attributes of the ideal helper. What are your personal strengths that might help you as a helper? How realistic are your expectations about what you will be doing as a helper?
- What are your thoughts about selecting an educational and professional route to pursue? Write a bit on factors you will need to consider in choosing your own career path.

8. Attend a professional state, regional, or national conference offered by one of the various professional organizations. Attending as a student has numerous benefits, such as developing a network for jobs, field placements, and meeting colleagues with similar interests

9. Bring your completed self-assessment inventory to class to compare your views with those of others in the class. Such a comparison might stimulate some

debate and help get the class involved in the topics to be discussed. In choosing the issues you want to discuss in class, circle the numbers of those items that you felt most strongly about as you were responding. You may find it instructive to ask others how they responded to these items in particular.

10. At the end of each chapter we provide some suggestions for further reading. For the full bibliographic entry for each of the sources listed, consult the References and Reading List at the back of the book. For a discussion on a wide array of issues confronting those in the helping professions, see Kottler (1993, 1997, 2000). For comprehensive coverage of topics such as development of a professional identity, ethical standards, basic process skills, approaches to counseling, and the making of a professional counselor, see Neukrug (1999) and Kottler and Brown (2000). Consult Hutchins and Cole Vaught (1997) and Doyle (1998) for an overview of strategies for helping and the building blocks of the interview, along with skills in the helping process.

InfoTrac College Edition Resources

For additional readings, explore InfoTrac College Edition, our online library. Go to http://www.infotrac.college.com/wadsworth and select these key word searches:

   social W2 profession
   social W2 career
   social W1 work
   clinical W1 psychology
   counseling W1 psychology
   school W1 counseling
   pastoral W1 counseling
   rehabilitation W1 counseling
   self W1 concept
   marriage and family therapy

Key words are listed in a form that enables the search engine to locate a wider range of articles in the online university library. Key words should be entered exactly as shown, including asterisks, "W1," "W2," "AND," and other search engine tools.

CHAPTER 2

Getting the Most From Your Education and Training

Focus Questions

Aim of the Chapter

Creating Meaning in Your Education

Making the Most of Your Fieldwork

Profiting From Your Supervision

By Way of Review

What Will You Do Now?

InfoTrac College Edition Resources

Focus Questions

1. How would you describe yourself as a learner? Would you like to change your style of learning? If so, how?

2. What can you do to make your educational program more meaningful? How can you derive the maximum benefit from your academic courses?

3. What can you do to maximize your learning from fieldwork placements?

4. How can you better profit from your supervision? If you are not getting the quality of supervision you need, what steps can you take?

5. What are some ways to challenge your self-doubts in both your academic courses and your fieldwork placement? How can you change your fears into assets and opportunities for learning?

6. What are some possible benefits of sticking with a field placement that is not to your liking?

7. In meetings with your supervisor and fellow students, what attitude can you assume that will lead to maximizing your learning? What specific steps can you take to confront any difficulties you are experiencing in your field placement?

8. What are your thoughts about receiving personal counseling as part of your sessions with your supervisor? What advantages and disadvantages do you see with this arrangement?

Aim of the Chapter

You will get far more from your program of studies and your fieldwork activities if you assume an *active stance* in your education. So often we hear students complain about their department, their professors, and their supervision. There are faults in any educational system, but it is more useful in the long run to look beyond these faults to see how you can get the most from your education. Rather than concentrating on all that you cannot do, for whatever reasons, take responsibility for your education.

Many systems impose limitations, but the challenge is to learn how to work creatively within that system to attain your key goals without sacrificing your integrity by "selling out." We often hear both students in college and professionals in human services systems argue that they could be more creative and productive "if it weren't for . . ." Here is a list of some common assertions. See how many of them sound familiar to you.

For students: "I would be a good learner if it weren't for . . .

- the professors who don't care."
- the long hours I work that cut into studying."
- my spouse, who won't support my efforts in going to college."
- my children, who take up so much of my time and interrupt my studies."
- an educational system that kills any creativity."
- so much reading and so many papers to write, leaving me no time to be concerned with what I'm learning."
- the unmotivated students in my classes."
- the unrealistic requirements and the pressures placed on me by my professors."

For professional helpers: "I would be productive, dynamic, and creative if it weren't for . . .

- my burned out colleagues, who infect me with their cynicism."
- the director at my agency, who is too demanding."
- the managed care system."
- my resistant clients."
- the lack of funding of our community program."
- all the paperwork, bureaucratic demands, and politics."
- my large caseload."
- my family, who make demands on me when I get home."
- supervisors who don't support my ideas."

These lists could easily be extended, but the point we want to make is that you could eternally create reasons outside of yourself to justify why you are not being productive. As long as you focus on "them out there," you are powerless to change your situation until someone or something else changes. We agree that these factors can hamper your efforts to find meaning at school and work; the challenge is to avoid letting these external barriers block you from attaining your goals.

Exercising a measure of freedom within external demands and restrictions entails accepting responsibility for doing what you can do, rather than focusing on what you cannot do. In this chapter we encourage you to assume a more powerful role in choosing an appropriate educational program, working in meaningful fieldwork placements, demanding adequate supervision, and continuing your learning after graduation.

Creating Meaning in Your Education

Learning to Cope With the System

There are real problems in working within any system. The reality of an educational program is grades, requirements, courses, and evaluation. Although students often balk at being evaluated and feel that grades are unfair, this system of evaluation does exist. Moreover, it is a mistake to assume that grading stops when you graduate from a university. There are reviews and evaluation practices on all levels in the professional world. In a business, for example, your supervisors rate you and determine whether you get a promotion or a raise. If you are a professional, your clients rate you by the business they bring to you or take away from you.

Students sometimes assume that there are worlds of difference between the roles they play in college and the roles they will assume as professionals. Many of the traits that you have as a student will no doubt carry over into your behavior as a worker. If you have great difficulty in showing up for classes regularly, for example, you are likely to carry this habit into your work appointments. Getting a position in a community agency is a highly competitive effort. If you hope to gain entry into the professional world, it is essential that you be prepared to cope with the realities of the marketplace. You are not being treated kindly if little is expected of you and if you are allowed to get by with minimal effort.

Students in the human services sometimes expect that their professors will make fewer demands on them or give them better grades because of the informal relationships established in the classroom. Many human services instructors are friendly, care about their students, and interact with them in a personal way. Some students have problems in knowing where to establish boundaries. They mistakenly assume that there should be no limits and that no demands should be placed on them because of this relatively close relationship. From our perspective a humanistic approach to education can be balanced with reasonable standards and expectations. Developing these academic standards is one basic way of preparing students to cope with the demands of the job market.

We asked some human service practitioners to comment on the degree to which both their undergraduate and graduate programs had prepared them for their jobs. We also asked them to say how much power they had had to provide input or to make meaningful changes in their educational program. Here are some of their responses:

- "Undergraduate studies prepared me well for counseling and proposal writing. Because I was a student representative to the program I was part of, I had a lot of power to provide input. I felt that my ideas were considered and that I had a voice."

- "I would have liked to have more administrative-type classes that dealt with how to best manage people. I often felt that I had the power to provide input, but I did not exercise this very often."

- "The kind of education and training that I most value is the practical and applied. Some of our professors asked us to relate our own issues with the course work. For example, in my graduate program in social work, we studied our own families. More than just learning material about families, we were encouraged to apply personal issues with the academic. We had a behavior class that consisted of weekly treatment cases. Vignettes on psychosocial problems were presented for us to analyze and discuss. We also talked about our job experiences, which proved to be useful."

- "It [the program] was a challenge! It gave me a wonderful foundation for the helping professions. It made me learn and believe in myself and my abilities."

- "My undergraduate program made me stop and take a look at who I was and what I wanted to do with my life, both personally and professionally. So many times I hear students say that their classes are not relevant to the real world. Fortunately, this was not the case for me with my program."

Investing in Your Education

At the beginning of your educational program you may feel that you will have to remain in school forever to do what you want professionally. However, if you are enjoying and gaining from the experience, you will likely be surprised at how soon you complete your program. The key is that you are personally involved in your educational program and that you can see a connection between your formal studies and your personal and professional goals. Think about how much time and energy you are prepared to devote to making your education meaningful. It may help to consider your education as an investment, and then decide what you can do to get the most from this investment.

Investments are often evaluated by their cost-benefit ratio. The cost of your educational investment includes not just money but your time and energy too. Look at the potential benefits of this investment, including what you hope you will gain from your investment. Basically, evaluating the cost-benefit ratio of your investment involves asking yourself if what you are putting in (costs) is worth what you hope to get out of it in return (benefits). What are the benefits of putting a great deal of yourself into your formal studies? What will taking responsibility for your education cost you in terms of time taken away from other facets of your life?

It is most important to take responsibility for your own learning. Students who fail to see their own role in the learning process may find others to blame for their failures. If you are dissatisfied with your education, consider how much you are willing to invest to make it more vital. If you were dissatisfied with your earlier education, now is a good time to look at yourself and ask how much you are willing to invest to get more out of this experience. Are you waiting for others to do something for you? How much are you willing to do to change the things you don't like?

Regardless of the structure of the course in which you are using this book, you can find ways to become personally involved in the course. *You* can decide to be either actively engaged or marginally involved in applying the themes in this book and your course in your life. *You* can make this class different by applying some of the ideas provided in this chapter. Once you become aware of those aspects of your education that you don't like, *you* can decide to change your style of learning.

Becoming an Active Learner for Life

Most of us spend years acquiring information about the world around us. We may even equate learning with absorbing facts that are external to us. Although academic knowledge provides a foundation for becoming a helper, it is equally important to learn about yourself and about how to live fully. What you get from your educational program will depend on the degree to which you become an active agent in your learning. Here are some guidelines to help you develop this active stance.

1. *Preparing.* Many students have been conditioned to view reading as an unpleasant assignment, and they tolerate textbooks as something to plow through for an examination. As an active learner, however, you can selectively read this book, reflecting on those sections that have special meaning to you. Write brief reactions in the margins as you read, and come to class prepared to share your thoughts on these topics. Taking the time to think about the topics explored in this book and the personal meaning they have for you will enhance your learning experience. For those of you who enjoy using the computer, you could keep a journal of your reactions to the assigned readings on your computer.

2. *Dealing with anxieties.* Personal learning is not without anxiety. Anxiety is a response to fear. Some of the fears students often express include the fear of taking an honest look at yourself and discovering terrible things; the fear of the unknown; the fear of looking foolish in front of others, especially your instructor; the fear of being criticized or ridiculed; and the fear of speaking out and expressing your values. How you deal with your fears is more important than trying to eliminate all of your anxieties. Facing your fears takes both courage and a genuine desire to increase your awareness of yourself. In doing so, you take a big step toward becoming the kind of person who can make a significant difference in the lives of others.

3. *Taking risks.* If you make the choice to get personally involved in the course, you should be prepared for the possibility of some disruption in your life. You may find yourself changing certain values, beliefs, and behaviors. You may like many of the changes you make that are an outgrowth of your participation in a program designed to educate and train professional helpers. However, some

people may neither like nor appreciate your changes, and, indeed, some may be intimidated by you and stubbornly resist your attempt to step outside of old and familiar patterns.

4. *Establishing trust.* It is up to you to take the initiative in establishing the trust necessary for you to participate in this course in a meaningful way. If you become aware that you hold yourself back from getting verbally active in class discussions, consider seeing the instructor outside of class to talk about this.

5. *Self-disclosing.* Disclosing yourself to others is one way to come to know yourself more fully. It is also a good way to let others in your educational program know you. You can be open and at the same time retain your privacy by deciding what you will share and how much you will disclose. Although it may be new and uncomfortable for you to express your ideas and share learnings based on your life experiences, we hope you challenge yourself to express your thoughts and feelings to the degree that it is appropriate in all phases of your educational program.

6. *Listening.* One of the basic helping skills is being able to listen fully to others and respond to the core of their messages. To develop this skill, listen to what others are saying without thinking of what you will say in reply. The first step in understanding is to listen carefully without judging what you hear. *Active listening* (really hearing the full message another is sending) requires that you remain open and carefully consider what others say rather than rushing to give reasons and explanations.

7. *Practicing outside of class.* One way to get the maximum benefit from your educational program is to think about ways of applying what you learn to your everyday life. You can make specific contracts with yourself (or with others) detailing what you are willing to do to experiment with new behavior and work toward the changes you want to make.

Integrating Knowledge, Skills, and Self

In our view you need to integrate what you know, what you can do, and the person who you are. Knowledge alone is not sufficient, yet without it you cannot become an effective helper. If you focus mainly on acquiring skills but neglect theory and knowledge, these skills will be of little use. Furthermore, your ability to use the skills and knowledge you have is very much a function of your being sensitive to the interpersonal dimension of the helping process. You need to know yourself and your client to effectively apply helping skills. Helpers who have a low degree of self-awareness are at best skilled technicians, and we doubt that they will make a positive difference with clients. Helping is more than technique; it is an art that is an expression of who the helper is. The helping professions are based on scientific knowledge that practitioners are able to use in creative and personal ways. In short, helping is both an art and a science.

A view from practitioners.   We asked some practitioners what specialized knowledge and skills they saw as most important in their present job, and most commented on the value of internships and fieldwork placements. These supervised practical experiences had helped them learn about ways of working meaningfully within a system. The skills most practitioners felt they needed included counseling skills, supervisory skills, consulting skills, communication skills, the ability to interact with different levels of management, the ability to write a proposal, organizational skills, the ability to deal with crisis intervention, and networking skills. A number of the professionals pointed out the value of self-exploratory experiences, especially groups aimed at personal and interpersonal growth. These therapeutic experiences gave them opportunities to look at themselves and to deal with their own feelings and problems, activities that were seen as especially helpful in preparing them to relate to clients. Even those professionals who were primarily engaged in the administration of human services programs commented on the value of self-awareness and the understanding of interpersonal dynamics as tools they utilized in their managerial functions. Those in management pointed out that they would not be able to develop and coordinate their programs if they did not know how to work effectively with people.

A view from community agencies.   As part of the self-study program conducted by our department at the university, community agencies that offer fieldwork placements to our students were contacted and asked a number of questions regarding what they were looking for in hiring employees as well as their views on other relevant issues. Here are some of the questions we posed to agency personnel along with a representative sample of their responses to these questions.

1.   What special knowledge and skills do our students need in order to work effectively at your agency?

- Ability to work with diverse cultures
- Organizational and social skills; professionalism
- Understand ethics and confidentiality issues
- Good people skills
- Ability to communicate effectively with children as well as staff members
- Knowledge of state laws affecting minors
- Resourcefulness and ability to direct and give referrals
- Listening skills, case management skills, and counseling skills
- Take the job seriously
- Ability to be proactive rather than reactive

2. What knowledge, skills, and competencies do you consider most important for employees in your agency?

- A good deal of independence combined with responsible reporting of treatment plans, incidents, and therapeutic progress
- Able to identify personal and professional boundaries and maintain clear boundaries

- An outreach person who can organize a program from start to finish
- Must be creative, adaptable, and open-minded with an eagerness to serve the community in a nonjudgmental way
- Sensitivity to older adults
- Punctuality, reliability, and interest in the mission and goals of this agency
- A level-headed person who does well in social situations
- Awareness and acceptance of cultural diversity, including the immigrant experience
- Self-motivated individuals
- Key skills in time management and using resources
- Good organizational skills
- Ability to work with a disabled population in an educational environment
- Good understanding of basic functions of nonprofit organizations
- Flexibility and ability to work as a team
- Outgoing, comfortable working with low-income, disadvantaged and ethnically diverse schools
- Good problem-solving skills and a good innovator
- Crisis intervention skills
- Writing, communication, and computer skills
- Understands legislative issues

3. What trends do you foresee in the future for the field of human services?

- More networking of agencies and organizations to combine programs for a better impact on the people they serve
- Family preservation and preventive programs
- Expansion in services for the upcoming senior population explosion
- Short-term interventions
- More community outreach in assisting multi-ethnic communities with access to health care services
- Need to be adept at serving people with dual and often triple diagnoses
- Managed care models
- Treating not just the senior but other family members as well

Keeping Current

In looking at the knowledge and skills community agencies deem essential for both interns and employees, it is clearly a tall order to expect to acquire all of this knowledge and the desired skills during your academic program. Thus, it is essential that you discover ways to extend your education beyond graduation, for your knowledge and skills will soon be outdated unless you take steps to keep abreast of new developments. Some current issues in the helping professions that are receiving increased attention are methods of dealing with substance abuse; eating disorders; gay, lesbian, and bisexual issues; physical, psychological, and sexual abuse of children; abuse of the elderly and spouses; HIV/AIDS; conflict resolution skills; parent education; adolescent suicide; school violence; culturally diverse client populations; and legal and ethical issues. Avail yourself of in-service and continuing-education programs and challenge yourself to find ways to go outside the confines of your daily work and not to become encapsulated by its boundaries.

Although many professionals have mandatory continuing-education requirements for the relicensing or recertification of their members, we hope that you develop your own self-directed program and do not merely comply with the minimum requirements. You can do this by taking specialized courses and workshops that deal with particular client groups and newer techniques.

Reading is another good way to keep abreast of developments in your field. In addition to professional journals and books dealing with your specific subject of interest, novels and nonfiction works about other cultures are also of value in your continuing education.

Perhaps one of the best ways of keeping yourself up to date is to be involved in a professional network with colleagues who are willing to learn from one another as well as assume a teaching role. Colleagues can offer both the challenge and the support for practitioners to adopt a fresh perspective on problems they encounter in professional practice. Networking among professionals can also provide a consistent means of identifying and addressing sources of negative feelings and loss of objectivity. An excellent way to develop this network is by joining the professional organization that most interests you and by attending the state, regional, and national conferences offered by this organization.

Making the Most of Your Fieldwork

In the helping professions of counseling, social work, psychology, and couples and family therapy, most graduate programs have fieldwork and internship at their core. Most undergraduate programs in human services have a comprehensive fieldwork component, which is often the heart of the program. These activities provide a bridge between theory and practice. Students can compare their expectations of the field with the reality imposed by most agencies. Actual experience in a field placement gives students opportunities to learn first-hand about paperwork, agency policies and procedures, and the challenge of working with a wide range of client populations and problems. These are some of the goals of a fieldwork instruction program:

- Provide students with knowledge of the varied approaches and methods used in human services programs
- Help students extend self-awareness and achieve a sense of professional identity
- Broaden students' sociocultural understanding of the individual, the family, the community, and relevant social systems
- Assist students in recognizing and respecting cultural diversity and offer ways to use this understanding in practice
- Help students expand their awareness of professional role relationships within their organization as well as the agency's role in the community

Of course, before you can meaningfully participate in fieldwork and internship placements, you need theory courses, specific knowledge, and a range of helping skills. You can enhance your academic learning by volunteering to work in a community agency. It is the combination of academic course work, fieldwork placement, skills training, and personal development that makes for a sound program.

If you have some choice in selecting the place where you will be gaining supervised practical experience, take an active role in securing the best placement possible. One way of actively participating in securing a quality fieldwork placement is by asking questions of potential agency settings when you are going through the interviewing process for a field placement. Here are some questions you might ask:

- What are the goals and purposes of your agency or organization? What services are provided?
- Have you worked with student interns before? If so, what have been some of their activities?
- What internship opportunities are now available at this agency?
- What would be my specific responsibilities?
- Are there any special skills or requirements for the placement?
- To whom would I report? Who would supervise me? How often would I be able to meet with this person for direct supervision?
- Are there training or staff development opportunities at the agency? What kinds of training might I receive prior to and during my placement?
- Is there any videotaping equipment available?
- Is any travel involved? If so, will I be reimbursed for travel?
- Would I be covered by the agency for malpractice liability?

Sometimes students seek placements that are expedient, convenient, and not very challenging. We hope you value your education enough to strive for a placement where you will receive adequate supervision and where you will be exposed to a variety of problems that clients bring to a community agency.

If you are employed at a community agency and want to use this agency for your fieldwork placement, we recommend that you branch out to get as much variety as possible in your placements. If you already have volunteer or paid work experience in a particular setting, consider doing something different for your internship: do different tasks, occupy a different role, or work with another client population. Your fieldwork experience should provide you with a variety of settings in which to work and also with various supervising environments. Trying to accomplish double duty by using your work experience as a substitute does not seem to us to be getting the most from your fieldwork. Although it may be possible to combine some aspects of your employment with an internship, we hope you do not take the easiest and quickest path toward getting your degree. A wide range of opportunities exists within an agency. Secure training in areas new to you so you will be able to acquire new knowledge and skills. The more practical and supervised experience you can get the better. Commit yourself to becoming the most competent practitioner you can be.

When we talk with graduates of human services programs, they typically mention that they found their current job as a result of contacts they established at their fieldwork placement. In fact, most graduates report wishing they had been able to participate in even more fieldwork activities. Some regret not having had a broader range of experience in their internships. We recommend that you visit as many sites as possible before making your selection, if that is allowed in your program. Get job descriptions and arrange interviews with selected agencies.

The Value of Fieldwork Experiences

For a variety of reasons, students often do not derive the maximum benefit from fieldwork and supervision. Here are some practical strategies for getting the most value out of your fieldwork placements:

• Instead of limiting yourself to one kind of population, seek a variety of placements. Stretch your boundaries to help you to discover where your talents lie and the kind of population you would eventually like to work with. Through your internships you may learn what you do not want to do as well as what you would like to do. Some students who initially want to "do counseling" exclusively later find themselves in the role of an administrator or a supervisor.

• Take courses and workshops that will prepare you for the type of work expected of you in your placement. These workshops can be a useful resource for staying on the cutting edge of new developments with specialized populations.

• Let yourself fit into the agency, instead of trying to make it fit you. Be open to learning from the staff and the clients who come to the agency. Attempt to suspend your preconceived judgments about what you should be learning and focus instead on the lessons that are available to you. Learn as much as you can about the politics of the agency by talking with people who work there, by attending staff meetings, and by asking questions. All of your learning will not result merely from interacting with clients. You can learn a good deal about an agency by being attentive and by talking with co-workers.

• Be aware of the toll that your work might have on you both emotionally and physically. Certain aspects of your life that you have not been willing to look at may be opened up as you get involved with clients. Know that your increased awareness could lead to more anxiety in your life.

• Recognize the limits of your training, practice only within these boundaries, and put yourself in situations where you will be able to obtain supervised experience. Regardless of your educational level, there is always more to learn. It is essential to learn the delicate balance between being overly confident and doubting yourself.

• Strive to be flexible in applying techniques to the different client populations, but do so under supervision. Avoid falling into the trap of fitting your clients to one particular theory. Use theory as a means of helping you understand the behavior of your clients. Realize that diverse client backgrounds necessitate diverse communication approaches. Although it is essential to learn therapeutic skills and techniques, they should be applied in appropriate ways.

• Do not write off as a waste of time a placement that you do not particularly like. At least you are learning that working in a particular agency or with a specific clientele may not be what you want for a career. Determine what you don't find productive about the placement, and why. Then try to make your assignment more meaningful rather than just putting in your time to get your credit. Create learning opportunities and welcome all experiences as resources that can teach you what you will need to know in future situations.

• Make connections in the community. Learn how to use community resources and how to draw on support systems beyond your office. Talk to other professionals in the field, ask fellow students about their connections in the community, and develop a network of contacts. This kind of networking may well lead to a range of job opportunities.

• Keep a journal; record your observations, experiences, concerns, and personal reactions to your work. Your journal is an excellent way to stay focused on yourself as well as to keep track of what you are doing with clients.

• Be open to trying new things. If you have not worked with a family, for example, observe a family session or, if possible, work with a supervisor who is counseling a family. Avoid setting yourself up by thinking that if you do not succeed perfectly in a new endeavor you are a dismal failure. Give yourself room to learn by doing, at the same time gaining supervised experience.

• Look for ways to apply what you are learning in your academic courses to your experiences in the field. For example, one professional recalls having taken abnormal psychology as part of her graduate program and also having served as an intern in a state mental institution. Through this internship she was able to actually see some of the concepts she was studying come to life. One important lesson she learned was that many of the patients did not fit neatly into some diagnostic category.

• Be prepared to adjust your expectations. An agency is unlikely to give you responsibility for providing services to clients before it has a chance to know you. You will probably start your fieldwork in an observing role. Later you may sit in on a counseling group, for example, and function as a co-leader.

• Find ways to work cooperatively with other students and to combine your talents with theirs. Look for means of tapping into your own creativity. If you are talented musically, for example, look for a way in which you might incorporate music into your field placement activities. If a fellow student has talents in dance and movement, perhaps you can combine forces in an innovative therapeutic intervention.

• Treat your field placement like a job. Approach fieldwork in much the same way as you would if you were employed by the agency. Demonstrate responsibility, be on time for your appointments and meetings, follow through with your commitments, and strive to do your best. Although you may be in an unpaid placement, this does not mean you can be irresponsible on the job.

• Learn as much as you can about the structure of the agency where you are placed. Ask about agency policies, about the way the programs are administered, and about management of the staff. At some point, you may be involved in the administrative aspects of a social program.

• Think and act in a self-directed way by involving yourself in a variety of activities. If you merely wait for a supervisor or other workers to take the initiative and give you meaningful assignments, you may be less than satisfied with your placement.

The Challenge of Diversity

As we have suggested, it is a good idea to seek a placement where you will be challenged to work with a variety of clients and tasks. Your learning will be limited if you attempt to get placements with clients just like yourself or those with whom you already know how to work. By working with diverse populations, you can test out your interests and develop new ones. If you focus narrowly on the population or problem area you have chosen as a specialization, you are likely to close off many rich avenues of learning and also limit your possibilities of finding a job.

As a part of your fieldwork for internship placement, you usually receive on-the-job training and supervision. Therefore, you might not need expertise in counseling rape victims before being accepted for such a placement. You will learn from co-workers and supervisors some interventions in working with such clients. Thus, more important than knowing how to work with a specific population or a specific problem is having a general background of knowledge and skills and being open to acquiring more specific abilities.

Helping someone different from you.   One of our colleagues told us that her paralyzed client became upset and angry when she said to him, "I understand how you feel." His reply was: "How would you know? You can walk out of here, and I can't." On reflection, our colleague thought that she might have said: "You're right, I don't fully understand your situation. I can imagine your frustration and pain over becoming paralyzed at such a young age in a motorcycle accident. But I haven't been in your situation, so I don't know what you're thinking and feeling. I hope you will help me understand what this is like for you, and I hope I can help you work through your own feelings about being paralyzed."

Some interns make the mistake of clinging to the conviction that to help a person they must have had the same life experience. Thus, a male counselor may doubt his capacity to effectively counsel an adolescent girl who is struggling with what she wants to do about being pregnant. A counselor may doubt that she can work with a client of a different race. Or a counselor who has not experienced trauma may wonder about her ability to empathize with clients who have had pain in their lives. When these counselors are challenged by a client, they often tend to backtrack and become apologetic. We hope that you can see the value of drawing on your own life experience in working with clients who are different from you. You may not have had the same problem, yet you may be able to identify with the feelings of loneliness or rejection of your client. It is more important to be able to understand the client's world than to have had the identical problem. What is crucial is that you realize that some of your clients will view the world from a different perspective than you do. In Chapter 8 we deal with this topic of diverse worldviews in more detail.

Challenging your self-doubt.   Interns are often unsure, apologetic, and unwilling to credit themselves with what they know and are able to do. Ask yourself how you deal with your own feelings about what you know and don't know.

Consider how you might deal with a client who challenged you. At the initial session your client is surprised at your age. "Who are you to be helping me?" he asks. "You look so young, and I wonder if you have the experience to help me." Assume that this challenge opens up some of your own fears and doubts. Can you imagine saying any of the following things silently to yourself?

- "He's right. There are many years separating us. I wonder if I can understand his situation?"
- "This guy's attitude really makes me mad. He's not giving me a chance, and I feel attacked before I've even had a chance to know him."
- "Well, I don't feel comfortable with this confrontation, but I don't want to back down. I feel like letting him know that even though we differ in age we might have many similarities in our struggles. I'd like an opportunity to at least explore whether we can form a relationship."
- "He's right. What makes me think I have anything to offer him? Maybe I should have chosen another line of work."

Certainly as individuals we are all affected when someone challenges us, but as helpers we cannot afford to have a fragile ego. Helping is not about proving that we are "right." Stay focused on the best interests of the clients and address any challenges in a direct and honest manner. If you feel that you might have done something more effectively or sensitively, it helps to simply acknowledge this.

Most professionals have feelings of self-doubt and question their competence at certain times and in certain situations. The purpose of your supervised fieldwork is to provide you with a rich and meaningful learning opportunity. This is a place where you can acquire specific knowledge and where you can develop the skills to translate the theory you have learned into practice. We hope you have the courage to face your feelings of incompetence rather than running from them or pretending that they do not exist.

Profiting From Your Supervision

Be clear in your own mind about what you expect from your supervisors, and discuss your desires with them from the outset. This section suggests how to approach your supervision and actively participate in this process.

Be Open to Learning From Your Supervisors

Be open to input not only from supervisors but also from teachers, peers, colleagues, and clients. You will limit your opportunities for learning if you assume a know-it-all stance. Have the courage to admit your imperfections, and do not become frozen out of fear of making errors. Be willing to recognize mistakes, and talk openly with your supervisor about them. If you do not have the courage to acknowledge when you fail, you will not be willing to try anything new. You will be overly conscious about what you are doing and whether you are doing it "right." Take advantage of your student role; as a student, you are certainly not expected to know everything. Give yourself permission to be a learner. If you can free yourself from the shackles of trying to live up to the unrealistic ideal of perfection, your clients will become your teachers in some significant ways.

In our training of group leaders we typically find that the students approach workshops with considerable anxiety over looking incompetent in the eyes of their peers and supervisors. Early in the workshop we tell them: "Be active. One sure way not to learn much in this workshop is by being extremely self-conscious and critically judging most of what you want to say or do. No matter what happens, there is something to be learned. If a group session is unproductive, you can explore what specific factors contributed to that outcome."

When we give students these instructions, they usually react with relief and tell us they feel much less anxious. We let them know that we understand and empathize with their difficulty in being observed by their peers and by supervisors. It is not possible to escape from being watched by clients, supervisors, and fellow workers. Talking about our experience of being observed allows us to be in control of this process rather than being controlled by what others might think of us. Students often find it helpful to openly share their fears. Paradoxically, the fears of the students appear to be diminished by this act of acknowledgment.

Be able to say "I don't know."   Being willing to admit when you have a lack of knowledge or understanding about a situation with both your supervisor and your clients. If you feel intimidated because you have to tell a client that you do not know an answer to her problem, you can say something like this: "You know, I'm not sure what to say or how best to help you with your predicament. I realize that you are anxious and that you'd very much like me to tell you what you should do. I'd be willing to consult my supervisor and get some ideas that I can bring back to you in a couple of days." In this way you acknowledge your limitations to your client, but you keep the door open to providing her with information she can use in resolving her own problems.

Express your reactions.   In working with both students and professionals, we often find that they have many good reactions that they keep to themselves. We typically encourage our trainees to talk out loud more often rather than engaging in an internal monologue. In a recent workshop a group counselor was quiet throughout the group session. The supervisor asked her what was going on. "Well, I'm very aware that you, my supervisor, are present in this session," she replied. "I feel inhibited in following my hunches, because I'm wondering what you might think of what I'm doing. I'm afraid that you might be judging me and that

I might not be measuring up very well." Her supervisor told her that this was what would have been best for her to say aloud.

In another instance one trainee continually suggested one exercise after another during a particular group-training session. Later, when he was asked why he had introduced so many different exercises in such a short session, he replied: "Well, the group seemed to be getting nowhere. People seemed bored, and I felt responsible for making something happen! I was hoping to bring the group alive by trying some interaction exercises." We told the trainee that it would have been good to describe what he saw happening in the group. He could have talked about his feelings of responsibility and about how his perception of boredom affected him. Instead, he ignored expressing his own important reactions in favor of using techniques, which didn't work in the long run. We are not suggesting that you express your every fleeting reaction to your clients, but in your supervision meetings it is wise to talk about unrehearsed material.

Focus on both elements of supervision. Some approaches to supervision emphasize the client's dynamics and teach you strategies for intervening in specific problems. Others focus on your dynamics as a helper and as a person and on your behavior in relationship to your client. Adequate supervision must take both of these elements into consideration. You need to understand models of helping clients, and you need to understand yourself if you hope to form truly therapeutic alliances. If your supervision is focused solely on what your client is doing or on teaching you specific techniques for what to do next, it will be lacking in a most important dimension. A critical focus for discussion in supervision sessions is the degree to which you are as present as possible for your clients. If you are overly concerned about what to do about a client's problem, this concern will distract you from making connections with the person. A useful focus of supervision is the variables that define the quality of the relationship between you and your clients. In supervision, you can talk about what you are experiencing as you work with different clients. This focus will reveal a good deal about both you and your clients.

Learn, but don't copy. We have observed that some trainees limit their own development by trying too hard to copy the style of a supervisor or teacher. You are likely to watch carefully supervisors whom you respect, and you may tend to adopt their methods. It is important, however, to be aware of how easy it is to become a carbon copy of another person. To get the most from your supervision, try different styles, but continually evaluate what works for you and what does not. You might ask yourself: "What fits my belief system, both personal and theoretical? Do I have any conflicts between the theory or application of my supervisor's way and my own?"

If you pay too much attention to another person, you are likely to blur your own uniqueness. You need to be able to take what is good from your various supervisors and teachers, yet it is important to avoid being a clone. Be willing to learn from others, but don't feel that you need to *be* them. If you learn to listen to your own inner voice and to respect your inner promptings, you will eventually have less need to look to outside authorities.

Maximize your time in supervision.   You will get the most from your supervision if you take an active stance as a supervisee. Here are a few suggestions for benefiting from your supervision:

- Know the general purpose of supervision.
- Recognize that different supervisors will attempt to achieve the purpose of supervision in a variety of ways.
- Accept that a certain level of anxiety is to be expected in the supervision process.
- Clarify any aspects of your contract with your supervisor regarding the content of the supervision sessions.
- Strive to be as honest and open as possible during your supervision sessions.
- If you are not able to select your supervisor, do your best to work within the framework of his or her supervisory style.
- Clarify for yourself what you most want and need from supervision, and be willing to ask your supervisor for this.
- Take the time to prepare for your supervision session by identifying questions you want to explore and by bringing in examples you want to discuss with your supervisor.

Learn to Be Assertive

Define how you want to spend your time in an agency, and get the supervision you need. Don't wait passively to be told what to do. Think about what you would like to learn and what skills you would like to acquire. A placement typically involves a written contract signed by the student and the supervisor of the agency. This contract usually spells out the number of hours to be worked per week, the activities that will be performed, the learning objectives, the opportunities for training, the expectations for the intern, and the expectations for the supervisor. Before agreeing to your contract with your supervisor, discuss in some detail the ways in which you think you could be of greatest benefit to the agency. In collaboration with your supervisor, spell out what you would like to experience and learn before you leave. Although you may not always get what you want, if you have a clear idea of what that is, you will have a better chance of obtaining it.

The assertion skills you practice in getting adequate supervision will be useful in your relationships with both clients and colleagues. Being assertive does not mean being aggressive, which alienates most people. By bulldozing your way into an agency, you will needlessly put others on the defensive. Being passive-aggressive is not useful either, whether it involves rebelling against all authority, appearing bored, or consistently showing up for appointments or meetings late. Resisting in such passive ways is likely to shut you off from many opportunities to learn.

It helps to realize that supervisors are people too. They get bogged down with their own burdens. As their client load grows and pressures increase, they may not initiate the regular supervision sessions that they have promised. Furthermore, some practitioners do not volunteer to become supervisors but are told that they should add interns to their already heavy workload. At times their training for being a supervisor is minimal, and they are expected to "learn by doing." If you are able to understand the predicament of supervisors, you are more likely to establish a basis of communication with them. Within a climate of open communication, you can sensitively and assertively let them know that you need help. If you have a difficult case, you can say something like this: "I really feel stuck with Susan. For several weeks now, we have made little progress. For every suggestion I make, she has many reasons why it won't work. I suggested termination, and she got angry with me. Now I don't know what to do. Can I meet with you for a few minutes to talk about some alternatives?" If you merely complain that your supervisor is always too busy or fails to show up for appointments, all you will get is frustration. But by being clear, specific, and persistent, you are likely to have your needs met.

We suggest that you give your supervisors credit for wanting to do their best. If you approach them with a genuine attitude of letting them know what you would like from them, they are more likely to respond positively than if you keep your distance from them and expect them to do all the work. If you learn to be assertive in asking for what you need from your supervisors without being aggressive, you will be going a long way toward creating a positive fieldwork experience and using supervision to its fullest extent.

Unfortunately, many students have negative experiences with fieldwork and with supervisors. At a conference of human service educators, Tricia McClam of the University of Tennessee made a presentation on effective field supervision. She commented that 9 out of 15 students had reported negative first field experiences! The relationship between the field supervisor and the student seems to be a key variable in determining whether the student's reactions are positive or negative. Supervisors certainly play a key role in the student's learning, and it is part of the student's responsibility to communicate with them, even if they are less than ideal.

Students with positive reactions to supervisors made comments such as these: "She was available." "She was involved in my cases." "My supervisor clearly stated what he expected of me and what I could expect of him." "My supervisor was both supportive and flexible." Students with negative reactions to supervisors observed: "He was too busy to properly supervise." "My supervisor did not meet with me regularly." "My supervisor was not organized."

When students begin their fieldwork activity, McClam indicated that they need supervisors who are clear about their expectations and who provide support and guidance. Firmness coupled with flexibility is useful for beginning trainees. When students have gained some fieldwork experience, they still need support and guidance, along with feedback from their supervisors, but they can profit from experiences that will demand more intuition and skill. Most important is establishing regular communication between supervisors and supervisees. Take the initiative to communicate with your supervisor. This is particularly challenging in cases where you perceive your supervision to be inadequate, a topic we explore shortly.

Case example.   Picture yourself as an intern in this situation. Your supervisor asks you to counsel a family, consisting of mother, father, and two young boys. The supervisor tells you that the parents are primarily interested in learning how to manage their problem children and want to learn disciplinary techniques. In the supervisor's view a more important problem consists of the conflicts between the wife and husband. You have had very little course work or training in working with families, and you feel lacking in the competencies to do family counseling. Here is a sample of some of the things that might be going on inside your head:

- "Now what am I going to do? I feel overwhelmed, but I don't want to appear like a neophyte, so I'd better take this family on."
- "I'm unprepared to counsel a family. I haven't even had a single course on family dynamics or family therapy. But if I don't agree to see the family, my supervisor might get angry and might think less of me. What should I do?"
- "The thought of dealing with this family terrifies me. I wouldn't know where to begin. I'd like to sit in on some sessions with my supervisor and observe and participate as a co-therapist. Do I dare suggest this?"

This inner dialogue gives some sense of the struggle you might go through in dealing with a supervisor who asks you to go beyond what you consider to be the boundaries of your competence. Let your supervisor know your concerns, and the two of you can talk about alternatives. Consider the following dialogue, and see how you might say some of the same or different things as the trainee.

SUPERVISOR: We are short on personnel in the agency, and we really need you to work with some families.

TRAINEE: My first reaction is to feel flattered that you think enough of me to ask for my help in seeing families. Yet at this stage of my professional development, I am going to have to decline.

SUPERVISOR: Look, one way to learn is by jumping in and getting involved. Most of us have hesitations when we begin working with new populations.

TRAINEE: In my case it is more than feeling anxious and having self-doubts. I have yet to take a single course in family therapy. It just does not seem ethical for me to undertake this task now.

SUPERVISOR: Well, I don't want you to do something that doesn't seem ethical to you. But I would be available for supervision, so you won't be without any guidance.

TRAINEE: I appreciate your offer for supervision. Perhaps I could observe your work with a family, with their permission of course, and then we could talk about your interventions after the session.

SUPERVISOR: If I had the time that would be great, but that would be adding one more thing to an already overbooked schedule.

TRAINEE: After I take the family therapy course next semester, perhaps I'll be in a better position to assist in this kind of work. For now, I need to work within my own limits.

This example is realistic in the sense that most organizations use interns as relatively "free" staff. The problem is not so much using interns to fill critical service needs but being unwilling to provide adequate supervision for trainees. Student interns do need some minimal theoretical foundation and knowledge competencies in working with families before they are able to effectively participate in actual clinical work with families. Certainly, when trainees are moving into a new area, they will need to acquire practical skills that will enable them to work effectively in this new setting. Good supervision enables trainees to apply their knowledge while acquiring these intervention strategies.

If you were the trainee in the situation we have described, would you have considered working with a family if you were not qualified to do so? Might you have given in to pressure, especially with the offer of some supervision? How might you have looked for ways on the job to acquire the knowledge base that would enable you to work with a family? How would you like to be able to respond to this supervisor?

Dealing With Supervision That Is Less Than Ideal

Realistically, there are times when you will have to deal with supervision that is far from ideal. How can you recognize inadequate supervision? What assertive courses of action are open to you in dealing with it?

Recognizing the effective supervisor.   Although there is no one way of conducting clinical supervision, there are established standards for counseling supervisors. The "Ethical Guidelines for Counseling Supervisors" (Association for Counselor Education and Supervision [ACES], 1993) are designed to help supervisors (1) observe ethical and legal protection of clients' and supervisees' rights; (2) provide training for supervisees in ways that are consistent with clients' welfare and requirements of the program; and (3) establish policies, procedures, and standards for implementing programs. The supervisor's main functions are to teach trainees, to foster their personal and professional development, and to assist in the provision of the effective delivery of counseling (helping) services. An underlying assumption of the ACES guidelines is that "supervision should be ongoing throughout a counselor's career and not stop when a particular level of education, certification, or membership in a professional organization is attained."

The ACES guidelines describe these characteristics of effective supervisors:

- Counseling supervisors are themselves effective counselors.
- Professional supervisors demonstrate personal characteristics that enable them to carry out their roles and functions. For instance, supervisors are encouraging and optimistic, sensitive to individual differences, able to demonstrate a sense of humor, comfortable with the authority of their role, and committed to updating their own skills as counselors and supervisors.
- Supervisors are knowledgeable about ethical, legal, and regulatory aspects of the profession.
- Supervisors inform supervisees of the goals, policies, theoretical orientations toward counseling, training, and supervision model on which the supervision is based.

- Supervisors demonstrate knowledge of individual differences with respect to gender, race, ethnicity, culture, sexual orientation, and age and understand the importance of these characteristics in the supervision process.
- Supervisors possess appropriate levels of empathy and respect genuineness, concreteness, and self-disclosure.
- Professional supervisors have training in supervision prior to initiating their role as supervisors.
- Supervisors set clear and explicit goals and use these goals to guide them in using various teaching techniques; they state the purposes of the supervisory relationship and explain the procedures to be used.
- Supervisors demonstrate knowledge and competency in case conceptualization and management.
- Supervisors of counselors meet regularly in face-to-face sessions with their supervisees.
- Supervisors provide supervisees with ongoing and immediate feedback that is closely tied to a supervisee's behavior. This feedback is systematic, objective, accurate, timely, and clearly understood.

The picture of the effective supervisor that emerges from the research is derived primarily from findings regarding supervisee satisfactions and preferences. The effective supervisor is one the supervisees most prefer, respond to positively, find satisfactory, and are able to trust. Some of the personal attributes of supervisors that have been consistently identified as helpful include humor, empathy, respect, genuineness, ability to confront, immediacy, concern for supervisee growth and well-being, concern for clients' welfare, availability for self-reflection, flexibility, courage, tolerance, and openness to various styles of learning. In short, good supervisors tend to be available, accessible, affable, and able. The general picture of the effective supervisor is a technically competent professional with good human relations skills and effective organizational and managerial skills.

You may meet and work with supervisors who demonstrate effectiveness in some of these areas. But other supervisors may feel ill equipped to do what is expected of them, and some may be as insecure in their supervisory role as you are in your new role as an intern. It is up to you to get the most from your supervisors, despite any limitations that may exist.

Accepting different styles of supervision.   You can benefit from learning how to function under a range of supervisory styles, both now as a student and later as a helping professional. One supervisor may believe harsh confrontation is a way to cut through a client's stubborn defenses. Another treats clients as victims who are not responsible for their problems. Another provides unlimited advice for clients and promotes a problem-solving orientation for every client problem. There are supervisors who foster a supportive and positive orientation exclusively. Other supervisors seem to thrive on crises and problems and tend to escalate such situations rather than defuse them. Some supervisors work very hard at establishing collegial relationships with their interns, whereas others create a professionally aloof relationship. Be open to supervisors with various orientations, and learn to incorporate their viewpoints into your style of helping. Do not be too quick to criticize a style different from yours, but consider it an opportunity for learning. As a supervisee, recognize that at different stages in your professional development you may require different styles of supervision.

If you do have trouble with a supervisor, the answer is not always merely finding a new one. You can learn a great deal by working with supervisors who have perspectives different from yours and from supervisors who may initially appear to be difficult for you to make contact with. When you experience conflicts with a supervisor, it is a good idea to discuss them and do all that you can to work them out. Rather than convincing yourself that your supervisor will not be cooperative, assume that he or she will be open to your suggestions. Later, when you accept a position in an agency, you typically do not have the option of changing supervisors. What is more, you often do not have choices in who your co-workers will be. Thus, it is important to learn the interpersonal skills necessary in working out differences while the stakes are not so high.

Our style of supervision. When we supervise, we pay attention to the relationship between our trainees and ourselves, as well as the dynamics and relationships between supervisees and their clients. Here we see a parallel process operating between a practice model and a supervisory model. Supervisees can learn ways to conceptualize what they are doing with their clients by reflecting on what they are learning about interpersonal dynamics in the supervisory relationship. Rather than placing emphasis exclusively on assessing and treating a client's problems, we are very concerned with the interpersonal aspects that are emerging between the supervisee and his or her clients. In our view, supervisors do well to look beyond the cases that trainees bring to the supervisory sessions and focus on the interpersonal dimensions.

In our role as supervisors we attempt to help our supervisees develop their own insights and refine their clinical hunches. Rather than placing the emphasis on direct teaching with supervisees by giving them information, we strive to help them learn how to conceptualize a case and think about how they are likely to proceed with a given client and why. Instead of using our words with supervisees' clients, we hope supervisees will discover their own words and find their own voice. Our style of supervision is reflected by the following questions we typically explore:

- What are you wanting to say to your clients?
- What direction do you think is most appropriate to take with your clients?
- How are you reacting to your clients?
- How is your behavior affecting them?
- Which clients bring out your own resistances?
- How are your values manifested by the way you interact with your clients?
- How might our relationship, in these supervisory sessions, mirror your relationships with your clients?
- Are you feeling free enough to bring into these supervisory sessions any difficulties you are having with your clients?

What style of supervision do you think would be most useful for you at this stage of your development? What kind of supervisor do you think would be the most difficult for you to work with, and why? If it were impractical to change positions or change supervisors, what strategies could you use in constructively dealing with this supervisor?

Solving problems in your supervision. You may encounter a number of problems in working with a supervisor. Communication may not be open or encouraged. Some supervisors may poorly define what they expect of you. Some may fail to show up for appointments. Others may delegate their responsibilities to their secretary. There is also the supervisor who is insecure but disguises this insecurity by being overly controlling and autocratic. Some supervisors dump too much on an intern too soon or delegate menial work and unwanted jobs. Supervisors may be guilty of unethical practices. One supervisor had her supervisee do her work and then wrote up the proceedings as though she had seen the client. Some supervisors misuse power through a need to be seen as always right. There are supervisors who do not carry out their responsibility to give feedback. They keep the student intern in the dark and offer very little direction.

These are but a few possible conflicts you are likely to face in your internship. What do you think you might do if your supervisor were to give you very little feedback? Would you be willing to let the supervisor know that you wanted more response? Would you ask for it? Would you insist on it? What might you do if no feedback were forthcoming?

Supervisory roles and functions themselves can be detrimental to efforts to create an open relationship. Supervisors are responsible for and will evaluate you, the supervisee, so it is understandable that you might be anxious about being observed and evaluated. You can challenge yourself by converting your anxiety into productive energy. You can spend time thinking about what you want and begin to find ways to ask directly for it. It may help to accept that performance anxiety goes with the territory of being a supervisee. However, you can challenge your fears rather than allowing yourself to be frozen by performance expectations.

Informed consent in supervision. Informed consent should be a basic part of the supervisory relationship (ACES, 1993). McCarthy and colleagues (1995) provide a practical guide to informed consent in clinical supervision. They conclude that informed consent is an essential ingredient of effective supervision and that it should be clearly articulated through written documents and a discussion between the supervisor and supervisee. Accountability can be increased by developing a written contractual agreement for supervision. When expectations are discussed and clarified at the beginning of a supervisory relationship, the relationship will be enhanced, promoting quality client care. McCarthy and her colleagues identified seven topic areas that are significant to informed consent: purpose, professional disclosure, practical issues, supervision process, administrative issues, ethical and legal issues, and statement of agreement. When these issue areas are addressed in the informed consent process in supervision, both supervisors and supervisees have a clearer idea of the nature of their respective roles, rights, and responsibilities. Written informed consent documents, along with a discussion of their contents, are an excellent way for supervisors to model for supervisees an approach they can use with their clients.

Participating in Group Supervision

The value of group supervision is sometimes overlooked. In groups, trainees can benefit by listening to others and by discussing cases with their peers as well as with a supervisor. Our approach is to combine individual and group supervision when this is practical and possible. Although group supervision is widely practiced, it appears to be poorly understood (Prieto, 1996). Group supervision is a time-efficient and unique format that assists trainees in developing skills in conceptualizing cases and in implementing a variety of treatment interventions. One study suggests that group supervision is not only complementary to individual supervision but may be interchangeable with individual supervision (Ray & Altekruse, 2000). Other researchers have found that group supervision using audiotapes of a session may be more efficient than individual supervision in terms of rate of learning (Calhoun, Moras, Pilkonis, & Rehm, 1998). Crespi, Fischetti, and Butler (2001) contend that group supervision, using a case model approach, is a viable way to conduct supervisory sessions with school counselors. Although group supervision will cut into other service responsibilities of school counselors, Calhoun and colleagues (1998) believe group supervision can lead to greater accountability, improve outcomes and, in the long run, be more cost-effective than individual supervision.

If you participate in group supervision, you learn not only from your supervisor but also from fellow trainees. You have an opportunity to learn that you are not alone with your anxiety and concerns surrounding clinical work, and you are exposed to different perspectives of the helping relationship. In group supervision you are likely to have many opportunities to role-play challenging clients and to try on a variety of helper roles in a given situation. Role playing offers many possibilities, not only for you to become aware of potential countertransference issues but as a way to acquire alternative perspectives in working with clients you sometimes perceive as being "difficult." You can assume the role of your client by "becoming" the client while the supervisor demonstrates other approaches to dealing with a given client. Later, the supervisor can switch roles and become the client while you experiment with another way of dealing with your client. Of course, in a group context your peers can assume various roles for one another, which tends to enhance learning. Role-playing techniques tend to bring to life a concrete situation that all can witness, as opposed to merely talking about problems and concerns with clients.

It is important to talk to other interns and to share experiences and struggles. The group supervision model is enhanced when you make the process a personal one. You can do this by focusing on your own reactions and sharing them in your supervision group. What clients seem to trigger you? What clients do you hope won't show up next week? What clients threaten you? What clients do you find yourself especially liking? By focusing on your relationships with your clients and your own dynamics, you can increase your self-awareness through the feedback you get from others in the group.

It is also helpful to explore your values and attitudes in conjunction with your supervision. If you become aware that you have a tendency to seek gratitude from clients, for example, it could be useful to explore your own need for approval and your fear of rejection, either in your own personal therapy or in a group supervision session.

Supervision Versus Therapy

Supervisors play multiple roles in the supervision process, functioning as teachers, consultants, mentors, and, at times, counselors. This complexity of roles means that the boundaries are not always clear. The process of supervision has some similarities with instructor-student and therapist-client relationships, but there are also distinctions. It is essential to keep the primary purpose of supervisory relationships in mind—that is, to ensure that clients receive the best possible services.

The therapeutic role of the supervisor is certainly not the same as the role of the counselor, yet the distinction between these two roles is not well defined. Whiston and Emerson (1989) propose a model of supervision that includes an exploration of a supervisee's personal problems that lead to an impasse in the trainee's counseling work. However, once the personal issues of supervisees are identified in the supervisory relationship, they contend that the trainee must be given the responsibility for resolving these problems. The ACES (1993) ethical guidelines state that "Supervisors should not establish a psychotherapeutic relationship as a substitute for supervision. Personal issues should be addressed in supervision only in terms of the impact of these issues on clients and on professional functioning." One study suggests that exploring supervisees' personal issues in an appropriate manner does not necessarily affect the supervisory relationship negatively. Such supervisors confront their supervisees with personal issues that influence their work with clients, but in a warm and supportive instructional manner. As supervisees gain experience, they may be more able to benefit from identifying and exploring personal issues that affect their relationships with clients (Sumerel & Borders, 1996).

We do not attempt to make training sessions into counseling sessions, but the supervisory process can be therapeutic and growth-producing. One goal of supervision is to promote the supervisee's self-awareness. It is especially important to assist supervisees in recognizing personal characteristics that could have a negative impact on their therapeutic relationships with clients. The boundaries between supervision and counseling are not always clear, and Corey and Herlihy (1996) offer this general guideline on the proper focus of supervision:

> Because supervisory relationships are a complex blend of professional, educational, and therapeutic relationships, supervisors need to work to create and maintain an ethical climate for both skill development and self-exploration. Again, it is the supervisor's responsibility to help trainees identify how their personal dynamics are likely to influence their professional work, but it is not the supervisor's proper role to serve as a personal counselor to supervisees. (p. 277)

Supervisors are in a good position to recognize some of your blocks and countertransferences. They can help you identify attitudes, feelings, and behaviors that are likely to interfere with your handling of certain clients. If further exploration is needed, and if your difficulties with certain clients are rooted in your own dynamics, a supervisor may encourage you to get involved in some form of personal therapy. You should not misconstrue such a suggestion as an indication that you are not personally fit for the profession. Getting involved in the lives of clients in a placement is bound to open up some of your own psychological wounds, and unresolved conflicts are likely to surface. We strongly encourage personal therapy along with your supervision as an ideal combination (provided your supervisor and your therapist are not the same person). This arrangement prevents blurring of boundaries and allows the proper focus to be either on working with clients (in supervision) or on dealing with your personal issues (in personal therapy). We address the topic of the importance of personal therapy for trainees in more detail in Chapter 3.

By Way of Review

• Become active in getting the most from your education. No program is perfect, but you can do a lot to bring more meaning to your course of study.

• Just as you are graded in your educational program, you will be evaluated in the professional world. Evaluation creates stresses and strains, but it is still possible to find meaning within the system.

• Skills and knowledge are obviously important in becoming an effective professional, but your personal qualities are equally important in determining your success as a helper.

• Graduation from a training program does not signal the end of learning but merely the beginning of a process of professional growth and development. To maintain your effectiveness, continuing education is a necessity. One of the best ways of keeping on the cutting edge of one's profession is to become involved in a peer-consultation group that affords professionals opportunities to share their concerns and learn from one another. Through peer groups, helpers can actively contribute to their own personal and professional development and that of their colleagues.

• Your fieldwork courses are likely to be among the most important experiences you will have in your program. Select these experiences wisely and arrange for diversity in your placements. Realize that these placements can help you decide on your professional specialization.

• Treat your field placement like a job, even if you don't get paid for your internship.

• Don't burden yourself with trying to be a perfect intern. Fieldwork experiences are designed to teach you about the skills of helping, and you can learn much from your mistakes.

- In getting the most from supervision, learn how to ask for what you need from your supervisor. It is important that you learn your limits and communicate them to your supervisor.

- Supervisors have different styles, and no one way is right. You can learn a great deal from various supervisors, but be cautious about copying their style.

- The ideal supervisor may be hard to find. Supervisors are sometimes assigned to this role with little preparation or training. If your supervision is inadequate, be assertive in doing something about the situation. Identify what you need and take an active stance in asking for it

- Even though supervision is like therapy in some ways, there are important differences. Personal therapy can be a useful adjunct to supervision, but it is best that the supervisor and the therapist not be the same person.

What Will You Do Now?

1. If you have a supervisor (for your fieldwork or in your job), make up a short list of questions that you would like to discuss with him or her. What would you like to gain from supervision? Approach your supervisor before the end of the semester to discuss your desires.

2. Make it a point to visit several community agencies where you might work as an intern. Interview the director of the agency or the supervisors who make decisions about accepting fieldwork students. Learn to ask questions that will help you select a placement that will teach you about various client populations and a range of problems. Each student in your class could visit just one agency and then present the findings to the rest of the class.

3. Reflect on some of the following issues and use this as a basis for your journal writing. Remember to write whatever comes to mind rather than censoring your thoughts and the flow of your writing.

- Write about the kind of learner you see yourself as being. What does the concept of active learning imply to you? How can you become a more active learner as you read this book and take this course?
- Write about the ideal kind of fieldwork experience you would like to obtain. What can you do to get the best possible field placement?
- If you are already in a field placement, write at least briefly about the work you are doing. What are your reactions to the staff at the agency? What is it like for you to interact with clients? What is this experience teaching you about yourself?
- If you are in supervision currently, what are you doing to get the most from this process? What kind of relationship do you have with your supervisor? Write about any ideas for improving the quality of your supervision sessions. Are any personal issues emerging as a result of your work with

clients? (Consider bringing personal issues that pertain to your ability to work effectively with your clients into supervision. At the very least, write in your journal about any personal problems that are surfacing as a result of your field placement and supervision.)

4. The full bibliographic entry for each of these sources can be found in the References and Reading List at the back of the book. For a comprehensive book on clinical supervision, see Bernard and Goodyear (1998). Useful introductory texts in the human services field include Neukrug (2000) and Woodside and McClam (2002). For a practical and concise guide to the internship experience, see Faiver, Eisengart, and Colonna (2000). Refer to Kiser's (2000) human service internship handbook as a way to get the most from your internship experience, and see Baird's (1996) handbook for internship, practicum, and field placements for helpful suggestions on ways to get the most from a fieldwork experience. Refer to Alle-Corliss and Alle-Corliss (1998) for an orientation to fieldwork and Alle-Corliss and Alle-Corliss (1999) for practice in human service agencies.

InfoTrac College Edition Resources

For additional readings, explore InfoTrac College Edition, our online library. Go to http://www.infotrac.college.com/wadsworth and select these key word searches:

   fieldwork
   practicum
   internship
   superv* AND therapy
   superv* AND couns*
   clinical W1 superv*
   clinical supervisor* role*
   clinical AND supervisor* AND responsib*
   clinical supervisor* AND competence
   superv* AND multicult*

Key words are listed in a form that enables the search engine to locate a wider range of articles in the online university library. Key words should be entered exactly as shown, including asterisks, "W1," "W2," "AND," and other search engine tools.

CHAPTER *3*

Helper, Know Thyself

Focus Questions

1. What growth experiences do you seek? Do you value travel? Would you like to participate in personal psychotherapy, family therapy, or some form of group therapy? What importance do you place on self-exploration as part of your development as a helper?

2. How much do you know about your family of origin? What do you know about the life experiences of your parents? your grandparents? other relatives?

3. In what ways do you think your experiences with your family of origin have affected your other current relationships?

4. Should a course in the family of origin should be required of students in a counseling program? Why or why not?

5. How might your family experiences help you in your role as a professional helper?

6. Can you identify any unresolved issues between you and your family that are likely to make it difficult for you to work with certain problems? What steps can you take to resolve these issues?

Aim of the Chapter

All of us come from families, and many of the problems your clients will bring to counseling are grounded in events and learnings as children growing up in their families.* To be an effective helper, you need to recognize the ways your own family of origin has influenced your present relationships and how your early background will influence your professional work. Whether you plan to work with individuals, couples, or families, it is essential for you to become aware of your family-of-origin issues, because your perceptions and reactions to those whom you counsel are bound to be influenced by your personal experiences with your own family. If you are unaware of your sensitive areas, you are likely to misinterpret your clients or steer them in a direction that will not arouse your own anxieties. If you are aware of emotional issues that activate your resistances, however, you can avoid getting entangled in the problems of your clients.

The material we present in this chapter is personal and is designed to assist you in examining as many dimensions of your family as possible so you will not be overly susceptible to countertransference, which are your reactions and emotions toward a client that are based on your earlier experiences with significant others in your life. We cannot stress enough this message—helper, know thyself. If you hope to be a therapeutic agent in the lives of others, it is essential that you know yourself and are able to heal yourself.

In this chapter we invite you to unravel the mystery of your connection with your family of origin so you may develop a richer appreciation for the many ways you continue to play out patterns established during childhood. In helping you review your family history, we present the perspective we use in our professional work. In doing so, we draw from numerous approaches and methods that we have found helpful in giving clients a focus for their work.

The Value of Self-Exploration for the Helper

You are likely to discover that working with individuals or families resurrects themes in your life, some of which may previously have been outside your conscious awareness. If you are unaware of issues stemming from your family experiences, you are likely to find ways to avoid acknowledging and dealing with potentially painful areas with your clients. As your clients confront events that trigger their pain, memories of your own pain may come forth. For example, you may still have a great deal of hurt over your parents' divorce. You may believe the divorce was your fault and that you could have done something to keep your parents together. If you are counseling a couple considering divorce, you may steer them toward remaining married for the sake of their children. You are giving them solutions that originate from your reservoir of hurt. On some level, you could be protecting the children from the pain of your situation that you have yet

---

* We express our appreciation to James Bitter, of East Tennessee State University, for his role in critiquing and contributing to this chapter.

to fully realize or appreciate. It is important for you to recognize that your capacity to facilitate the healing forces in others lies in your willingness to experience your own wounds and to do what is needed to bring about healing for yourself.

Identifying and resolving unfinished business related to your family of origin is essential if you hope to establish relationships that do not repeat negative patterns of interaction. If you are encumbered by the excess psychological baggage of unresolved conflicts, this burden is bound to interfere with your ability to create different relationships in your personal life. As you review your family history in this chapter, you will no doubt gain some insights into unresolved conflicts and patterns that you have "adopted" from your family of origin. Your own therapy can aid you in coming to understand how these past conflicts are affecting you in the present.

As you begin to practice counseling, some of you might become aware that you are taking on a professional role that resembles the role you played in your family. For example, you may recognize a need to preserve peace by becoming the caretaker of others. During your childhood you may have assumed adult roles with your own parents by trying to take care of them. Now, as you begin your professional work, it is possible that you could continue the pattern of taking on most of the responsibility for the changes your clients make.

Transference and countertransference are common in the therapeutic process. *Transference* generally has roots in a client's unresolved personal conflicts with significant others. Because of this unfinished business, the client perceives the helping professional in a distorted way and brings his or her past relationships into the present relationship with the counselor. Transference can be a path that enables a client to gain insight into how he or she operates in a variety of relationships. The counterpart of the client's transference feelings toward a helper is the helping person's *countertransference* (or emotional reactions) toward a client. Broadly speaking, helpers may have unconscious emotional responses to a client that result in a distorted perception of the client's behavior. At times helpers may be triggered by certain clients, and if this is not recognized, it could get in the way of a helper's objectivity and could block progress in the helping relationship. Consider your own possible sources of countertransference. If you have fears about your own dying or the aging and death of your parents, for example, you can expect to encounter difficulty in working with older people. The struggles of these clients can activate unconscious processes in you, which if left outside your awareness will be likely to interfere with your ability to be fully present for clients who remind you of your pain.

Many situations in a family can plant the seeds of potential countertransference: growing up in a home with the unpredictability of violence, conflicts that were never addressed, secrecy that was protected at all costs, fears surrounding incest, absence of any boundaries, and significant events (such as grave illness or the death of a family member) that were ignored on a psychological level. If you felt that no matter how much you did, it was never quite enough to win your mother's approval, for example, you may now be very finely attuned to the judgments of women who remind you of your mother. If you allowed your father to completely affirm or deny your value as a person, you may be very sensitive to what male authority figures think about you. You may give them the power to make you feel either competent or incompetent. As a child, if you often felt rejected and on the outside, you may now create situations in which you feel like the one who is left out and just does not fit. Your own counseling can assist you to identify the source of your pain and to work through places where you may be psychologically stalled. (These issues are discussed in more detail in Chapter 6.)

Using Individual and Group Counseling for Self-Exploration

When you become aware of carrying patterns that originated from your personal experiences into your professional life, individual and group counseling can provide a safe place to explore and talk about the sometimes painful memories that are often associated with these personal experiences. Ideally, you will consider participating in a combination of individual and group therapy, because the two therapy types complement each other.

Individual therapy provides you with an opportunity to look at yourself in some depth. As a part of your internship experience, you may experience a reopening of old emotional wounds as you engage in intensive work with your clients. For example, your therapeutic work may bring to the surface feelings of unexpressed and unresolved grief over significant loss. If you are in personal counseling while you are doing your internship, you can productively bring such problems to your therapy sessions. According to Norcross (2000), the majority of mental health professionals have participated in their own personal therapy, and the vast majority of mental health professionals rate the outcomes of personal therapy quite positively: "Our studies consistently find that psychotherapists regularly recommend, seek, and value episodic personal therapy as constructive self-care" (p. 712).

Group therapy, in contrast, can offer you an opportunity to hear and consider feedback you receive from others. A group experience can help you become aware of your interpersonal style and give you a chance to experiment with new behaviors in a group setting. The reactions you receive from others can help you learn about personal attributes that could be either strengths or limitations in your work as a helper. Many of the patterns you acquired as a child may still be problematic for you today. For instance, you could do useful work in group therapy on any unresolved issues you have with your parents, with family rules that you have accepted, or with places where you feel stuck.

Therapy—be it individual, group, or family—is not just for treatment purposes or for curing deeply rooted personality disturbances. We see therapy as an avenue for continuing to deepen your self-understanding and for looking at the ways in which your needs are related to your work. Becoming involved in some form of intensive self-exploration therapy can stimulate you to assess your needs and motives for becoming a helper, which were outlined in Chapter 1. Through the process of self-exploration, you will get first-hand knowledge of what your clients are likely to experience. This process will increases your respect for clients as they face their fears, vulnerabilities, inner conflicts, and psychological wounds. It will be difficult to teach others about the joys and pains of growth that result from a therapeutic relationship if you have not experienced what it is like to be on the receiving end of this process. If you have not participated in the journey of self-exploration, how can you serve as a guide for others?

As a helper you can perhaps learn nothing more important than the ways in which you carry old feelings from the past into present situations. It is illuminating for you to consider that you are living out unfinished scenarios from the dance enacted by your parents, both as individuals and in their relationship with each other and their children. You are not free of the vestiges of what you experienced in your family. You have a set of convictions that structure your life, and you may be intent on confirming these assumptions even though some of them are self-defeating and no longer functional. For example, when someone in your family was angry, perhaps people got hurt, either physically or emotionally. As a child you made a decision that anger was a useless emotion, that you would never show this feeling, and that you would not even allow yourself to feel angry. This decision could have protected you at the time, when you felt helpless and did not know how to cope with destructive expressions of anger. But your extreme denial of anger now interferes with your significant relationships at home and at work. People find it difficult to trust you because you never express negative reactions to anything. If you have trouble accepting your own anger, you will have difficulty allowing your clients to express their anger and deal constructively with it.

We have found that helpers often would rather look at the dynamics of their clients than at themselves. Although there is nothing wrong in wanting to find better ways of working with clients, you can best learn how to do this by allowing yourself to be as open as possible to your own life experience. Thus, whenever you take measures to understand yourself more fully, you are at the same time preparing yourself to help others in their quest for self-understanding.

The Impact of Therapeutic Work on Your Personal Life

In talking with mental health providers, we find that many of them are not able to separate themselves from their work. Both new and experienced practitioners often find it difficult to make a clear distinction between their personal life and their professional life. Here is how one helper put it:

> My work takes a toll on me personally at times. In sad and difficult cases, such as working with clients who have been sexually abused, there is the danger of getting overly involved. I find that if I get a series of severe clients, then stress builds up.

Working intimately with others can also be a catalyst that enables helpers to look at their own lives in a new way. One helper put it this way:

> My work helps me feel that I'm out there contributing and helping people. I feel that I'm doing something worthwhile and feel a sense of accomplishment. My work helps me put my own struggles in perspective. I'm able to learn a lot about myself through my involvement in the lives of others.

Helpers need to understand how they are personally affected by their professional work if they hope to maintain their own psychological health and continue to be effective in reaching those whom they serve. Self-knowledge is an essential place to begin. Jaffe (1986) argues that health professionals must see that they cannot simply give and remain detached from their feelings. Instead, they must look inward at their personal needs. Jaffe decries the notion that healers are not supposed to have needs, that personal feelings are not relevant, and that helpers should learn to cut themselves off from their own pain as they work with others' pain, much as in the Greek myth of the wounded healer. Such healers were supposed to possess the wisdom of life and death, yet they were not able to heal their own incurable wounds. According to Jaffe, helping professionals need to recognize the impact on their own life of working with suffering people. They must become aware of their inner responses and learn to work through their own pain in a constructive manner to be effective in their professional work.

Kottler (1993) contends that most therapists understand that they are jeopardizing their own emotional well-being when they intimately encounter the pain of others. He observes that the client and the therapist change each other and that there are hazards to the therapist as a result of this intimate relationship:

> There are tremendous risks for the therapist in living with the anguish of others, in being so close to others' torments. Sometimes we become desensitized by human emotions and experience an acute overdose of feeling; we turn ourselves off. Other times we overreact to personal incidents as a result of lingering dissonance created during sessions. (p. 12)

Unless you have identified your own sources of vulnerability and to some extent worked through experiences that may have left you psychologically wounded, you may be constantly triggered by the stories of your clients. Your old wounds can be opened, affecting both your personal and professional life. It is clear that therapeutic practice can reactivate your earlier experiences and reawaken unresolved needs and problems (Farber, 1983; Guy, 1987, Kottler, 1993). It is essential that you be willing to deal with your personal issues that are triggered through your work with others.

Case example.   Nancy, a beginning counselor working in an agency, is asked to co-lead a group of adults who are in some stage of grief over a significant loss. Nancy feels that there is a real need for this work, and she is enthusiastic in accepting the co-leadership role. She lost her husband through a tragic death, yet she feels that she has allowed herself to fully experience the pain of his death and has accepted the loss. She works very well with the members in her group. She can be compassionate, supportive, and empathic, and she is able to help them work through some of their pain.

After a few weeks Nancy notices that she is no longer looking forward to going to the group. She feels somewhat depressed and finds herself becoming apathetic toward the members. Although some of her old wounds were healed, exposure to the intense pain of so many other people has reopened these wounds. Thus, the only way she could survive was to numb herself from feeling the others' pain. This numbing led to her depression and her inability to work effectively with her clients. She has ignored her vulnerability to the pain of her loss and her need to express and work through this pain as it is being reexperienced.

Simply because Nancy reexperiences her old pain does not necessarily mean that she will become ineffective in working with this type of group. Quite to the contrary, if she accepts the fact that she is still wounded and explores these feelings, she can heal her own wounds at the same time that she is facilitating the healing process in others. She can model the ongoing nature of grief work and teach the members that although the pain will never be completely erased it can become less controlling. If at times her own pain feels overwhelming in the group, she can share it with the members. She can use her experiences as a bridge to connect with the struggles of others. Alternatively, Nancy can choose to seek personal therapy. If she repeatedly puts her own emotions "on hold," either in or out of the group, she is bound to become ineffectual as a helper, and if she continues this type of involvement over a long period, the chances are that she will burn out. The challenge for Nancy is to learn to pay attention to her inner experience and to use it as a road to her growth and as a way of making contact with others.

Working With Your Family of Origin

We know of one doctoral program in clinical psychology that requires a course on the family of origin. The assumption is that future practitioners need to know how their own family of origin influences them presently before they engage in professional work with individuals, couples, and families. Some states mandate such a course as a requirement for licensure as a couples and family therapist. We hope other training programs will follow this lead. Some writers suggest that training programs provide family-of-origin work for students as part of growth group experiences (Lawson & Gaushell, 1991; Wilcoxon, Walker, & Hovestadt, 1989). Other authors discuss how family-of-origin work can be used for personal-growth training for couples and family counselors (Getz & Protinsky, 1994), ways that early childhood family influences are related to counselor effectiveness (Watts, Trusty, Canada, & Harvill, 1995), and ethical considerations when using the family autobiography in training counselors (Goodman & Carpenter-White, 1996). Most hold that a practitioner's mental health, as defined by relationships with his or her family of origin, has implications for professional training. Helpers can benefit from exploring the dynamics of their family of origin because this significant knowledge enables them to relate more effectively to the families they will meet in their clinical practice.

Getz and Protinsky (1994) point to growing clinical evidence that a family-of-origin approach to supervision is a necessary dimension of training helpers who want to work with families. They contend that the reactions of helpers to their clients' stories tend to reactivate helpers' old learned patterns of behavior and unresolved problems. By studying their own families of origin, students are able to improve their ability to counsel families.

Lawson and Gaushell (1991) recommend that training programs address candidates' family issues before admitting them to a program. They suggest requiring a family autobiography as part of the application materials. This would yield useful information concerning intergenerational family characteristics that would have a relationship to a helper's ability to work with families. Lawson and

Gaushell emphasize these intergenerational family characteristics of counselor trainees:

- Clinicians who have resolved negative family experiences are better able to assist their clients, especially those with whom they have issues in common.
- It is essential that trainees be given assistance in identifying and addressing their own problematic family issues to enhance their psychological functioning and their effectiveness as helpers.
- Unmet needs in early family experiences later manifest themselves in intense and conflicting ties with these family members.
- Helpers' early roles as peacemakers create later ambivalence regarding intimacy with significant others.
- Counselor trainees' experiences in their families of origin can lead to difficulties in their current relationships.

Identifying Your Issues in Your Family of Origin

Family therapists generally assume that it is inevitable that they will meet parts of their family in every other family with whom they have a professional relationship. If you do not understand the patterns of interpersonal behavior learned in your family of origin, you will repeat these patterns with clients. Virginia Satir, one of the pioneers in family therapy, used to say that if she walked into a room with 12 people she would meet everyone she ever knew. When you are counseling a couple or a family, a roomful of people are participating in this interaction. In other words, you are not always perceiving individuals whom you meet with a fresh and unbiased perspective. The more you are aware of your patterns of interacting with your own family members, the greater is the benefit to your clients. It is crucial that you know to whom you are responding: to the individual in front of you or to a person from your past.

Try this exercise that Satir used to demonstrate that people are constantly revisiting friends and loved ones in their lives. Stand in front of someone (Person A) in your current life who interests you or with whom you are having some difficulty. This individual might be a client, an associate, a family member, or a friend. If the person is not present, you can imagine him or her. Take a good look at this person and form a picture on the screen of your mind. Now, let a picture of someone in your past come forward (Person B). Who comes to mind? How old are you, and how old is Person B? What relationship do you, or did you, have with this individual you are remembering? What feelings are linked with this relationship? What did you think about Person B? Now, examine again your reactions to Person A. Do you see any connection between what Person A is evoking in you and the past feelings evoked by Person B? You can apply this exercise by yourself through the use of imagery when you have intense emotional reactions to other people, especially if you do not know them well. This exercise can help you begin to recognize how your past relationships may sometimes affect here-and-now responses. Perhaps what is most important is simply to be aware of ways in which you are carrying your past into present interactions.

In this section we invite you to identify as many family-of-origin experiences as possible and also to reflect on how these life experiences are likely to have an influence on *who* and *what* you are at this point. Goldenberg and Goldenberg (2000b) have written a workbook designed to provoke students into thinking about how their roles in their family of origin and their current family continue to play out in maintaining their attitudes, values, and behavior patterns. In the preface they write: "By learning more about yourself, especially by adopting a family perspective, we believe you can help others, future clients, see themselves within the contexts of their family lives" (p. 5). You are not necessarily determined by your earlier experiences, and they do not have to serve as the template for your current significant relationships. You can shift your perspective, but only if you have recognized and dealt with your experiences. If you are working with a family, moreover, you will have an experiential starting point to invite them to look at their functioning as a system and as individuals within the family.

Much of the remainder of this section is based on our perspective on family history, which is a modification and integration of material taken from several sources: (1) Adlerian lifestyle assessment methods (see Corey, 2001a; Mosak & Shulman, 1988; Powers & Griffith, 1986, 1987; Shulman & Mosak, 1988); (2) Satir's communication approach to working with families (Satir, 1983, 1989; Satir & Baldwin, 1983; Satir, Bitter, & Krestensen, 1988; see also Bitter, 1987, 1988); (3) concepts of family systems (see Goldenberg & Goldenberg, 2000a, 2000b; Nichols & Schwartz, 2001); (4) genogram methods (see McGoldrick, Gerson, & Shellenberger, 1999); and (5) family autobiography methods (see Lawson & Gaushell, 1988). As you read the following material, we encourage you to personalize the information. We are primarily providing you with ways to understand and work with your own family material and secondarily offering you a basis for understanding the individuals and families in your professional work.

Your family structure.   The many patterns of family life include nuclear, extended, single-parent, divorced, and blended. The term *family structure* also refers to the social and psychological organization of the family system, including factors such as birth order and the individual's perception of self in the family context. Expand your awareness of your family of origin by thoughtfully answering these questions:

• In what type of family structure did you grow up? It might be that the structure of your family changed over time. If so, what were these changes? What were some of the most important family values? What most stands out for you about your family life? How do these experiences continue to influence who you are today?

• What is your current family structure? Are you still primarily involved in your family of origin, or do you have a different family structure? If you do, what roles do you play in your current family that you also enacted in your original family? Have you carried certain patterns from your original family into your current family? How do you see yourself as being different in the two families?

• Draw a picture of your family of origin. Include all the members, and identify their significant alliances. Identify the relationships with each person that you had as a child and your relationships with each member now.

- Make a list of the siblings, from oldest to youngest. Give a brief description of each (including yourself). What most stands out for each sibling? Which sibling(s) is (are) most different from you, and how? Which is most like you, and how?

- Review some key dimensions of your experiences as a child growing up in your family. How would you describe yourself as a child? What were some of your major fears? hopes? ambitions? What was school like for you? What was your role in your peer group? Identify any significant events in your physical, sexual, and social development during childhood.

- Identify one of your personal problems. How has your relationship with your family contributed to the development and perpetuation of this problem? Besides blaming your family for this problem, what options are open to you for making substantial changes in yourself? What are a few ways in which you can be different in your family?

- What is at least one strength you have, and how has your family contributed to the development of this strength?

Parental figures and relationships with parents.   Your parents were central figures in your development, and your interaction patterns with them have set the stage for many of your present relationships. A father or mother may have been absent from your early family life. If so, did any substitute figures emerge? If you grew up in a single-parent family, did this one parent play the role of both mother and father? What did your parent or parents teach you, mainly through the behavior they modeled, about marriage and about family life? Spend some time thinking about your parental figures and your relationships with them. Focus on what you learned from observing and interacting with your parents, on what you observed in their interactions with each other, and on how each parent interacted with each sibling. Remember how each of your siblings viewed and reacted to your parents.

Describe your father (or the person who substituted for him). What is he like as a person? What are his ambitions for each of the children? How did you view him as a child? How do you view him now? How are you like him? How are you unlike him? What does your father say when he compliments you? when he criticizes you? What was his main advice to you as a child? What is his main advice to you now? What could you do to disappoint him? What can you do to please him? What was his relationship to his children? What is his current relationship to your siblings? What sibling is the most like your father, and in what ways? What did your father tell you (either directly or indirectly) about you? life? death? love? sex? marriage? men? women? your birth?

Now describe your mother. Use the same list of questions and ask each of them about your mother (or the person who substituted for her). Give a sketch of how you viewed your mother.

Your parents have been the "air-traffic controllers" of your life. They launched you, guided you, and helped you survive. They are the people on whom you depended for survival, and you may feel less than grown up in relation to them. You may find yourself acting the way you did as a child when you are with them as opposed to functioning as a psychological adult. It is important to remember that for many people the last relationships they work out are those with their parents.

Becoming your own person. A healthy person has achieved both a psychological separateness from and a sense of intimacy with his or her family, which is often known as *individuation.* This process of individuation involves the balance between belonging to and separating from your family of origin. The increasing differentiation from the family enables you to accept personal responsibility for your thoughts, feelings, perceptions, and actions. Individuation, or psychological maturity, is not a fixed destination that you reach once and for all; rather, it is a lifelong developmental process achieved through reexamination and resolution of internal conflicts and intimacy issues with loved ones. You do not find yourself in isolation; rather, the process of self-discovery is bound up with the quality of your relationships to others in connection. Becoming your own person does not mean "doing your own thing" irrespective of your impact on those with whom you come in contact. Instead, being autonomous means that you have questioned the values you live by and made them your own; part of this process includes concern for the welfare of those people you love and associate with.

It is possible to assume responsibility by doing for yourself what you expected others to do for you as a child. Becoming your own person does not mean that you are indifferent to what others need or want from you, nor does it imply an exaggerated sense of independence. If you are becoming a separate being, you are vitally concerned with maintaining connections, reaching out to others, sharing with them, and giving yourself in your relationships. Being an integrated person requires that you recognize the many and varied aspects of your being, that you accept both positive and negative sides, and that you do not disown parts of yourself.

The notions of individuation, independence, autonomy, and self-determination are Western values, and not all cultures pay homage to such values. This emphasis on independence and self-determination tends to reduce the importance of the family of origin. Sue (1997) points out that in Chinese American families the notion of filial piety is a strong determinant of how children behave, even as they move to adulthood. Obedience, respect, obligation to parents, and duty leave little room for self-determination. For example, allegiance to one's parents is expected from a man, even after he marries and has his own family. The concept of individuation and separation from his family can easily lead to conflicts in his family relationships. For example, a son may have difficulty with the notion of being his own person beyond the limits of his family role. He may always think of himself as first a son and in the line of his family tree. For such a person, individuation is neither ideal nor particularly functional. He will discover who he is more easily within the family context than outside of it. It is quite clear that cultural values play a key role in adopting behaviors that reflect an individualistic or collectivistic spirit. At this point, reflect on these questions:

- What cultural values influenced the degree to which you have striven toward autonomy? Which values that stem from your culture do you want to retain? Which do you want to challenge or modify?

- In what significant ways, if any, do you see yourself as having a distinct identity and as being psychologically separate from your family of origin? And in what ways, if any, are you psychologically fused with your family of origin? Are there any aspects of this relationship that you want to change?

The concept of *boundaries* is used in family therapy to refer to emotional barriers that protect and enhance the integrity of members of a system. It also refers to a delineation between members that is governed by implicit or explicit rules. Apply the notion of boundaries to your development. In growing up in your family, what boundaries existed between you and your parents? between your parents and your siblings? among your siblings? between your parents? What did you learn about boundaries from the members of your family? Do you have any problems with boundaries today?

Coping with conflict in the family. If you have difficulty dealing with conflict in your current relationships, one reason may be that conflict was not addressed in direct ways in your family of origin. Perhaps you were taught that conflict was something to be avoided at all costs. If you observed that conflict had no resolution in your family of origin or that people would simply not speak to each other for weeks after a conflict, you are bound to be intimidated when conflicts emerge. Conflicts belong to the whole family, although parents often make their children into scapegoats. The key to successful relationships lies not in the absence of conflict but in recognizing its source and being able to cope directly with the situations that lead to conflict. Conflicts that are denied tend to fester and strain relationships. Reflect on what you learned about conflict in your family. How was it expressed and dealt with? What were its sources? What was your role? Were you encouraged to resolve conflict directly with your antagonist? Did you feel safe in recognizing and dealing directly with disputes between you and members of your family?

The Family as a System

Families have certain rules governing interactions. These *family rules* are not simple commandments, such as what time children need to be home after a date. They also include unspoken rules, messages given by parents to children, injunctions, myths, and secrets. These rules are often couched in terms of "do's" or "don'ts." When parents feel worried or helpless, they tend to dictate rules in an attempt to control any situation. These family rules initially assist children in handling anger, helplessness, and fear. They are intended to provide a safety net for children as they venture into the world (Satir et al., 1988). It is impossible for children to escape growing up without such rules or injunctions, and on the basis of them, children make early decisions. They decide either to accept family rules or to fight against them. Here are some examples of family rules: "Never be angry with your father." "Always keep a smile on your face." "Don't confront your parents, but do what you can to please them." "Don't talk to outsiders about your family." "Children are to be seen but not heard." "Have fun only when all the work is finished."

Rules or messages that were delivered by our parents and parent substitutes are often couched in terms of "do this or that." Consider the following "do" messages: "Be obedient." "Be practical at all times." "Be the very best you can be." "Be appropriate." "Be perfect." "Be a credit to your family." "Be better than we are."

Consider some of the major do's and don'ts that you heard growing up in your family and your reactions to them.

- What are a few messages or rules that you accepted?
- What are some rules that you fought against?
- What early decisions do you deem most significant in your life today? In what family context did you make these decisions?
- Do you ever hear yourself giving the same messages to others that you heard from your parents?

If you grew up in your family thinking "I am never enough," how has this conclusion played out in your current relationships? Consider for a moment the overall impact of the messages that you have received, both from your parents and from society. How have these messages influenced your self-worth? your view of yourself as a woman or as a man? your trust in yourself? your ability to be creative and spontaneous? your ability to receive love and give love? your willingness to make yourself vulnerable? your sense of security? your potential to succeed?

As children we receive rules in a less than clear manner, often learning by observing the behavior of our parents. When rules are presented without choice and as absolutes, they typically present problems for us. For example, you may have accepted a family rule that "I must never get angry." The "must" limits choice completely, and the "never" is an absolute that proves impossible to live by. As a small child, you may have decided to accept this rule and live by it for reasons of both physical and psychological survival. When you carry such a pattern into your adult interactions, it can become self-defeating and dysfunctional. When you live by an absolute rule that "I must never get angry!" it loses its functional nature and inevitably breaks down, and stress in the family goes up.

Rather than trying to get people to give up these survival rules in their lives, Satir suggests helping people transform rules that were not useful into something useful and functional. For example, if Satir were working with your rule that "I must never get angry!" she would broaden the range of choice and challenge you to rid yourself of the impossibility of living up to "always" and "never" standards. She would ask you to first try the statement "I can never get angry." Although this rule still isn't realistic, the word *can* implies more choice than the word *must*. Then she would ask you to try "I *can sometimes* get angry." This statement has both choice and possibility. To make the element of choice more salient, Satir would ask you to think of three situations in which you could imagine getting angry. Through this process, a dysfunctional survival rule can be transformed rather than being attacked.

In healthy families the number of rules is small, and rules are applied consistently. The rules are humanly possible, relevant, and flexible (Bitter, 1987). According to Satir and Baldwin (1983), the most important family rules are those that govern individuation (being unique) and sharing information (communication). These are the rules that influence the ability of a family to function in open ways and to allow all members the possibility for changing. Satir notes that many people develop a range of styles as a means for coping with stress resulting from the constrictions of family rules.

Bitter (1987) contrasts a functional family structure with one that is dysfunctional. In functional families each member is allowed to have a separate life as well as a shared life with the family group. Different relationships are given room to grow. Change is expected and invited, not viewed as a threat. When differentiation leads to disagreements, the situation is viewed as an opportunity for growth rather than an attack on the family system. The structure of the functional family system is characterized by freedom and flexibility and by open communication. All the family members have a voice and can speak for themselves. In this atmosphere, individuals feel support for taking risks and venturing into the world.

By contrast, dysfunctional families are characterized by closed communication, by the poor self-esteem of one or both parents, and by rigid patterns. Rules serve the function of masking fears about differences. They are rigid and are frequently inappropriate for meeting a situation. In unhealthy families, the members are expected to think, feel, and act in the same way. Parents attempt to control the family by using fear, punishment, guilt, or dominance. Eventually, the system breaks down because the rules are no longer able to keep the family structure intact.

When stress is exacerbated because of the breakdown of the family system, members tend to resort to defensive stances. Satir (1983) and Satir and Baldwin (1983) identify four universal communication patterns that express these defensive postures or stress positions: placating, blaming, being overly reasonable, and being irrelevant.

- Individuals who use *placating* as a style for dealing with stress pay the price of sacrificing themselves in their attempt to please others. Because they do not feel an inner sense of value and feel helpless without others, such people say and do what they think others expect of them. Out of their fear of being rejected, they strive to be too many things to too many people.
- People who adopt a *blaming* posture will sacrifice others to maintain their view of themselves. As they point the finger of blame at others, they avoid dealing with the deeper issues of their lack of self-worth and meaninglessness. They frequently say "if it weren't for you, . . ." They attribute responsibility to others for the way they are.
- People who become *overly reasonable* tend to function much like a computer. They strive for complete control over themselves, others, and their environment. In their attempt to avoid humiliation and embarrassment, they keep their emotions tightly in check. Of course, they pay a price of isolation and distance from others for being overcontrolled.
- *Irrelevant* behavior is manifested by a pattern of distractions in the mistaken hope that pain will diminish. Such people appear to be in constant motion. Because they are frightened of stress, they avoid taking a clear position lest they offend others.

Is there an alternative to dealing with family rules other than taking one of the four defensive postures described here? How does a healthy person deal with the stress of meeting family rules? Bitter (1987) describes how congruent people cope with this stress. They do not sacrifice themselves to a singular style in dealing with it. Instead, they transform stress into a challenge that is met in a useful way. Such people are centered, and they avoid changing their colors like a chameleon. Their words match their inner experience, and they are able to make direct and clear statements. They face stress with confidence and courage, because they know that they have the inner resources to cope effectively and to make sound choices. They feel a sense of belongingness and a connectedness with others. They are motivated by the principle of social interest, which means that they are not interested merely in self-enhancement but are aware of the need to contribute to the common good.

We encourage you to think about this discussion of how family rules are manifested in both functional and dysfunctional family structures. Rather than labeling your own family as "functional" or "dysfunctional," think about specific aspects within your family system that may not have been as healthy as you wish. Also think about those aspects of your family life that were helpful, functional, and healthy. Apply the discussion of family structures and family rules to your own experiences. We recommend several books that will provide you with more detailed information on this topic: Satir (1983), Satir (1989), and Satir and Baldwin (1983).

Changing the rules.   It is a mistake to assume that once decisions have been made they are cemented forever. Even children are not completely helpless in responding to the messages sent to them. If there are two children in a family, for example, each may react very differently to the same message of working hard that is modeled by their parents. The daughter decides to have more fun in her life than her parents and places little value on work. The son decides to outdo his parents and work even harder, becoming a workaholic. Children are not passively programmed, although they frequently develop patterns in reaction to what they see their parents doing.

On some level, children cooperate in making the early decisions that direct their lives, which means that they have the capacity to make new decisions that are appropriate to changing life circumstances. Apply the notion of early decisions and making new decisions to yourself. How have some of your early decisions served you? How have they interfered with your present significant relationships? Can you think of any early decisions that you have modified? If so, what are some new decisions that you made, and how has this redecision process affected your life today?

Various family members take on roles that influence the interactions within that family. For instance, your youngest brother may have assumed a role of victim, whereby he typically felt picked on and was constantly seeking protection. It could be that you assumed the role of keeping peace within the family. Even at an early age, others in your family may have looked to you as their counselor or expected you to take care of family difficulties. Your father may have taken on the role of the stern taskmaster and disciplinarian, whereas your mother may have assumed a nurturing role. What roles did you play in your family as a child? as an adolescent? And what are some key roles that you are playing today in your family and in your work?

Family secrets can also influence the structure and functioning of a family. Secrets can be particularly devastating, because that which is hidden typically assumes greater power than that which is out in the open. Generally, it is not what is openly talked about that causes difficulty in families but what is kept hidden. If there are secrets in the family, children are left to figure out what is going on in the home. Did you suspect any secrets in your family? If so, what was it like for you to perpetuate the secrecy? to divulge the secrets? What do you think that secrecy did to the family atmosphere?

Significant developments in your family.   You might find it useful to describe your family's life cycle. Chart significant turning points that have characterized your family's development. One way to do this is to look at family photo albums to see what the pictures reveal. Let them stimulate memories and reflections. As you view pictures of your parents, grandparents, siblings, and other relatives, look for patterns that can offer clues to family dynamics. In charting transitions in the development of your family, reflect on these questions:

- What were the crisis points for your family?
- Can you recall any unexpected events?
- Were there any periods of separation due to employment, military service, or imprisonment?
- Who tended to have problems within the family? How were these problems manifested? How did others in the family react to the person with problems?
- In what ways did births affect the family?
- Were there any serious illnesses, accidents, divorces, or deaths in your family? If so, how did they affect individual members in the family and the family as a whole?
- Was there a history of physical, sexual, or emotional abuse?

Proceed With Caution

Simply reflecting on the questions we have raised that deal with your family history can be therapeutic by itself, even though it may be accompanied by turmoil. If you decide to carry the process a step further and interview members of your family, being sensitive to their feelings and reactions will go a long way toward reducing the chances of your meeting with resistance and alienating family members.

In Chapter 8 you will learn that it is essential to be sensitive to cultural themes in the lives of your clients and their families and that you might lose certain clients if you do not demonstrate an understanding of how their culture affects their choices and actions. Apply this general principle as you approach members of your family. Be sensitive to the cultural rules of your family structure, and consider how concepts such as roles, rules, myths, and rituals operate in your family. In some families, a mother or father would feel offended if a child were to seek information from an aunt or uncle. A Japanese graduate student approached his father to interview him as part of his family autobiography assignment. The father was reluctant to engage in any significant sharing of family material despite the student's insistence that getting this knowledge was important for him. Explain to family members your reasons for asking these questions.

In doing a review of your family history, be prepared for the possibility of a crisis erupting, either in you or within your family. Doing this level of work may lead to a number of surprises and discoveries for which you are not prepared. One student discovered that she had been adopted. She was faced with dealing with anger and disappointment over not having been told. You may learn of family secrets, or you may learn that your "ideal family" is not as perfect as you thought. You may well find that your family has both functional and dysfunctional aspects. Many of the students who were enrolled in a personal-growth group with one of us (Marianne) became anxious or depressed by what they were learning about both themselves and their family system and felt a need to talk about how they were being affected.

You may well discover that the sources of information are scarce, even about your grandparents. For example, I (Jerry) know precious little about my father's life before he and my mother married. From my father, I have some knowledge about his difficult beginnings in this country. At the age of 7, he and his brother came from Italy to New York. His father (whom I know almost nothing about) brought the two children to this country after his wife died. Again, there is scant information about my father's mother. I don't even know how she died. Apparently, my grandfather's intentions were to have a relative in this country care for his boys, yet this relative was unable to do so because of other family responsibilities. This led to my father's placement in an orphanage. I recall some stories he told me about the loneliness of his childhood in the institution and how difficult it was coming to this country not being able to speak a word of English. What is striking to me is how little I do know about my father's side of the family, and this in itself reveals how much material was denied and was kept secret. Because my father died 35 years ago, I have had to look for bits of information that my mother remembers about my father's history and also to relatives who knew something about his life.

In contrast, Marianne's family history is easily traced back to the early 1600s. For many years, I (Marianne) have heard rich stories that formed the tapestry of my family's history. As I grew up in an extended family in a German village, many relatives and townspeople revealed information about several generations. I did become aware of one pattern from my father's side. Someone in the family would typically get angry, and an emotional cutoff would result in which certain people would never speak to each other again. It saddens me to see how this pattern unfolds even with one of my brothers, who, in spite of my efforts to form a closer relationship, seems to be following the tendency of keeping himself distant. This experience is teaching me that family patterns repeat themselves and that we cannot change another person. But we do have power over how we allow ourselves to be affected by the actions and decisions of others.

Doing this level of self-exploration is a must if you intend to work with families. Committing yourself to this arduous task will better enable you to appreciate what client family members go through when they are in therapy with you. We encourage you to stick with the process of discovery, preferably under supervision. It helps to be able to talk to someone about what you are learning.

Growth does not come about without some pain, and it can be anxiety-producing. Moreover, your commitment to exploration and change may bring discomfort to significant people in your life. Being involved in a training program as a helper involves some risks to your current relationships. Your parents, siblings, husband, wife, children, or other relatives may well be threatened by some of your changes. You may believe in the value of recognizing pain and dealing with it, and as a result of your changed perspective you may want your parents or siblings also to adopt a new outlook and change their ways. Perhaps they have avoided pain and are not interested in disturbing this pattern. Even if facing their situation could lead to basic changes and a fuller existence, it is not for you to decide that they should be any different than they are.

As a result of what you are learning about human relationships in your program, along with positive changes you are making in your life, it is bound to be difficult for you to witness people you love settling for a dull existence, if not a destructive lifestyle. You might ask, "How can I help other families in trouble if I cannot help my own family?" If you burden yourself with the thought that it is your mission to change members of your family, you are bound to wind up feeling frustrated.

A graduate student in a counseling program approached one of us and said he felt burdened in putting to use in his own family what he was learning in his courses. Asked what he hoped to accomplish for a weekend therapeutic group aimed at self-exploration, he said: "I feel an urgency to clean up all my problems with my family by the end of this weekend workshop. After all, how can I help my future clients solve their problems if I have problems within my family?" Although this student was to be encouraged in his attempt to deal with his problems, he was setting himself up for failure by trying to meet an unrealistic expectation. Even more of a burden was his belief that it was his place to get significant people in his life to change. If people within his family were not motivated to make certain changes, he needed to realize that he would never be able to do it for them—no matter how talented he was. What he could do was to focus on himself and tell them about himself, which in itself could be an invitation for them to change. He could talk about the changes he had made and what they meant to him. He could also let others know how he was affected by some of their behaviors and, as well, what kind of relationship he would like with them.

The point is to avoid adopting a zealous attitude that others should be different and then attempting to convert them to your way. Above all, patience is critical. To make changes in your life, you probably had to get through layers of your own resistances that masked your fears. It took both time and patience for you to allow yourself to become more vulnerable and open to new possibilities. Allow this space for others in your life to consider your invitations.

Avoid Blaming, and Keep the Focus on Yourself

As you learn about the effect that your family of origin has had on the person you have become, there is a danger of getting stuck in a blaming stance. If you are not careful, you could get sidetracked by believing "If only you had done____, I would be different." A blaming posture will keep you frozen in your attempt to make significant changes, both in yourself and in your relationships. Regardless of the quality of your experiences in your family and no matter how horrible your childhood years may have been, you do not have to remain a victim of your circumstances. It may well take your involvement in personal therapy to work through some of your feelings, so that you can eventually make peace with your past and more freely choose a new direction.

Through our work in group counseling, we have learned time and again that the tendency of many who participate in our groups is to put the focus on the other person in the relationship rather than emphasizing their own role. For example, a college student is quick to tell his mother that she should change and that then they would get along better. He puts considerable energy into searching for her faults, judging her for what she did to him or failed to do for him, and trying to get her to think, feel, and act in ways that he thinks she should. He does his best to control her, so that he is more comfortable in his relationship with her. It is good for couples to realize that it is almost impossible for one partner to control how the other will behave, but there is a wide range of possibilities when it comes to controlling your own life.

When we warn clients about the dangers inherent in blaming people and setting out to change others, they invariably resist changing their perspective. For many, focusing on others does serve the purpose of preserving their self-image. Paradoxically, however, many of our clients find that when they do stop trying to change another person and concentrate more on revealing themselves, the other person is more open to change.

If you are caught up in blaming others for the way that you are, in your counseling you will probably allow clients to blame others for their misery. From our perspective, a mistake that many helpers make is to listen endlessly to their clients recounting stories about how others have mistreated them. Helpers actually form a coalition with such clients, keeping them in a powerless position instead of confronting them on the ways in which they are avoiding taking responsibility for themselves.

When individuals devote a great deal of energy to denying aspects of their being that are not ego-enhancing, they are vulnerable to becoming possessed by the side that they refuse to recognize in themselves. A task of helpers is to provide a climate that invites clients to become excruciatingly honest, which allows them to recognize in themselves what they are projecting outward. This process helps clients focus on what they can do for themselves, as opposed to expecting others to adapt to their expectations. Effective therapy helps clients assume this stance.

By Way of Review

• One of the major contributions of the systemic approaches is that neither the individual nor the family is blamed for a particular dysfunction. Blaming others rarely leads to growth. Rather, it tends to cement the individual into a pattern of helplessness. Family therapy helps each family member change relationship patterns that are not working well and helps the family create new ways of interacting.

• Some training programs offer family-of-origin work for students as a way for them to come to a fuller appreciation of how their family experiences have influenced who and what they are. This training enables helpers to relate more effectively to the families they will meet in their clinical practice.

• To increase your effectiveness when working with families, it is essential that you unravel the mystery of your connection with your family of origin and that you become aware of ways you continue to play out patterns established during childhood.

• When interpreting the meaning of your experiences growing up in your family, it is useful to think about the structure of your family, your relationships with your parents and siblings, key turning points for your family, and the messages your parents conveyed.

• Personal counseling, both individual and group work, is of value in increasing a helper's self-awareness. Healthy individuals who want to help others can profit from professional assistance, especially in gaining increased insight into personal issues that could intrude in their work.

• Family therapy and personal therapy can illuminate your own areas of transference and countertransference and broaden your vision of how your family-of-origin experiences have served as a template for later interpersonal relationships. Your experience with the therapeutic process can increase your awareness of certain patterns of thinking, feeling, and behaving.

What Will You Do Now?

1. As a basis for discovering more about your family of origin, interview your parents and any others who knew you well as you were growing up. You can ask each of these people a specific list of questions about yourself. The point of this exercise is for you to gather events or situations that can assist you in getting a fuller picture of your childhood. What does each person remember the most about you? Are you able to detect any themes in what the people you interview recall about you?

2. Develop a list of questions to help you understand what it was like for your parents as they were growing up. For example, you might ask your parents what their relationships with their parents were like at ages 6, 14, or 21. The aim of the exercise is not to put them on the spot or to get them to divulge secrets, but to better understand the hopes, goals, concerns, fears, and dreams your parents had as children, adolescents, and young adults. You might talk with your parents about how their early experiences influenced them as parents. Discuss with them any patterns you see between them and yourself.

3. Consider interviewing your grandparents. Again, in thinking about questions you would like them to address, be sensitive to how they might respond to

sharing personal facets of their lives. You might simply ask them to share any events or memories that they would feel comfortable disclosing. Rather than simply asking them questions, consider sharing with them significant memories you have of them as you were growing up. What did they teach you? What similar patterns do you see that have been handed down from your grandparents, to your parents, to you, and to your children, if any?

4. Consider making a personal journal that will compile significant information about your family of origin. In putting this journal together, focus on the self-exploration questions raised in this chapter. You might even have short chapters illustrating turning points in your life. In doing this project, it would be useful to include pictures of you and your parents, siblings, grandparents, other relatives, and friends. Include any input from your parents, grandparents, and other relatives that will provide details of your family-of-origin experiences. Look for themes and patterns that will give you a clearer picture of the forces that still influence you today.

5. Much of this chapter provides you with material for reflection about how your family-of-origin experiences influence the person you are today. Spend some time thinking about what you learned about yourself *personally* by reading this chapter. Are there any personal issues that you see as being unresolved and that you are committed to exploring? If so, in your journal write about this unfinished business. How might your own unresolved personal issues affect your ability to work with individuals who are struggling with concerns pertaining to their family?

6. For the full bibliographic entry for each of these sources, consult the References and Reading List at the back of the book. Thomlison (2002) is a good source as a family assessment workbook. Satir (1983) elaborates on communication theory as it applies to working with families. One of the best sources of information for doing a lifestyle analysis is Powers and Griffith (1987). See Loeschen (1998) for a treatment of the systematic training in the skills of Virginia Satir.

InfoTrac College Edition Resources

For additional readings, explore InfoTrac College Edition, our online library. Go to http://www.infotrac.college.com/wadsworth and select these key word searches:

    family of origin
    system* approach

Key words are listed in a form that enables the search engine to locate a wider range of articles in the online university library. Key words should be entered exactly as shown, including asterisks, "W1," "W2," "AND," and other search engine tools.

CHAPTER 4

Understanding Life Transitions

Focus Questions

1. From which of your life experiences can you draw as you attempt to understand the diverse range of client problems you will encounter?

2. At this point in your life, how well do you think you have dealt with the effects of key transition periods in your life? How have some of your earlier experiences influenced the person you are today?

3. Your current life is largely a result of the earlier choices you have made. What choices have particularly affected the person you are today?

4. As you think about your childhood and adolescent years, how do you see those experiences as continuing to influence your present behavior?

5. What have you learned from dealing with a crisis in your personal life that could help you better understand clients who come to you in a state of crisis?

6. As you reflect on developmental patterns in your life, what have been some of the most significant events that have influenced your present attitudes and behavior?

7. Where are you in the process of achieving a healthy balance between independence and interdependence in your life? How might this balance influence your ability to provide help to others?

Aim of the Chapter

Meeting the challenges of life transitions, whether your own or your clients', entails making an assessment of personal assets (strengths) and liabilities (weaknesses). If you expect your clients to make an honest self-assessment, you must be committed to this same quest for self-awareness.

In this chapter we discuss major life themes at the various stages of human development from infancy through old age. Our hope is that you will reflect on critical turning points in your own life along with significant decisions that you have made at those junctures. This can also be a time to review any personal crises you may now be facing to assess how well you are using both your internal and external resources to meet the challenges of ending one stage of life and moving into the next phase of your development.

Personal transformation demands an awareness of how you dealt with developmental tasks in the past and how you are now addressing these issues. By drawing on your own life experiences, both past and present, you are likely to be in a better position to appreciate the struggles of your clients. To help you explore your personal struggles, we provide many case examples that illustrate problems clients are likely to bring to you. We focus on how awareness of your own life experiences can be a useful instrument when you intervene to help your clients.

Focus on Your Life Transitions

It takes courage to work through an upheaval such as marriage or divorce, the birth or death of a child, losing a job, or retiring. All of these transition points test your ability to handle uncertainty, to leave what is known and secure, and to begin a new course in life. A transformation to a more mature level of personal growth entails your willingness to suffer and to learn life-giving lessons through that suffering. If you are tethered to personal comfort at all costs, you could miss rich opportunities to become more of the person you were meant to become.

One way we train beginning helpers is to assist them in focusing on their own development as a person. As a result, we structure our training sessions for counselors around personal issues. We ask trainees to read about certain life themes, to think about their own development and turning points, and to recall key choices they have made. Some of these themes include dealing with childhood, adolescent, and adult struggles; love and intimate relationships; loneliness and solitude; death and loss; sexuality; the choice of a lifestyle; and the meaning in life. These are also some of the main themes clients will bring into counseling sessions. Helpers will be affected by the problems clients discuss in these areas. If helpers themselves have limited awareness of their own struggles with these themes, they are not likely to be very effective. In training workshops the participants can discover what impact their life experiences have on their clients and, in turn, how their clients' life experiences affect them. We ask you to reflect on how the themes we discuss pertain to your life.

By understanding the challenges at each period of life, you will be able to understand how earlier stages of personality development influence the choices you continue to make later in life. In reality there is great variability among individuals within a given developmental phase. Your family of origin, culture, race, gender, and socioeconomic status all have a great deal to do with the manner in which you experience the developmental process. Chronological age is only one index in considering emotional, physical, and social age.

A Theoretical Basis for Understanding Life Stages

There are many theoretical approaches to understanding human growth and development, each of which provides a somewhat different conceptualization of the stages from infancy to old age. These theories provide a road map to understanding how people develop in all areas of personal functioning. As you read the specifics of the individual's life cycle, think about how what is written either fits or does not fit for you.

Although the various theoretical frameworks offer alternative perspectives on lifelong personality development, we address only two of them in this chapter. We describe a model that draws on Erik Erikson's (1963, 1982) psychosocial theory of human development. We also highlight some major ideas about development from the self-in-context approach, which emphasizes the individual life cycle in a systemic perspective (McGoldrick & Carter, 1999). The systemic perspective is grounded on the assumption that how we develop can best be understood through learning about our role and place in our family of origin. The systemic view is that individuals cannot really be understood apart from the family system of which they are a part.

We describe nine stages of development from infancy to old age by pointing out the psychosocial tasks for each phase. We also briefly describe potential problems in personality development if these tasks are not mastered. With each stage of development we present a case illustration to give you some practice in thinking about how to approach given clients. We also encourage you to recognize how your own development in each of these areas can be either an asset or a liability as you help others. How well have you mastered some of the major psychosocial tasks at each period of your development?

Erikson's model is holistic, addressing humans inclusively as biological, social, and psychological beings. Psychosocial theory provides a conceptual framework for understanding trends in development; major developmental tasks at each stage of life; critical needs and their satisfaction or frustration; potentials for choice at each stage of life; critical turning points or developmental crises; and the origins of faulty personality development, which lead to later personality conflicts. Erikson's theory holds that we face the task of establishing an equilibrium between ourselves and our social world at each stage of life.

Erikson describes human development over the entire life span in terms of various stages, each marked by a particular crisis to be resolved. For Erikson, *crisis* means a turning point in life, a moment of transition characterized by the potential to go either forward or backward in development. These moments point to both dangers and opportunities: crises can be viewed as challenges to be met or as catastrophic events that simply happen to you. Each developmental stage builds on the psychological outcomes of earlier stages, and individuals sometimes fail to resolve the conflicts and thus regress. To a very large extent, an individual's current life is the result of earlier choices; life has continuity.

McGoldrick and Carter (1999) have criticized Erikson's theory of individual development for underplaying the importance of the interpersonal realm and connection to others. Contextual factors have a critical bearing on our ability to formulate a clear identity as an individual and also to be able to connect to others. The self-in-context perspective, as described by McGoldrick and Carter, takes into account race, socioeconomic class, gender, ethnicity, and culture as central factors that influence the course of development throughout the individual's life cycle. These factors influence a child's beliefs about self and ways of being emotionally connected with others. For healthy development to occur, it is necessary to establish a clear sense of our unique selves in the context of our connection with others at each stage of life.

Infancy

In infancy, birth to age 1, the basic task is to develop a sense of trust in self, others, and the environment. The core struggle at this time is between trust and mistrust. If the significant persons in an infant's life provide the needed warmth and attention, the child develops a sense of trust. This sense of being loved is the best safeguard against fear, insecurity, and feelings of inadequacy. Children who receive love from parents or parental substitutes generally have little difficulty accepting themselves.

If there is an absence of security in the home, personality problems tend to occur later. Insecure children come to view the world as a potentially hostile place. They have a fear of reaching out to others, a fear of loving and trusting, and an inability to form or maintain intimate relationships. Rejected children learn to mistrust the world and view it largely in terms of its ability to do them harm. Some of the effects of rejection in infancy include tendencies in later childhood to be fearful, insecure, jealous, aggressive, hostile, and isolated.

Daniel Goleman (1995) believes that infancy is the beginning point for establishing *emotional intelligence,* which he defines as the ability to control impulses, empathize with others, form responsible interpersonal relationships, and develop intimate relationships. He identifies the most crucial factor in teaching emotional competence as timing, especially in our family of origin and in our culture of origin during infancy. He adds that childhood and adolescence expand on the foundation for learning a range of human competencies. Later development offers the critical windows of opportunity for acquiring the basic emotional patterns that will govern the rest of our lives.

Case example. Imagine that you are working with a child with a history of being abused. As a result of her experiences, she is frightened and distrustful of the world. Some of her experiences stir up your own memories of difficult periods in childhood. Although you were never physically abused, you suffered much psychological cruelty from two alcoholic parents. Your reason for becoming a helper was to make the world a better place. In working with children like this, you become aware that some of your old cynicism and distrust of the world, which you thought you had successfully dealt with, is resurfacing. You find it increasingly difficult to work with abused children.

This case illustrates how your personal involvement (or countertransference) can render you ineffective in working with a child whose pain reminds you of your own pain. This is especially true if you have not resolved your early conflicts between trust and mistrust. However, such early experiences do not necessarily have to be a liability. If you are aware of your vulnerability in trusting and have worked through this negative conditioning to the point that you are now able to trust, your countertransference can actually be an asset. By drawing on your own life experiences, you can empathize with abused children and assist them in learning to trust the world.

Reflections and application.   As you reflect on the developmental tasks during this stage, think about the foundation you had during your earliest years and how these experiences either prepared you or handicapped you for the tasks you now face in your life. Particularly consider what you learned about trusting the world. Most of the decisions you made in infancy were unconscious and preverbal. Nevertheless, such decisions were powerful shapers of the way you viewed the world later. Consider these questions: "Do you have difficulty trusting others? Are you able to trust yourself and your ability to make it in the world? Do you have fears that others will let you down and that you have to be very careful about how much you show of yourself? What did you learn from your family of origin about how to be in the world?"

Early Childhood

The most critical task of early childhood, ages 1 to 3, is to begin the journey toward autonomy. The core struggle at this time is between self-reliance and self-doubt. By progressing from being taken care of by others to being able to care for one's own needs, children increase their understanding of interdependence and develop a sense of emotional competence, which involves delaying gratification.

Children who fail to master the task of establishing some control over themselves and coping with the world around them develop a sense of shame and feelings of doubt about their capabilities. Parents who do too much for children hamper their development. If parents insist on keeping children dependent, these children will begin to doubt the value of their own abilities. During this period it is essential that feelings such as hostility, anger, and hatred be accepted rather than judged. If these feelings are not accepted, children may not be able to accept their negative feelings later on. They will become adults who feel they must deny all of their "unacceptable" feelings.

Case example.   Your supervisor has asked you to co-lead a group of involuntary clients. Much anger is being expressed in the room. You find that you are working very hard to deflect this anger. At one point you tell a client that he doesn't have to get so angry. He responds by shouting "You don't understand me, so why don't you just shut up!" You feel scared and instinctively leave the room.

Reflections and application.   If you were the helper in this situation and thought about why it was so hard for you to be the recipient of intense anger, you might come up with several answers. Perhaps you grew up in a sheltered and protected environment where your parents made all of your decisions and you never had to struggle with deciding for yourself. You experienced your parents as very loving and kind. In your family nobody ever got angry. Even when your parents unexpectedly divorced, no one expressed anger or hurt. Basically, you were taught messages such as "Be happy and look at the brighter side of things." "Don't get angry." "We will always be there for you." "If you can't say something nice, don't say anything at all."

Some helpers have trouble recognizing or expressing angry feelings. Thus, they also have trouble allowing their clients to have these "unacceptable" feelings. They might talk their clients out of these feelings. If any of this situation fits you, are you able to see any alternatives besides withdrawing from anger? One way you could behave differently is to remain in the room as a client directs his anger toward you. Later, during a supervision session, you can deal with the fears that are evoked in you. If these feelings and attitudes get in the way of your dealing with clients, you may need to deal with them in your personal therapy as well.

Preschool

During the preschool years, ages 3 to 6, children seek to find out what they are able to do. The core struggle at this time is between initiative and guilt. Preschoolers may imitate others, begin to develop a sense of morality, and increase the circle of people who are significant to them. They also learn to give and receive love and affection, learn basic attitudes regarding sexuality, and begin to learn more complex social skills. Preschoolers take more initiative, and they increase their capacity to use and understand language. According to Erikson, the basic task of the preschool years is to establish a sense of competence and initiative. If children are allowed realistic freedom to choose their own activities and make some of their own decisions, they tend to develop a positive orientation characterized by confidence in their ability to initiate and follow through. According to the self-in-context perspective, this stage ushers in the awareness of "otherness" in terms of gender, race, and disability. A key task is to increase trust in others (McGoldrick & Carter, 1999).

If children are unduly restricted or not allowed to make decisions for themselves, they develop a sense of guilt and ultimately withdraw from taking an active stance toward life. Parental attitudes toward children are communicated both verbally and nonverbally, and children often develop feelings of guilt based on negative messages from their parents. Strict parental indoctrination tends to lead to rigidity, severe conflicts, remorse, and self-condemnation. Children may pick up subtle messages that their body and their impulses are unacceptable, for example, and thus they soon begin to feel guilty about their natural impulses and feelings. Carried into adult life, these attitudes can prevent them from enjoying sexual intimacy.

During this period the foundations of gender-role identity are laid. Children begin to form a picture of appropriate masculine and feminine behavior. The models that children have are important in determining whether their self-concepts are healthy. At some point both women and men may want to broaden their conception of what kind of person they want to be. However, early conditioning often makes the expansion of the self-concept somewhat difficult. Many people seek counseling because of problems they experience in regard to their gender-role identity.

Case example.   You are doing an intake interview with Paula, age 14, who was sent to you by her parents. She has had an abortion, is sexually promiscuous, is regularly abusing drugs, and is failing in school. You gather information about her developmental history, and it appears that many of her problems originated during her preschool years. The parents tell you that she was a model child who never gave them any trouble. They were strict disciplinarians. The children she was allowed to play with were all selected by her parents. Paula was an unusually pretty child, and her parents worried about her sexual development and communicated a distrust of boys to her. During the preschool years, when most children are given some freedom and some room for making decisions, Paula was highly controlled by her parents. She had no room to maneuver. Because no freedoms were granted to her, she never had the opportunity to develop self-responsibility. Her mother went to work when Paula was 12 years old, and she immediately began to take advantage of being on her own several hours a day. It was then that she made friends of whom her parents disapproved. With time she became increasingly rebellious toward the rigid climate in her home. She seemed determined to become everything her parents did not want her to be.

On the basis of this knowledge about Paula's situation, there are a number of directions in which you might proceed as her counselor. You could become an ally of her parents and take the role of attempting to present her with advice. You can see that she is heading down a destructive path, and you could attempt to influence her to give up her irresponsible ways of behaving.

From another perspective, you could become Paula's ally. You have empathy for her situation in that you see her oppressive background as largely contributing to her present behavior. You could decide to bring in the family, since you see the problem as being related to the parents' need to control. Do you think you could make sure that everybody in the family was being listened to? Would you be tempted to take sides?

Reflections and application.   As you reflect on the case of Paula, how do you think you would fare as a helper in this situation? What do you think you would do? Might you focus on the parents? on Paula? on both? Are you aware of any of your attitudes that would influence your interventions? How might your own struggles for independence with your parents affect you? If you have children, how might your relationship with them influence the way you would work with Paula or her parents?

As you read and apply the developmental tasks of this stage to your own life, look for patterns in your present attitudes and behavior that could be traced to your preschool years. Pay special attention to how these preschool patterns operate today in your life, either positively or negatively. Also, note how your life experiences either contribute to or detract from your ability to be helpful to Paula. Consider some of these questions: "Do you have a clear sense of your own gender-role identity? Are you the kind of woman or man you want to be? Where did you acquire your standards of appropriate gender-role behavior? Are you comfortable with your own sexuality? with your body? with giving and receiving in a sexual relationship? Are there any unresolved conflicts from your childhood that affect you today? Do your present behaviors and current conflicts indicate areas of unfinished business?"

Middle Childhood

Erikson states that the major struggle of middle childhood, ages 6 to 12, is between industry and inferiority. The central task is to achieve a sense of industry; failure to do so results in a sense of inadequacy. Children need to expand their understanding of the world and continue to develop an appropriate sex-role identity. The development of a sense of industry includes focusing on creating goals, such as meeting challenges and finding success in school.

From the self-in-context view, this is a time when children increase their understanding of self in terms of gender, race, culture, and abilities. There is an increased understanding of self in relation to family, peers, and community. A key task is developing empathy, or being able to take the perspective of others (McGoldrick & Carter, 1999).

Children who encounter failure in their early schooling often experience major handicaps later in life. Those children with early learning problems may begin to feel worthless. Such feelings often dramatically affect their relationships with their peers, which are also vital at this time. Problems that can originate during middle childhood include a negative self-concept, feelings of inferiority in establishing and maintaining social relationships, conflicts over values, a confused sex-role identity, dependency, a fear of new challenges, and a lack of initiative.

Case example. José and Maria are a middle-aged couple who come to you for marital counseling. One issue that has caused trouble in their marriage is the fact that José continually changes jobs, and as a result they are always financially strapped. Maria insists that her husband seeks jobs that are far below his capabilities. José basically agrees with Maria. During the interview you learn that he had many academic difficulties in elementary school. His parents were migrant farmers, and as a result he attended many different schools. When he started school, he did not speak English, and he recalls that his teachers were not understanding of him. Most of the time he felt like a failure and an outcast, he hated school, and he decided that he was unintelligent. As the years went on, his feelings of inadequacy progressed. He always reacted with surprise when some of his teachers told him that he was performing below his abilities. Even though he realizes that he is not stupid, he has decided that it is too late to overcome some of these earlier obstacles. Out of his fear of failure and limited self-confidence, he avoids pursuing jobs that are more challenging and that could be potentially more satisfying.

Assume that you are a white, upper-middle-class counselor. You are impatient with José, for you see him blaming the system and making chronic excuses for his failures. You have a hard time understanding why he has not overcome the obstacles that he faced so long ago. If this is your frame of reference, do you think you would be able to provide him with encouragement to explore his deeper problems, such as self-doubt and inadequacy?

Now consider that you understand how his early experiences in grade school are continuing to affect his self-confidence. Could you work with him on modifying his self-limiting assumptions and changing some of the decisions he made about himself as an early learner? With José you formulate a plan for change that includes participating in remedial courses in adult education. The crux of your work involves getting him to see that his early failures stemmed from unfortunate circumstances and not from the fact that he was unintelligent.

Reflections and application.   If you had a client like José, how might your own life experiences either hinder or enhance your ability to counsel him? What were some of the highlights of the first few years in school for you? In general, did you feel competent or incompetent as a learner? Did you see school as an exciting place to be or as a place that you wanted to avoid? What were some of the specific ways in which you felt that you were successful or that you were a failure? What attitudes did you form about your competence as a person during your early school years? Think of some significant people in your life at this time who affected you either positively or negatively. Attempt to recall some of their expectations for you, and remember the messages they gave you about your worth and potential. What connections do you see, if any, between the assumptions you made then and the assumptions that influence your life today?

Adolescence

Adolescence, ages 12 to 20, is a period of searching for an identity, continuing to find one's voice, and balancing caring of self with caring about others. The core struggle is between identity and identity confusion. From the self-in-context perspective, key developmental tasks include dealing with rapid body changes and body image issues, learning self-management, developing one's sexual identity, developing a philosophy of life and a spiritual identity, learning to deal with intimate relationships, and an expanded understanding of self in relation to others (McGoldrick & Carter, 1999).

For Erikson, the major developmental conflicts of adolescence center on the clarification of who you are, where you are going, and how you are getting there. The struggle involves integrating physical and social changes. Adolescents may feel pressured to make career choices early, to compete in the job market or in college, to become financially independent, and to commit themselves to physically and emotionally intimate relationships. Peer-group pressure is a major force, and it is easy to lose one's self by conforming to the expectations of friends. With the increasing stress experienced by many adolescents, suicidal ideation is not uncommon.

During the adolescent period a major part of the identity-formation process consists of separation from the family system and establishment of an identity based on one's own experiences. The process of separating from parents can be an agonizing part of the struggle toward individuation. Although adolescents may adopt many of their parents' values, to individuate they must choose these values freely as opposed to accepting them without thought.

Case example.   Adam is an adolescent who is referred to you by the school counselor. When you ask him what brings him to your office, he first tells you abruptly that his counselor has made him come to see you. After overcoming his initial resistance, he eventually tells you this about his problems: "I used to be a good student, but about a year ago I lost interest in school because I felt the pressure of having to get A's in all my classes. I want to go to college, but I'm afraid I won't make it because I've been failing some of my classes. My parents are very disappointed in me. We used to have a great relationship, but now I don't even want to talk to them. I'd much rather stay in bed than get up and go to school. My friends tell me I've become a bore to be around, and I don't want to be around them either. What really hurt me was when my girlfriend broke up with me. When I'm not at school, I spend most of my time alone in my room listening to music. I don't know anymore what I want to do. There's nothing I look forward to, and sometimes I wish I could go to sleep and never wake up."

Reflections and application.   If you were Adam's counselor, how able would you be to hear his hopelessness, his feelings of desperation, and his possible suicidal intentions? How might you be able to interact with him? Did you ever feel a sense of hopelessness and a belief that your future would never be any better? Feelings of hopelessness and suicidal thoughts are among the most difficult issues that you will have to explore with your clients. It will probably be most difficult to remain objective and not get lost in the client's hopelessness. You may feel afraid when your clients express the depths of their despair and their desire to end it all. At these times you will feel much pressure and responsibility in wondering what to do to be helpful. At some point in your life you may have struggled with finding a sense of meaning and not seen much hope for change in your life. How you recognized and dealt with these feelings will greatly influence the way you intervene with clients who see little hope.

Take a few moments to review some of your adolescent experiences. How did you feel about yourself during this time? In reviewing these years, how might your experiences work for or against you in dealing with Adam? Think about your degree of independence and interdependence during your adolescence. Focus on what gave meaning to your life. Also ask yourself these questions: "At this time in my life, did I have a clear sense of who I was and where I was going? What major choices did I struggle with during my adolescent years?" As you review this period, focus on how your adolescent experiences affected the person you are today.

Early Adulthood

According to Erikson, we enter young adulthood, ages 20 to 35, after we master the adolescent conflicts over identity. Our sense of identity is tested anew in adulthood, however, by the core struggle between intimacy and isolation. The ability to form intimate relationships depends largely on having a clear sense of self. One cannot give to another if one has a weak ego or an unclear sense of identity. Intimacy involves sharing, giving ourselves, relating to another based on our strength, and a desire to grow with that person. If we think very little of ourselves, the chances are not good that we will be able to give meaningfully to others. The failure to achieve intimacy often results in feelings of isolation from others and a sense of alienation. Erikson's concept of intimacy can be applied in any kind of close relationship between two adults. Relationships involving emotional commitments may be between close friends of the same or the opposite sex, and they may or may not have a sexual dimension.

The major aim of this period of life is being able to engage in intimate relationships and find satisfying work. Some developmental issues include caring for self and others, focusing on long-range goals, nurturing others physically and emotionally, finding meaning in life, and developing tolerance for delaying gratification to meet long-range goals (McGoldrick & Carter, 1999).

During their 20s, young people are challenged to make many critical choices. They wrestle with the choice of clinging to security or leaving those things that bring a secure existence. They struggle with the costs and benefits of developing relationships with a few people. Career choice becomes an important part of this time of life. Whether to marry and to become a parent is another issue. Young people are creating dreams and wondering about how they can translate their dreams into real life. Because of the many areas of choice pertaining to work, education, marriage, family life, and lifestyle, it is not uncommon for young adults to wonder what it is they really want. At this time of life, some allow others to decide for them what their standards and choices will be.

The struggle toward autonomy. As we leave adolescence and enter early adulthood, our central task is to assume increased responsibility and independence. Although most of us have moved away from our parents physically, not all of us have done so psychologically. To a greater or lesser degree, our parents will have a continuing influence on our lives. Cultural factors play a significant role in determining the degree to which our parents influence our lives. For example, in some cultures developing a spirit of independence is not encouraged. Instead, these cultures place a prime value on cooperation with others and on a spirit of interdependence. In some cultures, parents continue to have a significant impact and influence on their children even after they reach adulthood. Respect and honor for parents may be values that are extolled above individual freedom by the adult children. In these cultures the struggle for autonomy may be to define one's place in the family rather than to separate from it.

The struggle toward autonomy entails choosing for yourself and working for your own approval rather than living your life for the approval of your parents or others. Making decisions about the quality of life you want for yourself and affirming these choices are partly what autonomy is about. Autonomy also entails your willingness to accept responsibility for the consequences of your choices rather than placing the responsibility on others if you are not satisfied with the way your life is going. Furthermore, achieving a healthy balance between independence and interdependence is not something you do at a given time once and for all. The struggle toward autonomy and interdependence begins in early childhood and continues throughout life.

In writing about genuine maturity from the self-in-context perspective, McGoldrick and Carter (1999) remind us that the ultimate goal is to develop a mature, interdependent self. We are challenged to establish a solid sense of our unique self in the context of our connection to others. This systemic perspective is based on the assumption that maturity requires the ability to empathize, communicate, collaborate, connect, trust, and respect others. McGoldrick and Carter maintain that the degree to which we are able to form meaningful connections with people who differ from us in terms of gender, class, race, and culture "will depend on how these differences and connections were dealt with within our family of origin, within our communities, within our culture of origin, and within our society as a whole" (p. 28).

Transition from the 20s to the 30s.   The transition from the late 20s to the early 30s is a time of changing values and beliefs. Inner turmoil increases for many during this period. However, many others choose to delay making a commitment about relationships and careers. It used to be quite common for young people in their late 20s and early 30s to have a family and to be firmly established in a career. Now, taking on these responsibilities is often delayed, and it is not uncommon for couples to begin having children in their later 30s. During this transition people often take another look at their earlier dreams. They may reevaluate their life plans and make significant shifts. Some become aware that their dreams have not materialized, and they wonder what kind of future they want for themselves and others in their lives. Although this recognition often brings anxiety, it can spur the necessity of making new plans and working hard to attain them.

Case example.   Becky, 23, comes to you for counseling on the urging of a concerned friend. She tells you that she has been in a relationship with a young man for more than 5 years, yet she has never really been satisfied with it. Although she has tried to break off with him a number of times, she typically resumes seeing him when he begins to "treat her so nice" and when she begins feeling guilty. If she were to give him up for good, she fears she would have no man in her life. She concludes that having him is better than having nobody. In most aspects of her life Becky has allowed her parents to make her choices for her. Under parental pressure she pursued a teaching major and is currently in student teaching. She discovered that she really is not interested in teaching, yet she does not trust herself to follow her own interests. Becky has a great deal of talent in dancing, and she wanted to become a professional dancer. She abandoned this idea because she could tell that her parents did not support this choice. She is aware that she has been both financially and emotionally dependent on her parents. Although she would like to choose for herself, she stops herself from doing so out of her fear of making poor decisions. At this time in her life she feels a great deal of pressure within herself to please her parents, yet she realizes that she cannot please both them and herself.

Reflections and application.   Put yourself in the position of being Becky's counselor. Imagine that you have had a different kind of life from hers. You had few problems establishing goals and following them. You knew what you wanted to do, and you pretty much did it. With a minimum of help from your parents you attained most of your goals. If this were the case, do you think you would be able to empathize with Becky? Would you be able to identify with any of her struggles and thus help her find a way to move ahead?

If you are a middle-aged or older person, what decisions did you make in early adulthood, and how do you think those decisions would influence the way you work with Becky? Do you have any regrets about the choices you made? If you are unhappy about some of these choices, might you be inclined to be another person who would influence her to move in a particular direction?

How do you think your own struggles or lack of them would affect you in working with clients like Becky who have problems deciding for themselves what they want to do personally and vocationally?

Middle Adulthood

Middle adulthood, between ages 35 and 55, is characterized by a "going outside of ourselves." The core struggle at this time is between generativity and stagnation. It is a time for learning how to live creatively with ourselves and with others, and it can be the time of greatest productivity in our lives. This is a period when people are likely to engage in a philosophical reexamination of their lives, which may result in reinventing themselves in their work and in their involvement in the community (McGoldrick & Carter, 1999). A task of this life stage is solidifying one's philosophy of life. Other tasks include nurturing and supporting one's children, partner, and older family members. A challenge is to recognize accomplishments and accept limitations. Generativity includes more than fostering children. It includes being creative in one's career, finding meaningful leisure activities, and establishing significant relationships in which there is giving and receiving.

During middle age there is sometimes a period of depression. When people begin to see that some of their visions have not materialized, they may give up hope for a better future. Some women who married and made a family their main priority may begin to wonder if this is all there is to life. At this time many women will choose to return to college or to work full time or to combine the triple roles of homemaker, student, and worker. Some men begin to wonder if they want to stay in their career. They may have to cope with depression when they realize that they have not reached some of their important dreams.

As is true with any stage, there are both dangers and opportunities during this time. Some of the dangers include slipping into secure but deadening ruts and failing to take advantage of opportunities for enriching life. Many individuals experience a midlife crisis, when their whole world seems to be unstable. A few of the events that lead to such a crisis include the realization that youthful dreams will not come about; an illness or the onset of the aging process; the death of one's parents; the realization of one's ultimate aloneness in this life; the realization that life is not always fair and just; a marital crisis or the breakup of a long-established relationship; children leaving the nest; or losing one's job. A problem of this period is the failure to achieve a sense of productivity, which then leads to feelings of stagnation. What is important is that individuals realize the choices they have in their life and see the changes they can make rather than giving in to the feeling that they are victims of life's circumstances.

According to Carl Jung, we are confronted with major changes and possibilities for transformation as we begin the second half of life. Jung's therapy clients consistently revealed signs of experiencing a pivotal middle-age life crisis. Although they may have achieved worldly success, they typically were challenged with finding satisfaction in projects that had lost meaning. Many of his clients struggled to overcome feelings of emptiness and flatness of life.

Jung believed that major life transformations are an inevitable and universal part of the human condition at this juncture in life. He maintained that when the zest for living sags, this can be a catalyst for necessary and beneficial changes. To undergo such a transformation requires the death of some aspect of our psychological being so new growth can occur that will open us to far deeper and richer ranges of existence. To strive for what Jung called *individuation*—a condition of integration of the unconscious with the conscious and of psychological balance—people during their middle years must be willing to let go of preconceived notions and patterns that dominated the first part of their lives. Their task now is to be open to the unconscious forces that have been influencing them all of their lives and to deepen the meaning of their lives.

Jung believed people could bring unconscious material into awareness by paying attention to their dreams and fantasies and by expressing themselves through such avenues as poetry, writing, music, and art. Individuals need to recognize that the rational thought patterns that drove them during the first half of life represent merely one way of being. At this time in life, they must be willing to be guided by the spontaneous flow of the unconscious if they hope to achieve an integration of all facets of their being, which is part of psychological health (Schultz & Schultz, 2001).

Case example.　Ernie, age 49, has been referred to you by his minister. Ernie, who has been married for 24 years, has done everything with his wife. They have never spent a night apart. He did not make any close friends, either male or female, because his wife is very jealous and is threatened by any attempts to do so. He has totally surrendered to his wife's exaggerated fear of his having an affair. Ernie says that until recently there were no grounds for her fears. Although he had not questioned his marriage and life before, he finds himself growing more and more disenchanted with the boredom and predictability of his life. He feels caught in a rut, yet he hesitates to get out. Although he has a good job, it, too, has lost its appeal. He feels a lack of excitement in his work in much the same way that he feels a dullness about his marriage. He hates to go to work, and he hates to come home. He complains about a lack of sleep, waking up in the middle of the night and ruminating about his life situation.

A few months ago Ernie found that he enjoyed talking to one of the women at work. She listened to him, and they shared some common concerns. They developed a friendship, which he carefully kept a secret from his wife. Eventually Ernie and his friend became involved in a sexual relationship. Although he finds his time with her exciting and very much values her as a friend, he cannot imagine himself leaving his wife to live with her. She is also married, and she has several small children. He says that he still loves his wife, yet he is not ready to quit seeing the other woman. Although he feels caught in deadening ruts at home and at work, he is not ready to quit his job or seek a divorce. He is in much turmoil, for, as he puts it, he is going against his own values. He comes to you because he is in a great deal of pain and does not know what to do next.

Reflections and application. If you were counseling Ernie, what life experiences of yours do you think might help you in understanding him? Assume that you have been hurt by an affair, and consider your capacity for remaining objective as you work with Ernie. He wants someone to help him figure out what to do. Would you be willing to help him find the answers? Which of the following themes in his life would you tend to focus on: his affair? his marriage? his dissatisfaction with his job? the meaninglessness in his life?

If you have reached middle adulthood, what struggles and decisions could you draw on as a resource? If you have not yet reached middle age, what would you most want to be able to say that you have accomplished in your life by this time? What would you hope to have in your relationships? What would you want from your work? How might you go about keeping yourself alive and avoiding predictable ruts?

Late Middle Age

Erikson does not differentiate between middle age and late middle age, but instead has one general stage that spans the period between the ages of mid-30s to mid-60s. McGoldrick and Carter (1999) differentiate between these two phases of middle age. For them, late middle age, age 55 to 70, is a time when many adults are beginning to consider retirement, pursuing new interests, and thinking more about what they want to do with the rest of their lives. It is a period for taking up new interests, which may be increasingly possible because of being freed up from child rearing or financial responsibilities. During this time people become more aware of the reality of death, and they may reflect more on whether they are living well. It is a time for reevaluation and a time when people are at the crossroads of life. They may begin to question what else is left, and they may establish new priorities or renew their commitments. Late middle age is a period when people reach the top of the mountain and become aware that they must begin the downhill journey. They might painfully experience the discrepancy between the dreams of their younger years and the harsh reality of what they have actually accomplished with their life so far. A challenge during this period of life is coming to terms with the reality that not everything could be done. People must let go of some of their dreams, accept their limitations, stop dwelling on what they cannot do, and focus on what they *can* do (McGoldrick & Carter, 1999).

When people reach their mid-50s, they often begin the process of preparing for older age. Many are at their peak in terms of status and personal power. This can be a satisfying time of life, because now they do not have to work as hard as they did in the past, nor do they have to meet others' expectations. They can enjoy the benefits of long struggle and dedication rather than striving to continually prove themselves. It is likely that child rearing and work are moving toward a culmination. Adults at this stage often do a lot of reflecting, contemplating, refocusing, and evaluating of themselves so they can continue to discover new directions.

Sheehy (1995) suggests that we look at the positive and creative dimensions of late middle life, including the sources of love, meaning, fun, spiritual companionship, sexuality, and sustained well-being. Although many women may experience this as an exciting time, they are often challenged to cope with both the physical and psychological adjustments surrounding menopause. Some women, fearing that menopause means losing their youthful looks, sink into depression. For many, menopause represents a crisis. In *The Silent Passage*, Sheehy (1992) suggests that, far from being a marker that signifies the beginning of the end, menopause is better seen as a gateway to a second adulthood. Sheehy addresses the stigma of aging in a youth-obsessed society.

For men, the 50s and 60s can be a time for the potential awakening of their creative side. Instead of being consumed with achievement strivings, many men are opening up human facets of themselves beyond their rational thinking that can result in a richer existence. But men, too, are challenged to find new meaning in their lives. Projects that once were highly satisfying may now lack luster. Some men become depressed when they realize that they have been pursuing empty dreams. They may have met goals they set for themselves, only to find that they are still longing for a different kind of life. For both women and men in their 50s and 60s, examining their priorities can often lead to new decisions about how they want to spend their time.

According to Sheehy (1995, pp. 350–352), the vast majority of people in their 60s are quite able, both physically and mentally, to function independently. Most people in their 60s have reached a stage where maximum freedom still coexists with a minimum of physical limitations. What Sheehy claims to be true about people in their 60s is also true of people in their 70s, according to Rowe and Kahn (1998).

Case example. Cedric was picked up by the police after he was found wandering around, lost and disoriented. He was brought to the community mental health center where you work as an intern. You notice that he is unkempt and is talking incoherently. After some time on the ward he improves to the point of being able to join a therapy group. In this group he recalls many sad times in his life. He talks about his regrets. About 2 years ago he lost his wife, who died after a long illness. He feels lost without her, and he says that most of his will to live vanished after she died. Her medical bills ate up his savings. Because the company he worked for went bankrupt, he is left with few benefits for his retirement. He has five children and 15 grandchildren, but he has no contact with any of them because they are spread around the country. One of his major regrets is that he never really established meaningful ties with his children or grandchildren, and now he feels that it is too late. At age 64 he just does not see much sense in going on with his life. He never took the time to develop hobbies or friends and he finds life now to be boring and meaningless.

Reflections and application.   How do you think you would be affected by working with Cedric? What clues does Cedric provide that would call for an assessment of suicidal thoughts and intentions? What questions would you ask him to determine how serious he was about suicide? If you decided that he was suicidal, what course of action might you take? What help do you think you would offer him? Would you agree that his state was hopeless and that there was little he could do to change his life at this late stage? Or would you see hope for him? What alternatives might you pose to him about ways of finding meaning in his life? If you experienced countertransference in working with Cedric, what steps would you take to work through your own reactions? For a moment, reflect on a few personal and professional accomplishments you would most want to realize by the time you reach late middle age. If you could create a new direction at this time in your life, what might this look like?

Late Adulthood

Late adulthood, age 70 onward, is characterized by the core struggle between integrity and despair. Encountering the death of parents and losses of friends and relatives confronts us with the reality of preparing ourselves for our own death. A basic task of late adulthood is to complete a life review in which we put our life into perspective and come to accept who we are and what we have done. This is also a time in life when spirituality may take on a new meaning and provide us with a sense of purpose, even as we face a growing dependence on others (McGoldrick & Carter, 1999). Prevalent themes for people during late adulthood include loss; loneliness and social isolation; feelings of rejection; the struggle to find meaning in life; dependency; feelings of uselessness, hopelessness, and despair; fears of death and dying; grief over others' deaths; sadness over physical and mental deterioration; and regrets over past events. Today, many of these themes characterize people in their mid-80s more than people in their 60s and even 70s.

Late adulthood has changed just as dramatically as the earlier middle-age stages. As is the case for each of these developmental stages, there is a great deal of individual variance. Many 70-year-old people have the energy that many middle-aged people have. How people look and feel during late adulthood is more than a matter of physical age; it is largely a matter of attitude. To a great degree, vitality is influenced by state of mind more than by mere chronological years lived.

People who succeed in achieving ego integrity are able to accept that they have been productive and that they have coped with whatever failures they faced. Such people are able to accept the course of their lives, and they do not endlessly ruminate on all that they could have done, might have done, and should have done. In contrast, some elderly people fail to achieve ego integration. These people fear death. They develop a sense of hopelessness and feelings of self-disgust. They are able to see all that they have not done, and they often yearn for another chance to live in a different way. These people may feel that they have let valuable time slide by.

Case example.   Burt and Edith are a couple in their 80s who have been married for 60 years and who still enjoy each other's company. In addition to what they have as a couple, they are also blessed as individuals. They enjoy excellent health, live independently in their own home, are involved with a large extended family, enjoy many grandchildren and great grandchildren, and assume leadership roles in their church. They spend many hours doing volunteer work. Routinely, they make trips to another country where they provide assistance to an orphanage and a local church. Those who know them marvel at their ability to handle the strain connected with devoting countless hours to their work. What is most notable about them is their love for their family and their strong religious faith. Edith's quiet strength and gentleness blends nicely with Burt's incredible sharp wit and humor. You might not see a couple such as this, for it does not appear that they are in need of counseling. Yet it might be that you could include Burt and Edith in working with their children or grandchildren in some capacity. How might you be able to use them as resource people in assisting other family members?

Reflections and application.   If you have not reached old age, imagine yourself at that time of life. Think about what you would like to be able to say about your life. What kind of relationships would you most hope to be able to have established by this time in your life? Do Edith and Burt offer any kind of inspiration for you regarding your potential to create a meaningful life as an elderly person? Focus especially on your fears of aging and also on what you hope you could accomplish by this time. What kind of old age do you expect? What are you doing now that might have an effect on the kind of person you will be as you grow older? What things would you like to do during your later years? Can you think of any regrets you will be likely to express? As you anticipate growing older, think about what you can do today to increase the chances that you will be able to achieve a sense of integrity as an older person. Are you cultivating interests and relationships that can become a source of satisfaction in later years?

If you find yourself postponing many things that you would like to do now, ask yourself why. Assess the degree to which you are satisfied with the person you are becoming today. Finally, assess your present ability to work with elderly clients. If you yourself have not reached this age, what experiences could you draw on as a way of understanding the world of an elderly client? Even though you might not have had some of the same experiences, do you see how you can relate to some of their feelings that are very much like your own?

By Way of Review

• How you cope with crises in your own life is a good indication of your ability to help your clients work through theirs. If you face and deal with your problems with all the resources available to you, you can be present for clients who are in crisis. This is not to say that your way of coping with life challenges will be the same way your clients cope, nor that what has worked for you will necessarily work for them. Your understanding of finding internal resources can serve you as you guide clients in discovering their resources for change.

• Each of the nine stages of life represents a turning point when individuals are challenged with the fulfillment of their destinies. Both helpers and clients need to realize that personal transformation entails the willingness to tolerate pain and uncertainty. Growth is not generally a smooth process but involves some degree of turmoil.

• At each stage of life there are choices to be made. Your earlier choices have an impact on the kind of person you are now.

• Specific tasks and specific crises can occur from infancy through old age. Review your own developmental history so that you have a perspective in working with the developmental struggles of your clients. You will be in a better position to understand your clients' problems and to work with them if you have an understanding of your own vulnerabilities.

What Will You Do Now?

1. Write down a list of resources for personal growth and ways of increasing your self-awareness. Think of some avenues that would promote self-exploration on your part. Are you inclined to do something that will encourage you to reflect on the quality of your life?

2. Remember a time in your life that was either the most difficult (painful) or the most exciting (joyful). What did you learn from these experiences? If this time occurred during childhood, talk with someone you knew well as a child about what he or she remembers of you. What are the implications of these experiences in your own life for you as a helper? How might some of your life experiences affect you as you work with others who are like you? different from you?

3. Reflect on some of your life experiences that you think will facilitate your work with clients. In your journal write about a few key turning points in your life. Can you think of one or two times when you were faced with making a major decision? If so, how might this turning point still have an influence on your life? What lessons did you learn from making this decision, and how might this experience better enable you to identify with the struggles of clients?

4. For the full bibliographic entry for each of the sources listed here, consult the References and Reading List at the back of the book. See Erikson (1963) for a description of the psychosocial theory of development with a focus on the critical tasks of each of the life stages. For a description of developmental themes of the stages of adulthood, see Sheehy (1995). For a self-in-context developmental approach that emphasizes an individual life cycle in a systemic perspective, see McGoldrick and Carter (1999). For themes and choices dealing with childhood, adolescence, and adulthood, refer to G. Corey and M. Corey (2002).

InfoTrac College Edition Resources

For additional readings, explore InfoTrac College Edition, our online library. Go to http://www.infotrac.college.com/wadsworth and select these key word searches:

developmental W1 theme*
life W1 choice*
Erikson* psychosocial approach
emotional W1 intelligence

Key words are listed in a form that enables the search engine to locate a wider range of articles in the online university library. Key words should be entered exactly as shown, including asterisks, "W1," "W2," "AND," and other search engine tools.

Stages in the Helping Process

Focus Questions

1. What beliefs do you hold about the capacity of people to change? How can change best be facilitated? What constitutes effective helping? What is the best way to evaluate the degree of change in clients?

2. How are your views and beliefs about human nature related to your approach to working with people who seek your help?

3. What basic beliefs do you hold about the helping process? If a client asked you how you work or about your orientation to helping, what would you most want to say?

4. Which of your assets and resources can you draw on in establishing helping relationships? What liabilities or limitations do you have that might interfere with forming working relationships with certain clients?

5. What are the advantages and disadvantages of brief models of therapy? How do brief, solution-focused intervention strategies fit the requirements of managed care programs? How do these approaches fit with your beliefs about what constitutes effective helping?

6. How do you determine whether an intervention you are planning to use is for you or for the client?

7. What guidelines would you use in confronting clients? What is the purpose of confrontation? Can you think of anything that might get in the way of effective confrontation on your part?

8. How important is helper self-disclosure in the helping relationship? What guidelines would you use to determine when self-disclosure would be appropriate? Can you think of any difficulties you might have in engaging in self-disclosure?

9. What are your thoughts about working with clients collaboratively to formulate goals that will guide the helping relationship? How might you develop action plans in a collaborative way with your clients?

10. How would you best prepare clients for termination? Can you think of any factors that might make it difficult for you to end therapy with clients? What guidelines might you use for effective termination?

Aim of the Chapter

The purpose of this chapter is to help you clarify your role at various stages in the helping process. We look at the skills and knowledge you need at the various stages of helping, along with the personal characteristics that are required to apply your skills. Our basic assumption is that the kind of person you are and the attitudes you bring to the helping relationship are the major determinants of its quality. We also consider the role of theory as a guiding factor for practicing effectively. The model we describe is an integrative approach that emphasizes the role of thinking, feeling, and acting in human behavior. Your theoretical orientation provides you with a map for making interventions, but we stress the importance of developing a personal stance toward helping that fits the person you are and is flexible enough to meet the unique needs of the client population with which you work.

Orientations to Helping

Your orientation to the helping process is largely a function of your beliefs about human nature and about how people change. Before you accept a position in any setting, find out about the agency's theoretical framework. Sometimes an orientation will be imposed on you. For example, you might work in a state facility that employs behavior-modification strategies. Or an agency may make extensive use of a system of diagnoses, and you will be expected to conduct interviews and arrive at a specific diagnostic category for each client you see. If the methods of intervention are not compatible with your views of helping, you are bound to experience conflict in this institution. Clarify your thinking about helping by answering these questions: Who is responsible for change in the helping relationship? What focus is most likely to lead to change? a focus on feelings? a focus on insight? a focus on behavior? a focus on cognition? What is the best balance between providing a great deal of structure and providing only minimal structure? What is an appropriate balance between confrontation and support? Do you believe clients are capable of finding their own solutions to problems?

The Impact of Your Beliefs on Your Work

Your views and beliefs about human nature are very much related to the helping strategies you will employ with your clients. If you see people as basically good, for example, you will trust that your clients can assume responsibility for the direction of their lives. If you see human nature through negative lenses, you will adopt a role as a helper who attempts to correct people's flawed nature. To clarify your views about human nature, reflect on these statements. Use this scale: 5 = strongly agree; 4 = agree; 3 = undecided; 2 = disagree; 1 = strongly disagree.

____ 1. People need direction from an authority to resolve their problems.
____ 2. People have the capacity to find their answers within themselves.
____ 3. People create their own misery.

_____ 4. People are victims of outside circumstances.

_____ 5. People are basically good and are therefore trustworthy.

_____ 6. People are negatively inclined and therefore need a great deal of direction.

_____ 7. People are the product of their choices; that is, they are the architects of their lives.

_____ 8. People are shaped by fate.

_____ 9. People won't change unless they are in pain.

_____ 10. People are motivated by their goals.

_____ 11. People are determined by their early childhood experiences.

Review your choices and determine whether you have a positive or negative view of human nature.

If you expect the best in people, they are likely to give you their best. If you treat people as though they have the capacity to understand and resolve their problems, they are more likely to find answers within themselves. By developing a collaborative partnership with your clients, you are telling them that they can use the helping relationship as a pathway to re-creating their lives.

Effective helpers hold positive beliefs about people; have a healthy self-concept; ground their interventions in values; are respectful of cultural differences; are able to fully listen and understand; and possess empathy, congruence, warmth, compassion, genuineness, and positive regard. They test their beliefs and examine whether their interventions are expressions of their core beliefs and assumptions about how people change.

In contrast, ineffective helpers tend to hold rigid and judgmental beliefs about people. They tend to tell clients how they should think and how to solve their problems. Ineffective helpers do not believe their clients have the means to assume control of their own destiny. Ineffective helpers are not willing to challenge their own assumptions and tend to look for client behaviors that support their hunches and convictions. We have heard most of the following statements from students or professionals. As you review these examples of helpers' assumptions, ask yourself if you might have made some of these statements. Reflect on how you think your beliefs about people might lead to placing them in a category and judging them.

- "A sociopath is resistant to therapy and will never change."
- "Old people can't change. They should be given support but not challenged."
- "I'm 'color blind'—I can work equally well with any racial or ethnic group."
- "If clients don't change, it is their fault, not mine."
- "People who come to me need help, which means they are not able to direct their own lives. It is my job to provide them with a high degree of structure."
- "People who are on welfare are basically unmotivated and really don't want to work."
- "Most people don't want to change. They just want to learn how to manipulate people more effectively so they can get what they want."
- "People can't be depended on to follow through with their commitments."
- "The clients in this institution are highly resistant and want to hide their true feelings and thoughts."

- "The best way to get through the client's resistance is to employ very directive and highly confrontive techniques. You have to strip away a client's defenses."
- "If you are empathic and supportive, clients will merely use this against you by manipulating you."

We do not mean to imply that if you hold any one of these beliefs you are necessarily ineffective in helping others. If you worked with a difficult client population over a period of years, for example, you might begin to assume that people generally resist change. But, if you applied this generalization to all the clients you saw, they would be likely to exhibit resistance in response to the messages that they picked up from you. You would be fostering a self-fulfilling prophecy that reinforced your assumptions. A temporary mild cynicism does not mean that you will remain cynical forever. You might ask yourself questions such as "How rigidly do I hold certain assumptions? Am I quick to generalize on the basis of limited experience? Do I tend to form quick judgments about people and make generalizations? Am I willing to seriously examine the assumptions that I make, and am I open to changing some of them?" It is a positive sign if you demonstrate a willingness to question the origin of your assumptions and to modify them.

Learning to Challenge Your Assumptions

We provided a series of in-service training workshops at a state institution for the criminally insane and for mentally disordered sex offenders. Although we had the good fortune to meet and work with some dedicated and effective helpers, we also encountered some ineffective helpers. To us it seemed that they thought their patients could do no right. A few workers at the institution were quite outspoken in their beliefs that these patients were resistant to therapy, were not motivated to change, and were only putting in their time as ordered by the court. If the clients did not talk during the sessions, they were labeled "resistant"; if they did talk, they were often viewed as "manipulative."

In our training workshops we urged the staff members at least to suspend their judgments during the time they were providing therapy. We encouraged them to give their patients a chance to show something more of themselves than the problem with which they had become identified. Although a child molester does have severe problems, we suggested that he be viewed more broadly than as someone who has committed sexual crimes. If the staff members were open to discovering other facets of the patient's personality, they would discover that he had had pain and struggles in his life with which the helper could identify. We hoped that the helpers would challenge some of their assumptions that seemed nontherapeutic and be open to the possibility that they could begin to see clients and the helping process in a different light.

If you are making some of the assumptions we have described, think about how they are likely to influence the way you approach certain clients. Your beliefs about yourself, the people with whom you work, and the nature of the helping process are often more subtle than the assumptions we have highlighted. Whether your beliefs are subtle or extreme, however, you tend to behave on the basis of them. If you basically do not trust your clients to understand and deal with their problems, for example, you will use strategies to get them to accept your assessment and to follow your prescriptions.

After becoming aware of the attitudes and assumptions you hold, you can decide the degree to which your attitudes are being expressed in your behavior. Then you can assess how well such attitudes and behaviors are working for you and helping your clients. We hope you will examine the source of your beliefs about the good life, an individual's capacity to make substantial change, and the nature of the helper-client relationship. Think through, clarify, and challenge these beliefs, confirming them through a conscious process of self-examination.

You may not have clear beliefs about the helping process. You may have incorporated them in an uncritical and unconscious manner. It is possible that they are narrow and have not been tested to determine if they are valid or functional. If you have lived in a sheltered environment and have rarely stepped outside of your social group, you may not even be aware of your narrow belief system. It is possible to live in an encapsulated environment and thereby "see" only what confirms your existing belief system.

One good way to identify and clarify your beliefs is to put yourself in situations that might prove challenging. If you have limited contact with alcoholics and see them as individuals without willpower, for instance, consider attending some Alcoholics Anonymous meetings. If you have limited experience with certain cultural and ethnic groups, seek volunteer experiences or fieldwork placements where you will work with a culturally diverse population. If you are aware that you hold stereotypes about old people, volunteer to work with the elderly. If you have fears about working with people who have AIDS or are HIV-positive, consider challenging your fears by learning more about this disease or working with these people. Direct contact with populations that are unfamiliar to you is the best way to learn about people whom you might have stereotyped. Of course, it is essential that you approach these situations with an open mind and that you avoid simply looking for evidence to support your prior judgments. A stance of openness will enable you to develop a personal orientation to helping that will lend itself to modification as you gain experience.

Some Beliefs We Hold About the Helping Process

It took us some time to learn that there is no one right way to approach clients. Instead of looking for the right thing to do or say, we strive to follow what we think is an interesting path to pursue with a client. In this process we trust our intuition and develop our own ways of working. If our hunches about a client are incorrect, that quickly becomes apparent if we pay attention to the relationship. We continually relearn that it is important to talk with clients about what we think is going on between us. At times, when we have trouble relating to a particular client, this person is reflecting some dimension within ourselves that we are reluctant to accept. It can be helpful to consider our clients as mirrors that reflect some aspect of our being. We do not necessarily need to change anything, but it does help to simply recognize patterns that we have in common with our clients.

We do not accept the full responsibility for deciding what the focus of a help-ing relationship will be. Rather than working very hard to figure out what clients should want, we ask them frequently what it is they want. We often ask: "Is what you are doing working for you? If not, what are you willing to do to change it?" If their current behavior is generally serving them well, they may not feel a strong need to change a particular style. We still encourage them to look at the price they often pay for being the way they are, and then the decision whether to change is up to them. We do not see it as our job to decide for them how they should live their lives.

If clients appear to be getting little from the helping relationship, we still ex-amine our part in this outcome by asking ourselves about our involvement and willingness to risk with this client. Yet we also explore with the client his or her part in the lack of progress. We recognize that we cannot make clients want to change, yet we can create a climate where together we look at the advantages and disadvantages of making changes. We see helping as a mutual endeavor in which both parties share the responsibility for making change happen.

Choosing a Theoretical Orientation

Some helpers focus on feelings. They think that what clients need most is to iden-tify and express feelings that have been bottled up. Other helpers put emphasis on gaining insight, exploring the reasons for actions and interpreting clients' be-havior. Some helpers are not much concerned about having clients develop in-sight or express their feelings. Their focus is on behavior and helping clients de-velop specific action plans to change what they are doing. Other helpers like clients to focus on examining their beliefs about themselves and about their world. These helpers believe change will result if clients can eliminate faulty thinking and replace it with constructive thoughts and self-talk.

Helpers may focus on the past, the present, or the future. Begin to consider whether you see the past, present, or future as being most productive. This is more than just a theoretical notion. If you believe your clients' past is an important focus for exploration, many of your interventions are likely to be designed to assist them in understanding their past. If you think that your clients' goals and strivings are important, your interventions are likely to focus them on the future. If you are ori-ented toward the present, many of your interventions will focus your clients on what they are thinking, feeling, and doing in the moment.

Each of these choices represents a particular theoretical orientation. Attempting to practice without having an explicit theoretical rationale is like flying a plane without a flight plan. If you operate in a theoretical vacuum and are unable to draw on theory to support your interventions, you may flounder in your attempts to help people change.

Theory is not a rigid set of structures that prescribes, step by step, what and how you should function as a helper. Rather, we see theory as a general frame-work that enables you to make sense of the many facets of the helping process, providing you with a map that gives direction to what you do and say. Ultimately, the most meaningful perspective is one that is an extension of your values and personality. A theory is not something divorced from you as a person. At best, a theory becomes an integral part of the person you are and an expression of your uniqueness.

Our Theoretical Orientation

Neither of us subscribes to any single theory in its totality. Rather, we function within an integrative framework that we continue to develop and modify as we practice. We draw on concepts and techniques from most of the contemporary counseling models and adapt them to our own unique personalities. Our conceptual framework takes into account the *thinking, feeling,* and *behaving* dimensions of human experience. Thus, our theoretical orientations and styles of practice are primarily a function of the individuals we are.

We value those approaches that emphasize the *thinking* dimension. We typically challenge clients to think about the decisions they have made about themselves. Some of these decisions may have been necessary for their psychological survival as children but now may be clearly out of date. We hope that clients will eventually be able to make necessary revisions that can lead them to live more fully. One way we do this is by asking clients to pay attention to their "self-talk." Here are some questions we encourage clients to ask themselves: "How are my problems actually caused by the assumptions I make about myself, about others, and about life? How do I create problems by the thoughts and beliefs I cling to? How can I begin to free myself by critically evaluating the sentences I repeat to myself?" Many of the techniques we use are designed to tap clients' thinking processes, to help them think about events in their lives and how they have interpreted these events, and to work on a cognitive level to change certain belief systems.

Thinking is only one dimension that we pay attention to in our work with clients. The *feeling* dimension is also extremely important. We emphasize this facet of human experience by encouraging clients to identify and express their feelings. Clients are often stuck due to unexpressed and unresolved emotional concerns. If they allow themselves to experience the range of their feelings and talk about how certain events have affected them, their healing process is facilitated. If individuals feel listened to and understood, they are more likely to express feelings that they have kept to themselves.

Thinking and feeling are vital components in the helping process, but eventually clients must express themselves in the *behaving* or *doing* dimension. Clients can spend countless hours gaining insights and ventilating pent-up feelings, but at some point they need to get involved in an action-oriented program of change. Their feelings and thoughts can then be applied to real-life situations. Examining current behavior is the heart of the helping process. We tend to ask questions such as these: "What are you doing? What do you see for yourself now and in the future? Does your present behavior have a reasonable chance of getting you what you want now, and will it take you in the direction you want to go?" If the focus of the helping process is on what people are doing, there is a greater chance that they will also be able to change their thinking and feeling.

In addition to highlighting the thinking, feeling, and behaving dimensions, we help clients consolidate what they are learning and apply these new behaviors to situations they encounter every day. Some strategies we use are contracts, homework assignments, action programs, self-monitoring techniques, support systems, and self-directed programs of change. These approaches all stress the role of commitment on the clients' part to practice new behaviors, to follow through with a realistic plan for change, and to develop practical methods of carrying out this plan in everyday life.

Underlying our integrated focus on thinking, feeling, and behaving is our philosophical leaning toward the existential approach, which places primary emphasis on the role of choice and responsibility in the process of change. We challenge people to look at the choices they *do* have, however limited they may be, and to accept responsibility for choosing for themselves.

Most of what we do in our therapeutic work is based on the assumption that people can exercise their freedom to change situations, even though the range of this freedom may be restricted by external factors. It is important for helpers to do more than assume that clients are capable of changing their internal world. Helpers also have a role in bringing about change in the external environment that is directly contributing to a client's problems.

Individuals cannot be understood without considering the various systems that affect them—family, social groups, community, church, and other cultural forces. For the helping process to be effective, it is critical to understand how individuals influence and are influenced by their social world. Sue, Ivey, and Pedersen (1996) point out that people are not only thinking, feeling, behaving, and social beings but are also biological, cultural, spiritual, and political beings. Ignoring any one of these facets of human experience will limit our understanding of human behavior. Effective helpers need to acquire a holistic approach that encompasses all of human experience.

As we work with an individual, we are not consciously thinking about what theory we are using. We adapt the techniques we use to fit the needs of the individual rather than attempting to fit the client to our techniques. In deciding on techniques to introduce, we take into account an array of factors about the client population. We consider the client's readiness to confront an issue, the client's cultural background, the client's value system, and the client's trust in us as helpers. We have a rationale for using the techniques we employ, and our interventions generally flow from some particular theoretical framework. Our concern is to help clients identify and experience whatever they are feeling, identify ways in which their assumptions influence how they feel and behave, and experiment with alternative modes of behaving.

An Integrative Approach to Helping

One reason for the current trend toward an integrative approach to the helping process is the recognition that no single theory is comprehensive enough to account for the complexities of human behavior when the full range of client types and their specific problems are taken into consideration. Practitioners who are open to an integrative perspective may find that several theories play a crucial role in their personal approach. Each theory has its unique contributions and its own domain of expertise. By accepting that each theory has strengths and weaknesses and is, by definition, "different" from the others, practitioners have some basis to begin developing a counseling model that fits them.

At the May 2000 Evolution of Psychotherapy Conference we were struck with how many pioneers of a particular theoretical model had eventually come around to acknowledging the value of the diversity of theories. Some of these founders, now in their 80s, stated that during their early career they were more parochial in their practices. Although they still adhere largely to their own approach, they demonstrated more openness to the contributions of other theories to the field of psychotherapy.

We encourage you to remain open to the value inherent in each of the theories of counseling. Study all the contemporary theories to determine what concepts and techniques you can incorporate into your approach to practice. You will need to have a basic knowledge of various theoretical systems and counseling techniques to work effectively with diverse client populations in various settings. Functioning exclusively within the parameters of one theory may not provide you with the therapeutic flexibility that you need to deal creatively with the complexities associated with your practice.

Each theory represents a different vantage point from which to look at human behavior, but no one theory has "the truth." Because there is no "correct" theoretical approach, it is well for you to search for an approach that fits who you are and to think in terms of working toward an integrated approach that addresses thinking, feeling, and behaving. To develop this kind of integration, you need to be thoroughly grounded in a number of theories, be open to the idea that these theories can be unified in some ways, and be willing to continually test your hypotheses to determine how well they are working. If you are currently a student in training, it is unrealistic to expect to have integrated a well-defined theoretical model. This will take years of extensive reading and practice. Keep in mind that an integrative perspective is the product of a great deal of study, clinical practice, research, and theorizing. Developing your personalized approach that guides your practice is a lifelong endeavor that is refined with experience.

Of necessity, this discussion of theoretical orientations has been brief. For a more elaborate discussion of the various theoretical approaches, see *The Art of Integrative Counseling* (Corey, 2001a) and *Theory and Practice of Counseling and Psychotherapy* (Corey, 2001c).

The Stages of Helping

This section is designed to help you determine your assets and liabilities as a potential helper. We use the overall framework of Ivey and Ivey's (1999) model of intentional interviewing and counseling, describing the stages in the helping process and the major tasks facing helpers at each of these stages. We also draw from the conceptualization of skills-development approaches of Brammer (1993), Brems (2001), Cormier and Hackney (1999), Egan (2002), James and Gilliland (2001), Patterson and Welfel (2000), Teyber (2000), and Okun (2002). The skills-development model offers a general framework of the phases of the helping process and is not linked to any particular theoretical approach. You can apply any of the current theories of counseling (Corey, 2001a, 2001b, 2001c) to this model of helping.

The model of the helping process we will discuss here has five major stages, each with particular tasks to be accomplished. At each stage in this process, helpers face different challenges that require specific skills. The framework we provide will help you assess your ability to engage others in a helping relationship. The human relations skills we describe are crucial for all helpers.

In the first stage, the central task is to create a working relationship, or a collaborative partnership, that is based on trust and informed consent. This is a time for establishing and structuring the helping relationship. This initial phase sets the foundation upon which all other interventions are able to take root in later phases of helping.

During the second stage, the central task is to gather information, conduct an assessment, and identify the client's problems. Typically, people become clients when they recognize that they need outside help to understand and cope with their problems, or someone else thinks that professional intervention is required. Clients often need assistance in identifying and clarifying aspects of their lives that are not working for them. This task may include identifying problem situations or missed opportunities for full development.

In the third stage, the helper and the client collaboratively establish goals by determining the specific changes desired. If clients hope to make actual changes, they have to be willing to go beyond talking and planning; they must translate their plans into action.

The fourth stage of helping deals with exploring alternatives, identifying strategies for action, choosing which combination of strategies will best meet the client's goals, and putting these plans into a realistic action program. One of the tasks of this phase is to facilitate generalization and transfer of learning from the office to daily life.

Termination is the fifth stage, and it is here that clients consolidate their learning and make longer-range plans.

There is considerable overlap among the functions at each of these stages. Rather than thinking of this model as discrete steps that flow in linear order, it is best to think of it as a circular process of decision making. Ivey and Ivey (1999) point out that a circle has no beginning and no end and can sometimes be used as a symbol of an egalitarian relationship in which the client and the helper form a partnership in working on commonly agreed-upon concerns. Not all clients will feel comfortable with the stages as presented, regardless of cultural background. Furthermore, issues of rapport, structuring, defining problems, and establishing goals will be important for the duration of the helping relationship.

As we describe each of these stages, we focus on *you as a helper.* Assess your own qualities to determine your interest and ability in helping others. Realize that the helping relationship is not a mechanical process but a deeply personal human endeavor. As a helper you will be actively involved with those you are helping by drawing on what you know, by applying skills and interventions in a timely and appropriate manner, and by using yourself as a person in creating meaningful relationships with clients or others you help. This is true whether you are involved in the counseling or the administrative aspects of the human services. If you are unable to apply some basic human relations skills, the chances are slim that you will be able to create and maintain adequate rapport with those whom you are supposed to be helping. Although the focus of our discussion is on these skills as they apply to counseling relationships, you can also apply them to a variety of other interpersonal situations.

In this era of managed care, you will be challenged to work with clients in very few sessions. You will need to develop interventions tailored to short-term and specific behavioral change. Brief interventions stress time-limited, solution-focused, structured, effective strategies that empower clients by enabling them to make specific behavioral changes they desire. Furthermore, the requirements of managed care impose upon agencies and practitioners the expectation of being accountable. Increasingly, you will be expected to quickly assess the salient problems of your clients, formulate a short-term treatment approach, and then demonstrate the degree to which your interventions are effective. Therefore, the stages of helping will be described primarily from the vantage point of a relatively brief model rather than from the perspective of long-term therapy.

Stage 1: Establishing a Working Relationship

Helpers are expected to create a relationship in which clients can reveal their story, focus more clearly on what they want to change, and attain a new perspective in dealing with their problems. People often seek professional assistance when they realize they are not dealing with problem situations satisfactorily. Some clients seek counseling because they struggle with self-doubt, feel trapped by their fears, and suffer from some form of loss. Others seek help not because they feel plagued by major problems but because they are not living as effectively as they would like. They may feel caught in a meaningless job, experience frustration because they are not living up to their own goals and ideals, or feel dissatisfied in their personal lives. In short, most people who become clients are not managing their lives as well as they might. They are not dealing effectively with life problems, and they are not using the full range of their potentials or taking advantage of opportunities available to them. Two general goals of helping arise from these assumptions: one goal relates to clients' managing their lives more effectively and the other relates to clients' abilities to deal realistically with problems and develop opportunities (Egan, 2002).

Of course, not all clients come to you voluntarily. Involuntary clients will surely have some unwillingness to seeking help, and they may not even believe that you can help them. Working with involuntary clients is extremely challenging because of the degree of minimization and denial clients bring with them. Your task is to get through the initial intimidation such clients can present and to work in such a way that will increase the chances of their acknowledging their problems. A good place to begin is to ascertain why they are seeking help *now* and what they expect from you. Dealing with their hesitation and doubts, rather than ignoring these attitudes, is one of the best ways to begin with the reluctant client.

An essential task in addressing any barriers to creating a working relationship means that you can recognize the signs of resistance, both in your client and in yourself. It is important to understand the many meanings of client resistance and not to interpret it as a sign of your failure as a helper. If you are focused on defending yourself against the various forms of resistance you will encounter with clients, you deprive them of opportunities to explore the meanings of their behavior.

One way of not reacting defensively to a client's resistance and of exploring its meaning is illustrated by the following example. You are seeing an involuntary client for the first time. She is extremely hostile and lets you know that she neither wants nor needs your help. She attacks your abilities as a counselor. As an effective helper you cannot indulge yourself in feelings of rejection. However, in a nondefensive way you can explore with this client her unwillingness and her difficulty in seeing you. If you are patient, you may discover that this client has some very good reasons not to trust a professional like you. She may have felt betrayed by a counselor, and she may fear that the information she gives you will be used against her one more time. We discuss at greater length in Chapter 6 the topic of dealing with resistance.

Creating a climate for change.   In your work with both voluntary and involuntary client populations, your clients' willingness to engage in self-exploration will have a lot to do with the kind of climate you establish during the initial sessions. You can make the mistake of working too hard, asking too many questions and offering quick solutions. Your role is to create a collaborative partnership with your clients, which means that they assume a fair share of the responsibility for what takes place both inside and outside the session. During the early sessions you can greatly assist clients by teaching them how they can assess their own problems and search for their own solutions. In *The Elements of Counseling,* Meier and Davis (2001) suggest the following guidelines for the first session with clients:

- Make personal contact.
- Develop a working alliance.
- Explain the helping process to the client.
- Pace and lead the client.
- Speak briefly; at times silence is golden.
- Find a balance between confronting and supporting.
- Individualize your helping approach.
- Pay attention to resistance.
- When in doubt, focus on feelings
- Plan for termination at the beginning of the helping relationship.

Establishing the relationship.   To create an effective helping relationship, it is essential for the helper to assist clients in becoming aware of their assets and strengths rather than concentrating on their problems, deficits, and liabilities. For clients to feel free to talk about themselves, helpers need to provide attention, active listening, and empathy. Clients must sense your respect for them, which you can demonstrate by your attitudes and behaviors. You reveal an attitude of respect for your clients when you are concerned about their best interests, view them as able to exercise control of their own destiny, and treat them as individuals rather than stereotyping them. You actually show clients that you respect them through your behavior, such as actively listening to and understanding them, suspending critical judgment, expressing appropriate warmth and acceptance, communicating to them that you understand their world as they experience it, providing a combination of support and challenge, assisting them in cultivating their inner resources for change, and helping them consider the specific steps needed to bring change about.

In addition to demonstrating respect, you help clients tell their story through your own genuineness. Being genuine does not mean acting on any impulse or saying everything that you think or feel. You can be genuine with your clients when you avoid hiding yourself in a professional role; are open and nondefensive, even if you feel threatened; are willing to share yourself and your experiences with clients; and show a consistency between what you are thinking, feeling, and valuing and what you reveal through your words and actions. These questions are typically asked at the initial session:

- What brings you here?
- What has been going on in your life recently that prompted you to seek professional help at this time?
- What expectations do you have regarding the helping process?
- What are your hopes, fears, and reservations?
- What would you most like to accomplish in these sessions?

James and Gilliland (2001) describe the early stages involved in crisis intervention under the general framework of being able to listen. In crisis intervention work, the first step is to define and understand the problem from the client's point of view. To do this, helpers must possess listening and attending skills. Their capacity to understand and to respond with empathy, genuineness, respect, acceptance, and caring greatly influences their ability to help their clients clearly identify their problems. The next step involves ensuring the safety of clients who are experiencing a crisis. This involves making an assessment of lethality by determining the seriousness of the threat to the client's physical, emotional, and psychological safety. Another step consists of providing support for clients in crisis. Helpers best demonstrate their support not only by their words but even more so by their voice and body language.

Ask yourself how well you are able to pay attention to others, to fully listen to them, and to empathize with their situation. Assess the qualities you possess that will either help or hinder you in doing what is needed to assume the client's internal and subjective frame of reference. Consider these questions:

- Are you able to attend to what clients are telling you both verbally and nonverbally? Do you pay attention mainly to *what* (content) people tell you, or do you also notice *how* (process) they deliver their messages?
- Are you able to set aside your own biases for a time and attempt to enter the client's world? For example, if you consider yourself a liberated woman, are you willing to accept the client who tells you that she is satisfied in her traditional role as a housewife?
- As your client speaks, are you able to listen to and detect the core messages? How do you check with your client to make certain that you are understanding him or her?

- Are you able to keep your clients focused on issues they want to explore? Are you able to keep your own centeredness, even when your clients may seem very fragmented or are making demands on you?
- Are you able to communicate your understanding and acceptance to your clients?
- Are you able to work nondefensively with signs of resistance from your clients? Can you use this resistance as a way of helping them explore their issues more deeply?

Although it may seem deceptively simple to merely listen to others, the attempt to understand the world as others see it is demanding. Respect, genuineness, and empathy are best considered as a "way of being," not as mere techniques to be used on clients. Consider just a few ways in which you might interfere with allowing clients to express themselves. You could put forth too much effort in trying to be real and thus, in the process, actually be nongenuine. For example, you may want to prove to clients that you are a real person and that you struggle with your own problems. To demonstrate your "realness," you may take the focus away from your clients and put it on yourself by telling detailed stories about your life experiences. Ask yourself if your clients are getting what they need from their relationship with you if you do this.

Establishing a working relationship with clients implies that you are genuine and respectful in behavioral ways, that the relationship is a two-way process, and that the clients' interests are supreme. This means that you avoid doing for clients what they are capable of doing for themselves. For example, assume that an adolescent client tells you that he wants more time with his father but feels intimidated and shy around him. He is afraid to approach his father. You show respect for this client when you encourage him to risk approaching his father and teach him ways of taking this initiative. You demonstrate a lack of trust in his ability if you take it upon yourself to talk to his father, even if your client has asked you to intervene.

Educating clients and obtaining informed consent. Informed consent involves the right of clients to be made aware of what is involved in the helping relationship and to make autonomous decisions about it. The process of educating clients about how to get the most from the helping relationship, addressing their questions, and clarifying their expectations are routes to ethical and effective practice. What is necessary is to create a balance between giving clients too much and not enough information. Provide clients with the opportunity to talk about what they hope to gain from being in counseling. For clients to feel trusting enough to meaningfully express themselves, they need to have at least some minimal information about the nature of the helping relationship. During the early sessions, discussion should be guided by clients' concerns, interests, and questions. Many clients ask questions like these: How is confidentiality protected, and what are the limits of confidentiality? How does the therapeutic process work? What is your primary role as a helper? What is expected of me as a client? What is the approximate length of the counseling process? How will termination be handled? What are my main rights and responsibilities as a client? What are some of the main benefits and risks of counseling? Of course, not all these topics can be addressed in one session. Educating clients and obtaining informed consent begins at the first session and continues throughout the duration of the helping process.

Stage 2: Identifying Clients' Problems

At the second stage of the helping process, the main task is to assist clients in defining and clarifying their problems. This can best be accomplished by gathering information from the client and conducting an assessment. The purpose of this stage is to ascertain why the client has come for help and to listen to his or her story.

As soon as possible in the helping process it is crucial to teach clients how to identify and clarify problem areas and how to acquire problem-solving skills they can apply in a variety of difficult situations in everyday living. As a helper, your role is not to identify the nature of clients' problems but to assist them in doing this themselves. In a sense, from the very first meeting you can be most helpful to clients by encouraging them to look within themselves for resources and strengths they can draw on to better manage their lives. Effective helpers also put clients in touch with external resources within the community that they can utilize in meeting the demands of daily living. The confidence your clients have in you will increase if they are convinced that you appreciate the resources both within themselves and in their external world.

By understanding your client's cultural background, you are doing a great deal to build upon the therapeutic working relationship that was begun at the initial session. Although it is not necessary to have an in-depth understanding of your client's culture and worldview, you must have some understanding of your client's basic beliefs and values if you hope to be useful to this person. If you are not aware of the central values that guide your client's behavior and decisions, your client will soon pick up on this and likely not return for further sessions. A more detailed discussion of the importance of understanding clients' cultural values appears in Chapter 8.

Understanding the context. Clients may come to you not to resolve internal conflicts but to better understand and deal with external stressors in their environment. Some people who seek your services may need your guidance to link them to resources within their community. They may need legal assistance or your help in coping with day-to-day survival issues such as getting a job, arranging for child care, or taking care of an elderly parent. Clients in a crisis situation will require immediate direction in finding external resources to cope effectively with the crisis.

As you listen to your clients, do not assume that they simply need to adjust to problematic situations. They may feel frustration and anger due to societal factors such as being discriminated against in their workplace because of their age, gender, race, religion, or sexual orientation. You will do them a disservice if you encourage them to settle for injustices in an oppressive environment. Instead of merely solving the presenting problems of your clients, you can begin supporting your clients in their efforts to take action within their community to bring about change. Of course, to do this means that you must assume a variety of helping roles: educator, advocate, social change agent, and influencer of policymaking. A more detailed discussion of your role in influencing change within the community is presented in Chapter 11.

Conducting an initial assessment.   Assessment consists of evaluating the relevant factors in a client's life to identify themes for further exploration in the counseling process. This assessment does not necessarily have to be completed during the intake interview or even the early phase of helping, nor does it have to be a fixed judgment that the helper makes about the client. To obtain the most accurate results from an assessment, it is first necessary to have established rapport and structured the relationship, which is hopefully done during the first stage. Ideally, assessment is a collaborative effort that is part of the interaction between the client and the helper. Both should be involved in discovering the nature of the client's presenting problem, a process that begins with the initial sessions and continues until the professional relationship ends. Here are a few questions that are helpful to consider during this early assessment phase:

- What appears to be going on in this person's life at this time?
- What are the client's main assets and liabilities?
- On what support systems can the client rely in making changes? Who are the significant people in the client's life?
- Is this a crisis situation, or is it a long-standing problem?
- What is the client primarily seeking from the therapeutic relationship, and how can it best be achieved?
- What major internal and external factors are contributing to the client's current problems, and what can be done to alleviate them?
- In what ways can an understanding of the person's cultural background shed light on developing a plan to deal with these problems?
- What significant past events appear to be related to the client's present level of functioning?
- What are the prospects for meaningful change, and how will we know when that change has occurred?

Helpers will develop tentative hypotheses, which they can share with their clients as the process proceeds. At a later time, additional data are bound to emerge, which may call for a modification of the original assessment. This process of assessment does not necessarily have to result in classifying the client under some clinical category. Instead, helpers can describe behavior as they observe it and encourage clients to think about its meaning. In this way assessment becomes a process of thinking about issues with the client rather than a mechanical procedure conducted by an expert professional. From this perspective, assessment is vital to the therapeutic procedures that are selected, and it helps practitioners conceptualize a case.

Diagnosis, which is sometimes part of the assessment process, consists of identifying a specific psychological or behavioral problem based on a pattern of symptoms. A psychological diagnosis is a general term covering the process of identifying an emotional or behavioral problem and making a statement about the current status of a client. This process also includes identification of possible causes of the person's emotional, psychological, and behavioral difficulties, suggestions for appropriate therapy techniques to deal effectively with the identified problem, and estimates of the chances for a successful resolution. The fourth edition of the American Psychiatric Association's (1994) *Diagnostic and Statistical Manual of Mental Disorders* (DSM-IV) is the standard reference for distinguishing one form of psychological disorder from another. The rationale for the traditional diagnostic approach is to allow the therapist to plan treatments tailored to the special needs of the client.

Whether diagnosis should be part of psychotherapeutic practice is a controversial issue. Some mental health professionals see diagnosis as an essential step in any treatment plan, but others oppose a diagnostic model on the assumption that DSM-IV labels stigmatize people. Although you may not yet have had to face the practical question of whether to diagnose a client, you will probably need to come to terms with this issue at some point in your work because more and more agencies rely on initial assessments and a DSM-IV diagnosis for reimbursement purposes. Because most agency settings require some form of official assessment and diagnosis, being able to carry out these functions competently is likely to be an integral part of your job responsibilities.

In our view, diagnosis does not have to be a matter of categorizing clients; rather, practitioners can think more broadly, describe behavior, and think about its meaning. In this way, diagnosis becomes a process of thinking *about* the client *with* the client. Diagnosis can be viewed as a general descriptive statement identifying a client's style of functioning.

Ivey and Ivey (1998) propose reframing DSM-IV by paying special attention to the interface of multicultural issues, origin of problems, and treatment. Ivey and Ivey suggest that diagnostic systems need more balance and attention to the reality of human experience. In their developmental counseling and therapy model, psychological distress is viewed as the result of biological and developmental factors. Although the stressor may be located within the individual, this model calls for inclusion of the broader systemic and cultural contexts as a basis for meaningful assessment. For example, the distress of depression is generally the result of the interaction of the person in the environment. Depression in women or an ethnic minority group can result from cultural racism or sexism. Individuals who have been discriminated against may experience depression as a result of environmental factors. From the developmental perspective, the inclusion of culture-related issues such as race, ethnicity, gender, sexual orientation, and spirituality is essential for accurate assessment and diagnosis. Ivey and Ivey argue that "a diagnosis that is not culture-centered with awareness of multiple contextual issues is incomplete at best and potentially dangerous and misleading" (p. 336).

Even though you may not find diagnosis necessary or useful in your practice, it may behoove you to know enough about diagnosis to refer a client. For example, once you have made a diagnosis of a client who is chronically depressed with possible suicidal tendencies, you are in a position to make an appropriate referral if you do not have the competence to deal with this problem area.

Helping clients gain a focus.   Some people who come for help feel over-whelmed with a number of problems. By trying to talk about everything that is troubling them in one session, they also may manage to overwhelm the helper. It is necessary to provide a direction for the helping efforts, enabling both the client and the helper to know where to start. To achieve this focus, it is essential to make an assessment of the major concerns of the client. You could say to a client who pre-sents you with a long list of problems: "We won't be able to deal with all your prob-lems in one session. What was going on in your life when you finally decided to call for help?" Here are some other focusing questions: "At this time in your life, what seems most pressing and troublesome to you?" "You say that you often wake up in the middle of the night. What do you find yourself ruminating over?" "When you don't want to get up in the morning, what is it that you most want to avoid?" "If you could address only one problem today, which one would you pick?"

As a helper, you can be instrumental in encouraging clients to tell their story and to explore their key issues in terms of their experiences, feelings, and behav-iors. By focusing on what is salient in the present and by avoiding dwelling on the past, you can assist clients in clarifying their own problems and opportunities for change. A participant in one of our training workshops made the comment that she was beginning to see the fine line that exists between the therapeutic value of telling one's story versus overwhelming people by getting lost in talking about themselves. She also learned that the purpose of clients' sharing personal infor-mation is not to satisfy the helper's curiosity but rather to give enough of a sense of their struggles to enable the helper to develop understanding and know how to intervene.

Reflect for a moment regarding the degree to which you are able to facilitate the process of your clients' being able to tell some aspect of their life story. Do you let clients tell their story, or do you get impatient and want to talk too soon? Do you encourage clients to tell stories in great detail for the sake of your curiosity? Do you have a tendency to get lost in the details of their story and miss the es-sence of their struggle? Are you able to inquire with open-ended questions that lead clients to flesh out meaningful stories?

Identifying exceptions to one's problems.   As the helping relationship deep-ens and clients present you with information about their life, help them identify and overcome their own distortions. This is a good time to encourage clients to identify exceptions to their problem-saturated lives. Ask them what they can do and have already done to deal with their problems. Ask clients to focus on pos-sible solutions rather than having them define themselves in light of their present-ing problem. By reconceptualizing a particular problem, you can help clients ac-quire a new perspective that will lead to action. Help clients who see very few options to develop a variety of alternatives in coping with a given problem. You can help them distinguish between what they can do and what might be difficult for them to do, and you can challenge them to stretch their boundaries. Encourage clients to make choices for themselves and to develop the courage to accept re-sponsibility for their decisions. By providing clients with support and challenge, you can help them change.

Stage 3: Helping Clients Create Goals

During this stage, the aim is to help clients identify very specific goals that will guide the remainder of their work with you. To clarify goals, helpers often ask these questions: What would you like to achieve from our work together? Where would you like to be in your life at this time? What specific feelings, thoughts, and behaviors are you most interested in changing? What would you like to reduce or eliminate from your life? What qualities would you like to acquire that you do not now have? What do you imagine the ideal solution would be to the problems you have presented? How might things be different if you were able to eliminate a key problem from your life?

Clients need to state their goals in such a manner that both they and the helper will know what changes are desired and both will have a framework to assess the degree to which these goals are being attained. Establishing, refining, and revising goals takes time and continued effort, yet doing so will give direction to the helping process. After goals are collaboratively established, it is critical to devise alternative approaches to dealing with their problems. This is done by guiding clients in a brainstorming process to create perspectives that are in line with their values and can lead to action. It is important that these goals be measurable, be realistic in terms of the resources of the client, be chosen by the client, and be achievable in a realistic period.

Clients in crisis may feel immobilized and may fail to examine the options available to them. In fact, they may not see any options. Effective helping involves teaching clients to recognize that there are alternatives, some of which are better than others. James and Gilliland (2001) describe the following three strategies designed to help clients in crisis consider the options open to them: (1) *situational supports*, which include people in the client's life from whom they can draw strength during their crisis; (2) *coping mechanisms*, which are the actions, behaviors, or environmental resources that clients can use in getting through a crisis; and (3) *positive and constructive thinking patterns*, which can substantially change a client's perspective on a problem and can lessen stress and anxiety. Crisis workers are in a position to examine a number of possibilities for action, and they can enable their clients to develop a different perspective, especially if such clients feel that their situation is hopeless and that they are lacking in choices.

A case example.   Brian, a young worker, comes to you because he wants help in pursuing his goal of getting into college. He has put off applying to colleges for several years, and the thought of actually being accepted scares him. His job dissatisfaction is so great that it has begun to affect his personal life.

In his work with you, Brian discovers that he has accepted some early messages from his parents. They communicated to him that he was ignorant and would never amount to anything, and they attributed his early difficulties in school to laziness. Test results have shown that Brian is performing far below his intellectual abilities. His insight that he unconditionally accepted these early messages has been important. He realizes now that he must acquire better reading and writing skills before he can successfully compete in college. As a helper, you could make a mistake by focusing mainly on his feelings about his parents and himself and by endlessly exploring the reasons why he feels inadequate. At this stage he is aware of what has stopped him so far in accomplishing his goals. He knows specifically what he needs to do to make a change in his life. Now he has clarified a new set of goals, and his task is to identify the specific steps to take in accomplishing them.

Some problems with a problem-solving approach. The need of helpers to solve problems for others could easily block them from hearing what clients want to communicate. A common mistake we observe with trainees is their tendency to short-circuit the exploration of feelings of clients and provide them too readily with a solution to their presenting problem. This problem-solving focus aborts the struggle of clients in expressing and dealing with feelings and thoughts and eventually coming up with alternatives that are best for them.

If you are too intent on providing solutions for every problem, it is likely that you are focused on your own needs for being a competent helper who wants to see results. You may be uncomfortable with the client's struggle, and you may push for resolution long before thorough exploration has even begun. If you were the helper in the case of Brian, you would have spent no time listening and exploring his deep feelings of inadequacy. You would not have assisted him in examining what had kept him time and again from succeeding academically. With your problem-solving orientation, you would have urged him to apply prematurely for college. If Brian had not had enough opportunity to express and explore his fears and self-doubts and if he had not acquired any insights into his own part in setting himself up to fail, it is not likely that he would have succeeded in college.

Stage 4: Encouraging Client Exploration and Taking Action

Once the goals of the helper-client relationship have been identified, it becomes necessary to decide on the various avenues by which these goals can be accomplished. Knowing *what* you want to change is the first step, and knowing *how* to bring about this change is the next step. Helpers first assist clients in developing and assessing action strategies for making their vision a reality. To work toward changing a client's thoughts, feelings, and behaviors, it is generally necessary to explore alternatives and confront incongruities. This stage of helping may be the longest, and it at times involves a lengthy exploration of an individual's dynamics. The helper's task is to explore possibilities and to assist the client in finding new ways to act more intentionally in the world (Ivey & Ivey, 1999). Confrontation and self-disclosure are both very important aspects that can further client self-exploration, can lead to new insights, and can encourage clients to take action over doing what is necessary to achieve their personal goals. The crux of this stage also involves collaboratively creating a plan of action that is discussed in the sessions and carried out in daily life. After an action plan has been formulated, the steps need to be carried out, and then the plan must be evaluated (Egan, 2002).

Confronting (or challenging) clients. Clients typically experience a sense of being stuck in their lives. A helper needs to acquire the skills of caring and gentle confrontation of clients' behaviors as a way to enable them to get unstuck. Confrontation is a practice that is often misunderstood. It should not be viewed as aggressive or as destructive of a supportive relationship. Unfortunately, there are many misconceptions about the purpose and value of confrontation. Some helpers see it as producing defensiveness and withdrawal in clients. Or they may view it as an adversarial stance between them and their clients, which can lead to premature termination of the helping relationship. Helpers sometimes see confrontation as a negative act with destructive potential. Because of this connotation, they sometimes avoid it at all costs, when it is the very thing that they need to provide as the impetus for growth.

A lack of confrontation or challenge often results in stagnation. Without some degree of challenge, clients often remain stuck in self-defeating behavior and do not develop the new perspectives and skills needed to make changes. Helpers cease being effective catalysts to others' growth if all they offer is support and empathy. Confrontation can be viewed as "care-frontation" if it is done out of genuine concern and in a responsible way. Constructive and caring confrontation invites individuals to look at the discrepancies, incongruities, distortions, excuses, resistances, and evasions that are keeping them stuck in their lives.

Ask yourself if you are willing to challenge others. You may be timid and apologetic when it comes to being challenging. If you find that you have a hard time confronting others, it is important to understand what makes it difficult for you. It could be that you very much want to be liked and approved of by your clients. You might fear that they will turn on you or will not return. Even though challenging others might not be easy for you, it is a skill that you will need to acquire if you hope to move clients beyond a mere "talking-about" phase of their counseling. It may help to realize that it is not abnormal to feel anxious about challenging others or being confronted ourselves. Yet even though you may be uncomfortable, one of the ways to develop skills in confronting is by doing what is difficult. If you back down when a challenge is required, you are feeding the anxiety that can keep you in a rigid stance with others.

Challenging clients effectively entails focusing on their awareness of what they are thinking, feeling, and doing. If the challenge is successful, clients are able to overcome blind spots and develop new perspectives on their life situation, and they are also influenced to make changes based on this self-understanding. Thus, confronting aims at enabling clients to participate actively and fully in the process of helping themselves. Done with sensitivity, challenges from a helper can ultimately enable clients to develop the capacity for self-confrontation that they will need in working through their problems.

Here are a few suggestions for making confrontations effective. First of all, earn the right to confront. Know your motivations for confronting. Is it because you want to more deeply understand another, or is it because you want to control the other person? Do you care about your relationships with clients? Are you really interested in getting closer to them, and are you aware of what gets in the way of a closer relationship? Challenge clients only if you feel an investment in them and if you have the time and effort to continue building the relationship with them. If you have not yet established a working relationship with a client, your confrontation is likely to be received defensively. The degree to which you can confront your clients depends on how much they trust you and how much you trust them (Egan, 2002).

Be willing to be confronted yourself. If you model a nondefensive stance in the counseling relationship, your clients will be much more willing to consider what you tell them. Before you confront others, imagine being the recipient of what is said. The tone and your general manner of giving your message will have a lot to do with how others receive what you tell them. It is also useful to present your confrontations in a tentative manner, as opposed to issuing a dogmatic pronouncement. Confronting is your chance not to "put down" clients but to inspire them to look at what they most want to change in themselves and what seems to be blocking this change.

Confrontation is not intended to rip away the defenses of clients; rather, it invites them to challenge their defensive ways and keep moving toward more effective behavior. Confrontations should not be dogmatic statements concerning who or what others are. Here is an example of a confrontation that would be certain to arouse a client's defensiveness and evoke resistance: "I'm impatient with hearing you complain every week about how horrible your life is. I doubt that you will ever change."

A confrontation that could lead to a more productive exploration of the client's difficulties is as follows: "You have said time and again that most of all you want to be successful, feel good about yourself, and feel proud of your accomplishments. Yet much of what you do and say sets you up to fail and to get what you say you don't want. You've done this for a long time, and you tell me that not feeling good is very familiar to you. Your father has never given you his approval, and around him you feel insignificant. Let's talk about the possibility that your chronic failures have something to do with your relationship with your father."

Likewise, in counseling a couple it would be unhelpful to tell a husband to "Be quiet and listen to what she has to say!" This confrontation might shut him up for good. It would be more helpful to describe what you saw going on between the two of them: "You say you want your wife to tell you how she feels about you, but every time she has tried this in the last 10 minutes, you've interrupted her and told her all the reasons she shouldn't feel the way she does. Describe your wife's behavior, rather than labeling her. Talk to her about how you're affected by this behavior. Would you be willing for the next few minutes to let her talk and not think about what you're going to say in return? When she's finished, I'd like you to tell her how you're affected by what she has said. Instead of focusing on how your wife is, focus more on yourself, and tell her about yourself." People who are being confronted are less likely to be defensive if they are told what effect they have on others rather than simply being judged and labeled.

Some clients will have numerous excuses for the way they are. You can confront them to accept responsibility for what they are doing rather than relying on excuses for what they are not doing. With effective confrontation you can assist them in redirecting the focus from others to themselves. Other clients may operate on the assumption that they must have universal approval. Again, your challenge of their belief system can help them see where they picked up such a belief and whether it is now serving them well.

You can also challenge clients on the strengths they possess but are not fully using rather than limiting your confrontation to their weaknesses. It helps to be specific, avoiding sweeping judgments and focusing on concrete behaviors. Remember to describe to clients what you see them doing and how this behavior affects you. It is also useful to encourage a dialogue with clients, and your sensitivity to their responses is a key factor in determining the degree to which they will accept your confrontations.

Here is an example of a helper's challenge to a client who is not making the best use of her strengths: "For several weeks now you've made detailed plans to reach out to a friend. You say that when you do reach out to people they usually like you, and you have no reason to fear that this friend will reject you. Yet you have not made contact with her, and you have many reasons for not doing so. Let's explore the possibility that you don't want to make this contact. What is stopping you from contacting her?"

To make the issue of confrontation more concrete, we present examples of other styles of confronting. The first statement illustrates ineffective confrontation; this is followed by an effective confrontation alternative.

- "You're always so cold and aloof, and you make me feel distant from you." This could be changed to: "I feel uncomfortable with you because I'm afraid of you. Rather than avoiding you, I'd like to see if we can be different with each other."
- "You're a phony! You're always smiling, and that's not real." An effective confrontation is: "I find it difficult to trust you, because often when you say you're angry, you're smiling. I have a hard time knowing what you want."
- "If I were your husband, I'd leave you. You're full of hostility, and you'll destroy any relationship." A more effective statement is: "I find it difficult to be open with you. Many of the things you say really hurt me and distance me from you."

In the ineffective statements, the people being confronted are being told how they are, and in some way they are being discounted. In the effective statements, the helper doing the confronting is revealing his or her perceptions and feelings about the client and is reporting the effects of the person's behavior.

Using helper self-disclosure appropriately.   Sharing yourself can be a powerful intervention in making contact with clients and facilitating a process of their self-exploration. It is a mistake to think of self-disclosure in terms of "all" or "none"; it can best be viewed on a continuum. There is a distinction between a helper's self-disclosing statements (sharing personal information about oneself) and self-involving statements (revealing personal thoughts, feelings, and reactions to the client in the context of here-and-now aspects of the helping relationship). Strive to let your clients know how you are perceiving and experiencing them. You are bound to have many reactions to your clients in the therapeutic relationship. Frequently, sharing with your clients how you are affected by what they are saying and doing is more useful to them than limiting your disclosures to revealing aspects of your personal life. If you are having a difficult time listening to a client, for example, it could be useful to share this information. You might say: "I've noticed at times that it's very difficult for me to stay tuned in to what you're telling me. I'm able to be with you when you talk about yourself and your own feelings, but I tend to get lost as you go into great detail about all the things your daughter is doing or not doing." In this statement the client is not being labeled or judged, but the helper is giving his reactions about what he hears when his client tells stories about others. An example of an unhelpful response would be "You're boring me!" This response is a judgment of the client, and the helper assumes no responsibility for his own part in his boredom.

It can be therapeutic to talk about yourself if doing so is for a client's benefit, but it is not necessary to share detailed stories of your past to form a trusting relationship with others. Inappropriate sharing of yourself or indiscriminately revealing your personal problems to your clients can easily distract them from productive self-exploration. Examine the impact that your disclosures have on others, and develop an honesty about your own motivations and behavior. If you are distracting your clients from exploring their issues, this is the time that you could benefit from your own therapy. In your therapy sessions you can put the focus on yourself and work on your concerns.

Some helpers use self-disclosure inappropriately as a way of unburdening themselves. They make the mistake of pulling the focus away from the clients and directing it to their own concerns. If your feelings are very much in the foreground and inhibit you from fully attending to a client, it may be helpful for you and your client if you share how you are being affected. Depending on your relationship with the client, you might give some detail about your own situation, or you might simply reveal that what the client is struggling with touches you personally.

Identifying and assessing action strategies. Insight without action is of little value. Self-understanding and seeing a range of possible alternatives can be significant in the change process, but clients also need to identify specific actions they can take and are willing to carry out in everyday living. Clients often do not accomplish their goals because they rush into the first strategy that comes to mind or devise strategies that are unrealistically difficult. One function of helping at this stage is to assist clients in thinking of many possible routes to achieving their goals. Together, helpers and clients can come up with a wide range of alternatives for coping with problems, can assess how practical these strategies are, and can decide on the best plans for action. Helpers guide clients to recognize the skills they need to put their goals into action. If they don't have certain skills, they can acquire them during the helping sessions or learn about resources that are available to them.

At this stage of helping, the focus is on asking clients to come up with clear plans for what they will do today, tomorrow, and the next day to bring about change and to anticipate what might get in the way of their plans. In choosing action strategies, clients consider their internal and external resources and limitations and then determine which strategies are best suited to their capabilities. Helpers work with them to ensure that these strategies are specific and realistic, are related to their goals, and are consistent with their value system. This process is especially important in working with clients in crisis situations. In these cases it is helpful to work collaboratively with clients so that they will have some degree of responsibility for their plan. Even in crisis intervention, the critical element in developing a plan is that clients do not feel robbed of their power and independence (James & Gilliland, 2001).

The process of creating and carrying out plans enables people to gain effective control over their lives. This is clearly the teaching phase of the helping process, which is best directed toward providing clients with new information and assisting them in the discovery of more effective ways of getting what they want and need. Throughout this planning phase, the helper continually urges clients to assume responsibility for their own choices and actions. This is done by reminding them that no one in the world will do things for them or live their life for them.

Wubbolding (1988, 2000) writes about the central place of planning and commitment in any change process, emphasizing that when clients make plans and follow through they are taking charge of their lives by redirecting their energy and making action choices. According to Wubbolding, effective plans have the following characteristics:

- The plan should be within the limits of the motivation and capacities of each client. Plans should be realistic and attainable. Helpers do well to caution clients about plans that are too ambitious or unrealistic.
- Good plans are simple and easy to understand. Although plans need to be concrete and measurable, they should be flexible and open to modification as clients gain a deeper understanding of the specific behaviors that they want to change.
- The plan should involve positive action and should be stated in terms of what the client is willing to do.
- Helpers should encourage clients to develop plans that they can carry out independently. Plans that are contingent on what others will do lead clients to sense that they are not steering their own ship but are at the mercy of others.
- Good plans are specific and concrete. Clients can develop specificity when helpers raise questions such as "What?" "Where?" "With whom?" "When?" and "How often?"
- Effective plans are repetitive and ideally are performed daily. For people to overcome symptoms of depression, anxiety, negative thinking, or psychosomatic complaints, it is essential for them to replace these symptoms with new patterns of thinking and behaving. Each day, clients might choose a course that will lead to a sense of being in charge of their lives.
- Plans should be done as soon as possible. Helpers can ask questions such as "What are you willing to do today to begin to change your life?" "You say you'd like to stop depressing yourself. What are you going to do now to attain this goal?"
- Effective planning involves process-centered activities. For example, clients may state that they will do any of the following: apply for a job, write a letter to a friend, take a yoga class, substitute nutritious food for junk food, devote 2 hours a week to volunteer work, or take a vacation that they have been wanting.
- Before clients carry out their plan, it is a good idea for them to evaluate it to determine if it is realistic, attainable, and reflective of what they need and want. After the plan has been carried out in real life, it is useful to evaluate it again. Helpers can raise the question to the client "Is your plan helpful?" If the plan does not work, it can be reevaluated and alternatives can be considered.
- For clients to commit themselves to their plan, it is useful for them to firm it up in writing.

- Part of developing a plan for action involves a discussion of the main costs and benefits of each strategy as well as a discussion of the possible risks involved and the chances for success. It is the helper's task to work with clients in constructively dealing with any hesitations they might have to formulating plans or carrying them out.

Resolutions and plans are empty unless there is a decision to carry them out. It is crucial that clients commit themselves to a definite plan that they can realistically accomplish. The ultimate responsibility for making plans and following them through rests with the client. It is up to each client to determine ways of carrying these plans outside the helping relationship itself and into the everyday world. Effective helping can be the catalyst that leads to self-directed, responsible living.

Carrying out an action program.   Clients are encouraged to see the value in actively trying new behavior rather than being passive and leaving action to chance. One way of fostering an active stance by clients is to formulate clear contracts. In this way clients are continually confronted with what they want and what they are willing to do. Contracts are also a useful frame of reference for evaluating the outcomes of helping. Discussion can be focused on how well the contract is being met and what modifications of it are in order.

If certain plans do not work out well, this is a topic for exploration in a subsequent session. For example, if a mother does not follow through with her plan to deal with her unruly son who is getting in trouble in school, the counselor can explore with her what got in her way of carrying it out. Contingency plans are also developed. The counselor might role-play different ways the mother could deal with setbacks or with her son's lack of cooperation. In this way clients learn how to deal with reverses and how to predict possible roadblocks to their progress.

Stage 5: Termination

Just as the initial session sets the tone for the helping relationship, the ending phase enables clients to maximize the benefits from the relationship and decide how they can continue the change process. As a helper, your goal is to work with clients in such a way that they can terminate the professional relationship with you as soon as possible and continue to make changes on their own. In settings where brief therapy is the standard, it is especially important that termination and issues pertaining to restrictions on time be addressed at the initial session. If an agency policy specifies that clients can be seen for only six sessions, for example, they have a right to know this from the outset. Working in a short-term therapy approach, the final phase of the helping process should always be in the background. With brief interventions, the goal is to teach clients, as quickly and efficiently as possible, the coping skills they need to live in self-directed ways. Your overriding goal is to increase the chances that your client will not continue to need you. Kramer (1990) puts this well: "The therapist must be clear from the first contact, unless there are mitigating circumstances, that the intent of treatment is to help the patient function without the therapist" (p. 166).

In cases of structured, time-limited counseling, both you and your client know from the beginning the approximate number of sessions available. However, while clients may know cognitively that they have only 6 to 12 sessions, they may emotionally deny the reality that counseling will be short term. Termination should be discussed at the first session and be explored as necessary throughout the course of the helping relationship. In this way, the discussion of termination does not come as a surprise to the client.

The limitation of time can actually assist both you and your clients in establishing short-term, realistic goals of helping. Toward the end of each session, you can ask clients the degree to which they see themselves reaching the goals they have established. By reviewing the course of treatment, clients are in a position to identify what is and is not working for them in the helping process. Each session can be assessed in light of having a specific number of sessions devoted to accomplishing pre-set goals.

Basically, the interventions for endings pertain to assisting clients in consolidating their learning and determining how they can proceed once they stop coming in for treatment. Here are some considerations for effectively accomplishing these tasks:

• Remind clients of the approaching ending of the sessions with you. This should be done a couple of sessions before the final one. You might ask clients to think about any unfinished business they have and what they would most like to talk about in the final two meetings with you. You could even ask at a session prior to the last one, "If this were our last meeting, how would that be for you?"

• If you are not limited to a specified number of sessions, and both you and your client determine that termination is appropriate, one option is to space out the final few sessions. Instead of meeting weekly, your client might come in every 3 weeks. This schedule allows more opportunity to practice and to prepare for termination.

• Review the course of treatment. What lessons did clients learn, how did they learn them, and what do they intend to do with what they have learned? What did they find most helpful in the sessions with you? What did they think about their own participation in this process?

• Allow clients to talk about their feelings of separation. Just as they may have had fears about seeking help, they may have different fears about ending the work with you.

• Be clear about your own feelings about endings. Helpers often have ambivalence in letting go of clients. It is possible to hold back clients because of your own reluctance to terminate with a client, for whatever reason. It is essential that you reflect on the degree to which you may need your clients more than they need you. Clients are likely to give you positive feedback by letting you know how influential you have been in their lives. It is critical to remember that if you are a good helper you will eventually put yourself out of business—at least with your current clients. Your task is to get them moving on their own, not to keep them coming to you for advice. If you can teach your clients ways of finding their own solutions to problems, they can use what they learn in dealing not only with present concerns but also with any future problems they will meet.

• It is a good idea to have an open-door policy, meaning that clients might be encouraged to return at a later time should they feel a need for further learning. Although professional helping is best viewed as a terminal process, at a later period of development clients may be ready to deal with a new set of problems or concerns in ways they were not willing to do when they initially began counseling. Clients may need only a session or a few sessions to get refocused.

• Assisting clients to translate their learning into action programs is one of the most important functions during the action phase and the ending phase of helping. If clients have been successful, the ending stage is a *commencement*; they now have some new directions to follow in dealing with problems as they arise. Furthermore, clients acquire some needed tools and resources for continuing the process of personal growth. For this reason, discussing available programs and making referrals are especially timely toward the end of your work with clients. In this way the end leads to new beginnings.

By Way of Review

• Your orientation to the helping process is largely a function of your beliefs about human nature and about how people change. It is essential that you clarify your beliefs about what brings about change.

• Effective helpers hold positive beliefs about people; have a healthy self-concept; ground their interventions in values; and possess empathy, congruence, warmth, compassion, genuineness, and unconditional positive regard.

• Generalizations that helpers make about clients tend to foster a self-fulfilling prophecy within clients. If individuals are viewed by a helper as being highly dependent and unable to find their own way, they will most likely live up to this expectation.

• Examine your assumptions to determine whether they are helpful for clients. Challenge your beliefs and make them your own through this process of self-examination.

• A theoretical orientation that integrates thinking, feeling, and behaving provides the basis for developing interventions that can be used flexibly with clients at various stages of the helping process.

• Because there is no one "right" theoretical approach, you would do well to consider adopting an approach that is congruent with your personality and values.

- There are five stages in the helping process. Stage 1 is the time for creating rapport and structure in the relationship. Stage 2 consists of helping clients identify and clarify their problems. In Stage 3 the client and the helper collaboratively create goals. Stage 4 involves encouraging clients to engage in self-exploration and to develop an action plan aimed at change. This is a time to take action and to assist clients in translating what they have learned in counseling to everyday life situations. Stage 5 deals with termination and the consolidation of learnings. Specific helper strategies are required at each of these stages. Developing these skills takes time and supervised practice. Your own life experiences play a vital role in your ability to be present and to be effective in working with clients.

What Will You Do Now?

1. Identify a few of your key beliefs and assumptions that stand out after you have read this chapter. As a way of examining how you acquired these beliefs and assumptions, talk with someone you know who tends to hold similar beliefs. Then seek out somebody with a different perspective. With both of these people, discuss how you developed your beliefs.

2. Consider the skills needed for effective helping, and select what you consider to be your one major asset and your one major limitation, and write them down. How do you see your main asset enabling you to be an effective helper? How might your main limitation get in the way of working successfully with others? What can you do to work on your weak area? You might ask people you know well to review your statements about yourself. Do they see you as you see yourself?

3. Write a one-page essay that describes your personal view of what helping is about. You might imagine that a supervisor had asked you to describe your views about counseling or that in a job interview you had been instructed "Tell us briefly how you see the helping process." You could also imagine that someone who is not sophisticated in your field had said to you: "Oh, you're a counselor. What do you do?"

4. After reflecting on your beliefs about people and about the helping process, write some key ideas in your journal pertaining to the role that your beliefs play in the manner in which you might intervene in the lives of clients. How do your beliefs influence the suggestions you make to clients? How are your beliefs the groundwork for the strategies from which you will draw in dealing with client populations?

5. As you review the stages of the helping process, ask yourself what you consider to be your most important tasks at each of the different stages. Write in your journal about some of the challenges you expect to face when working with people at each of these stages. For example, might termination be a difficult process for you? Would you have difficulty appropriately sharing your life experi-

ences with your clients? Might you have difficulty confronting clients? What can you do to develop the personal characteristics and skills you will need to effectively intervene at each of the stages of helping?

6. For the full bibliographic entry for each of these sources, consult the References and Reading List at the back of the book. For comprehensive overviews of stages in the helping process, descriptions of systematic skill development, and intervention strategies, see Brammer (1993), Brems (2001), Doyle (1998), Egan (2002), Hutchins and Cole Vaught (1997), Ivey and Ivey (1999), Nelson-Jones (1993), Okun (2002), Patterson and Welfel (2000), and Teyber (2000). Consult James and Gilliland (2001) for an excellent survey text on crisis intervention strategies and Kanel (1999) for a practical guide to crisis-counseling techniques. Purkey and Schmidt (1996) address topics such as integrating approaches to counseling, ingredients of invitational counseling, beliefs about professional counseling, and characteristics of successful counselors.

InfoTrac College Edition Resources

For additional readings, explore InfoTrac College Edition, our online library. Go to http://www.infotrac.college.com/wadsworth and select these key word searches:

    helping W1 relationship*
    helping W1 skill*
    help* AND skill* AND couns*

Key words are listed in a form that enables the search engine to locate a wider range of articles in the online university library. Key words should be entered exactly as shown, including asterisks, "W1," "W2," "AND," and other search engine tools.

CHAPTER **6**

Common Concerns
of Beginning Helpers

Focus Questions

1. As a helper, how can you best deal with resistant clients? angry clients? unmotivated clients? clients who exhibit traits that are a part of your personality?

2. How can you handle your fear of angering clients when you confront them about inconsistent behaviors? How would you deal therapeutically with clients' resistance so they are more likely to look at their behavior than defend themselves?

3. How can you learn to avoid bringing the problems of clients home with you? How can you remain open and sensitive to your clients' struggles yet at the same time acquire some healthy distance from their problems?

4. How can you deal with your own reactions that are stimulated by working with a wide range of clients?

5. What client behaviors do you find most problematic? Why?

6. When you are faced with working with "difficult clients" (or difficult friends), what do you generally do?

7. Are you aware of any unfinished business from your past that is likely to affect your ability to work with certain types of clients? What have you done to heal your own psychological wounds?

8. What kind of clients would you be most likely to refer to another professional? What might this answer tell you about yourself?

9. What defensive behaviors do you employ when you feel personally threatened? How open are you to recognizing your patterns of resistance? If you had a caseload composed of clients like yourself, what do you think your job would be like?

Aim of the Chapter

As a helper you will encounter a range of special concerns throughout your career, but some problems will be particularly pressing when you begin helping others. One challenge you will face is learning how to deal effectively with the feelings that some of your clients have toward you and the corresponding feelings that they evoke in you. Even experienced helpers show an interest in learning creative ways to deal with difficult clients, especially those who exhibit great resistance to their interventions. In this chapter we address the important issues of transference, countertransference, resistance, and management of your own feelings as you work with difficult clients.

This chapter will probably raise more questions than it answers. There are no simple solutions to the many complex and challenging situations that you will encounter in your helping relationships. Our purpose is to introduce you to a range of common concerns that beginning helpers typically face.

Too often helpers become riveted on getting resistant clients to change, and they underplay the importance of being aware of their own dynamics and reactions as they interact with difficult clients. Pay attention to yourself at least as much as you do to your client. Don't overwhelm yourself with the belief that you should know exactly what to do in every helping situation. You are enrolled in a program in which you have many opportunities to learn and practice the skills that can be applied to challenging situations. Your supervised field placement activities and your supervisory sessions are ideal places to talk about many of the concerns raised in this chapter as well as to practice various intervention skills. If you are beginning your training program, you are certainly not expected to have the knowledge or skills to cope effectively with some of the cases we present. More important at this point is your capacity for being open to what is emerging inside of you as you confront resistant behavior in your clients. As you will learn in this chapter, your willingness to work on yourself is a good gauge of your ability to work with others.

Exploring Self-Doubts and Fears

Students in human services programs sometimes bring up fears, resistances, perfectionist strivings, and other personal concerns. For example, many students express their anxiety over the prospect of facing clients. They ask themselves: "What will my clients want? Will I be able to give them what they want? What will I say, and how will I say it? Will they want to come back? If they do, what will I do then?" It is possible to become so anxiety-ridden that an intern or a practitioner is not able to pay attention to the client. Another concern of many students and practitioners is their expectation that they must be the perfect helpers. They often burden themselves with the belief that they cannot afford to be less than perfect, lest they make a mistake, which would have dire consequences for both their clients and themselves. These become ethical concerns when they are dealt with in a manner that reduces the effectiveness of the helper.

In practicum and internship courses we frequently hear statements of self-doubt from those who are beginning to help others. Apply these statements to yourself, and decide to what degree you see them as your concerns. If a statement is more true than false for you, place a "T" in front of it; if it is more false than true for you, mark it with an "F."

_____ 1. I am afraid my clients will suffer because of my mistakes and my uncertainty in knowing what to do.

_____ 2. I demand perfection of myself, and I constantly feel I should know more than I do.

_____ 3. I would feel threatened by silences in counseling situations.

_____ 4. It is important for me to know that my clients are making steady improvement.

_____ 5. It would be difficult for me to deal with demanding clients.

_____ 6. I expect to have trouble working with clients who are not motivated to change or who are required to come to me for counseling.

_____ 7. I have trouble deciding how much of the responsibility for the direction of a counseling session is mine and how much is my client's.

_____ 8. I think I should be successful with all of my clients.

_____ 9. I expect to have trouble being myself and trusting my intuition when I am counseling.

_____ 10. I am afraid of confrontation and I think this might get in my way when helping others.

_____ 11. I worry that my clients will see that I am a beginner and wonder if I am competent.

_____ 12. I am concerned about how much of my personal reactions and my private life I should reveal in counseling sessions.

_____ 13. I tend to worry about whether I am making the proper intervention.

_____ 14. I sometimes worry that I may overidentify with my client's problems to the extent that they become *my* problems.

_____ 15. During a counseling session, I might find myself wanting to give advice.

_____ 16. I am afraid that I might say or do something that would greatly disturb a client.

_____ 17. I'm concerned about working with clients whose values and culture are different from my own.

_____ 18. I would be apprehensive about whether my clients liked and approved of me and whether they would want to come back.

_____ 19. I am nervous about videotaping my sessions.

_____ 20. I am concerned about ending a counseling session or a counseling relationship.

Now go back and select the issues that represent your greatest concerns. Begin to challenge some of the assumptions behind these statements.

Transference and Countertransference

In the questionnaire that you just took, you may have pinpointed several concerns and fears that could influence your ability to work effectively with clients. Certainly, a major concern of many helpers, both personally and professionally, is being able to deal constructively with clients' reactions to them. A central challenge you will face is identifying when your reactions are the result of your own internal conflicts that surface as you offer services to a range of clients.

Dealing With Transference Issues

Transference is the unconscious process whereby clients project onto a helper past feelings or attitudes they had toward significant people in their lives. Transference typically has its origins in the client's early childhood, and it constitutes a repetition of past conflicts. Because of unfinished business, the client perceives you in a distorted way. A client may view you with a mixture of positive and negative feelings, and at different times the same individual may express love, affection, resentment, rage, dependency, and ambivalence. You are likely to experience transference feelings from clients even if you limit your practice to brief counseling. It is essential that you understand what transference means and that you know how to deal with it skillfully.

Transference tends to evoke reactions in you as a helper. These reactions can become problematic if they result in countertransference. Your unconscious emotional responses to a client may result in a distorted perception of the client's behavior. It is important to be alert to the possibility of countertransference.

In our training workshops for students and mental health practitioners, we explore examples of difficult client behavior that participants present to us. We stress the importance of understanding the functions that resistive and defensive behaviors serve for individuals, examining the payoffs of a client's defensive style and understanding how resistance is an attempt to cope with anxiety. Rather than focusing on the dynamics of difficult clients and ways of dealing with them, we devote attention to assisting helpers in becoming aware of, understanding, and exploring their own reactions and potential countertransference. We encourage those whom we teach to approach resistance with interest and respect rather than with impatience.

Here are some examples of transference situations that you are likely to encounter. Ask yourself what your response might be to a client's feelings toward you and what feelings are likely to be evoked in you.

Clients who make you into something you are not. Some clients will want you to be the mother or father they never had but always wanted. These clients may have visions that you will take care of them and solve all their problems. They see you as an all-knowing being who can pull them out of the quandary they are stuck in. In considering clients who make you into a parent and want you to adopt them, ask yourself these questions: "Do I look to others to be the parents I never had? How comfortable or uncomfortable am I with clients who attribute to me traits such as being all-knowing and all-wise? How do I feel when clients expect me to make decisions for them? To what degree do I make it my responsibility to pull clients out of stuck places? What needs of mine could I be satisfying by assuming the role of parent for such clients?"

Other clients may immediately distrust you because you remind them of a former spouse, a critical parent, or some other important figure in their life. For example, consider the female client who is assigned to a male therapist and lets him know that she has no regard for men. All the men in her life have been untrustworthy, and because her therapist is male, he, too, will betray her. If you had a client who prejudged you on the basis of earlier experiences, how might you react? Are you able to recognize your client's behavior as a transference reaction and deal with it nondefensively? How might you go about showing this client that you are a different person from people in her past? How do you think you might react if your client insisted on treating you as she treated her father? How might you respond if no matter how you treated her, she deeply believed that you eventually would be "just like every other man"?

Some clients will not let themselves get emotionally close to you because they feel that as children they were abandoned by people they cared for. They are taking past experiences and superimposing them on the relationship with you. Assume that a client of yours comes from a divorced family. She is somehow convinced that a fault of hers caused her parents to separate. Because she was abandoned in the past and remembers the pain of that time in her life, she is leery of letting you into her life. If she gets too close to you, she fears that she will not know what to do and that you may also abandon her. In working with such a client, consider these questions: "Is there much I can do to convince her that I do not intend to abandon her? What are my reactions to being told that I am going to be like her parents? What might I do in such a situation?"

Clients who see you as a superperson.   Consider having this man as a client: He uses only superlative adjectives to describe you. He sees you as always understanding and supportive and as perfect in all areas of living. He cannot imagine that you might have personal difficulties. He is sure that you have the ideal marriage, that your children are ideally happy, and that you have the ideal career. This client gives you full credit for any changes that he has made. Might you be inclined to believe some of what such a client tells you about yourself? To what degree might you feel burdened by his perception? What do you think you might have to do to live up to his ideal? How would you deal with his giving you total credit for his improvement?

Clients who make unrealistic demands on you.   Some clients make no decisions without first finding out what you think. They want to know if they can call you at any time. They may frequently call you between their sessions, leaving detailed messages on your voice mail or answering machine, claiming to be in crisis. These are the clients who time and again want to run over the allotted time for their session. They want you to see them for no fee, with only the promise of paying later when they are in a better financial position. They feel close to you and would like to include you in their social life. They demand that you always be patient with them even when they do little to change. They expect you to accept them no matter what their behavior is during the session. They want you to affirm them and convince them that they are special in your eyes. If you fail to give them what they want, they are likely to be resentful and to react toward you with hostility. Even though you may intellectually understand the nature of these unrealistic demands on you, how do you imagine such demands would affect you emotionally? In what ways could you help such clients see the connection between how they are treating you and how they treated some significant person in their past? In what ways would you want to react to them differently than did significant persons in their past?

Clients who are not able to accept boundaries.   Related to clients who consistently make unrealistic demands on you are those who have problems understanding or accepting appropriate boundaries. As they were growing up, their home environment lacked boundaries, so they never learned the importance of not encroaching on the territory of others. The discipline in their home probably was inconsistent. One of their parents might have pampered and protected them from the other parent, who was overly severe in administering discipline. In their professional relationship with you, such individuals may treat you sometimes as an overprotective parent and at other times as an unduly harsh and punitive parent. Much of their behavior within the helping relationship may be aimed at testing you so that they know how far they can go with you. They will probably give you many excuses for why they fail to follow through on their commitments in the helping relationship. They are likely to be lost and to feel anxious because they are not certain where they stand with you. In working with such clients, it is essential that you do not fall into the trap of allowing them to treat you as they did a parent.

Clients who displace anger onto you.   Some clients will lash out at you with displaced anger. They will be annoyed with you if you dare to become impatient. These clients are basically telling you that because you are supposed to be helping them you have no right to express your own feelings. These clients also lack appropriate boundaries between themselves and other people. It is important that you not deny your own feelings by swallowing them or trying too hard to "remain objective." Recognize that you are probably getting more of this client's anger than you deserve, and avoid getting into a debate with the person. If you take what you are getting too personally, you are bound to begin to react defensively. With this kind of client, you may need to ventilate some of your own feelings in the safety of a supervised session or with a colleague whom you trust. As a helper, how do you deal with your feelings toward a person who behaves in this way? How do you react to clients who project anger onto you? How can you express your reactions to clients in a way that does not cause them to become closed? How do you know whether a client's anger expressed toward you is transference or a genuine feeling based on your behavior?

Clients who easily fall in love with you.   Some clients will make you the object of all of their verbal affection. They may tell you that there is nobody in the world whom they feel as much affection for as you. They may see you as the ideal person and want very much to become the person they see you as being. They are convinced that they could find a resolution to their problems if only they found a person like you who would love and accept them. How might you respond to being the object of adulation? Might you be inclined to solicit such ego-gratifying feedback? Could your client's reactions distort or enhance your self-perceptions?

Working With Transference Therapeutically

These illustrations of transference behaviors demonstrate how essential it is for you to gain awareness of your own needs and motivations. If you are unaware of your own dynamics, you will tie into your clients' projections and get lost in their distortions. You are likely to avoid focusing on key issues and instead focus on defending yourself. Paying attention to your own feelings about a client who imposes on you and makes unreasonable demands of you will give you a sense of how significant people in this client's life are affected by his or her behavior.

When clients appear to work very hard at getting the counselor to push them away, it can be useful to explore what they are getting from this self-defeating behavior or how what they are doing serves them. Handled properly, clients can experience and express feelings toward you that more properly belong to others who have been significant in their lives. When these feelings are productively explored, clients become aware of how they are keeping old patterns functional in many of their present relationships. By paying attention to how your clients behave and react in the helping relationship itself, you can begin to understand how they might react to others.

It is a mistake to think that all feelings your clients have toward you are simply signs of transference. At times clients may be realistically angry with you because of something you have done or said. Their anger does not have to be an irrational response triggered from past situations. If you answer your phone continually during a session with a client, for example, she may become angry with you over the interruptions and your lack of presence. Her anger could be a justifiable reaction and not one that should be "explained away" as a mere expression of transference.

Likewise, clients' affection toward you does not always indicate transference. It could be that they genuinely like some of your traits and enjoy being with you. Of course, many helpers are quick to interpret positive feelings as realistic and negative feelings as distortions. You can err both by being too willing to accept unconditionally whatever clients tell you and by interpreting everything they tell you as a sign of transference.

In a group setting we have found it useful to have the participants gradually become aware of their transference reactions to one another and to the group leaders. At the beginning of a group we ask members to pay particular attention to people in the room whom they notice most. We facilitate the process of members' increasing their awareness of others by asking the questions:

- Whom in this group are you most aware of?
- Are you finding yourself drawn to some people more than to others? Are there some people with whom you quickly identify?
- Are there some people who seem especially threatening to you?
- Are you finding yourself making quick assumptions about others and forming hasty impressions? For example, "He looks judgmental." "She's intimidating me." "I think I can trust him and will like him." "I definitely want to stay away from her." "It looks as if these three people are in a clique."

We pay particular attention to members who have strong reactions to another person whom they hardly know. It is common for people to "see" in others some of the very traits that they are disowning in themselves. This process of projection forms the basis of transference. Although we ask the participants to become aware of their first reactions to others, we do not ask them to reveal these thoughts or to respond to others too quickly. Instead, we suggest that participants share their reactions after they have had some chances for interaction. By disclosing such persistent positive or negative responses, they have rich opportunities to come to a deeper understanding of aspects of themselves that they are disowning. Through this process, participants often gain insight into their behaviors outside the group. This insight includes coming to an understanding of how they reacted to important figures in their childhood and how they now act around people who are important to them. With this new insight, people are able to catch themselves when old patterns become evident. Rather than responding automatically, they are now able to respond in different ways. Thus, an individual who treats most men in authority roles with deference can stop himself from making them into representations of his father. He can then respond to different men more as they really are.

Dealing With Countertransference Issues

The other side of transference is countertransference, or unrealistic reactions helpers have toward their clients that may interfere with their objectivity. If you hope to be effective in your helping efforts, it is essential that you consider countertransference as a potential source of difficulties. You do not have to be problem free, but it is crucial that you be aware of how your own problems or countertransference can affect the quality of your working relationships with clients.

Countertransference is not always harmful. You can use all of your reactions in therapeutic ways, assuming that you eventually become aware of the sources of your countertransference. Remember that we are considering countertransference from a broader perspective than the psychoanalytic view of countertransference as being merely a reflection of an individual's unresolved internal conflicts that need to be overcome as a prerequisite to working effectively with a client. Brockett and Gleckman (1991) conceptualize countertransference broadly to encompass all of the counselor's thoughts and feelings in reaction to clients, whether prompted by the clients themselves or by events in the helper's own life.

The helper's task is to attend to the feelings he or she is experiencing in relationship to the client and then to identify the sources of these emotional reactions. When counselors' personal issues are brought into awareness, the chances increase that their countertransference will be managed appropriately, which means that these reactions are less likely to interfere with the helping relationship. Brockett and Gleckman believe that supervision, honest introspection, and involvement in one's own therapy as a client are particularly useful ways of achieving awareness of countertransference phenomena.

Simply having feelings toward a client does not automatically mean that you are having countertransference reactions. You may feel deep empathy and compassion for some of your clients as a function of their life situations. Countertransference occurs when your needs become too much a part of the relationship or when your clients trigger old wounds of yours that may not have healed. Just as your clients will have some unrealistic reactions to you and will project onto you some of their unfinished business, so will you have some unrealistic reactions to them. Your own vulnerabilities will be opened up as you are drawn into some of the transference reactions of those you help.

As you reflect on ways that you may be emotionally triggered in working with certain clients, think about how you are affected by those clients you perceive as being especially difficult. How do you respond to the different forms of transference? What kind of transference tends to elicit your countertransference? Do you take the resistance of a client in a personal way? Do you blame yourself for not being skillful enough? Do you tend to become combative with clients whom you view as problematic?

We encourage you to look at how your own attitudes, behaviors, and reactions to clients may, at times, actually foster resistance in clients. Without blaming yourself, it is useful to examine your reactions to those with whom you work to determine how what you are doing can either decrease or escalate the resistances your clients manifest. As a helper, it is crucial that you be willing to look at your own part in contributing to the problems associated with resistive behaviors in clients.

Countertransference can have both positive and negative effects on the helping process. If your own needs or unresolved personal conflicts become entangled in your professional relationships and blur your sense of objectivity, your countertransference reactions will probably interfere with the client's capacity to change. If you use your own feelings as a way of understanding yourself, your client, and the relationship between the two of you, these feelings can be a positive and healing force. Even though you may be insightful and self-aware, the demands of the helping profession are great. The emotionally intense relationships that develop with your clients can be expected to bring your unresolved conflicts to the surface. Because countertransference may be a form of identification with your client, you can easily get lost in the client's world, and thus your ability to be helpful is limited. Here are some illustrations of countertransference:

• *"Let me help you."* Your client has gotten a raw deal from life. No matter how hard he tries, things typically go sour in spite of his best efforts. You find yourself going out of your way to be helpful to this client and even consider having him move in with a relative of yours.

• *"I hope he cancels."* You are intimidated by a client's anger directed at you or others. When you are in the presence of this client, you are not yourself but are self-conscious and guarded. When he cancels a session, you find yourself relieved.

• *"You remind me of someone I know."* Your clients will often remind you of significant people in your own life. Put yourself in each of these situations, and imagine how you would respond:

1. You are a middle-aged therapist, and your husband has left you for a 20-year-old woman. You are faced with a female client who is having an affair with a middle-aged married man. Next, consider that your client is the middle-aged man who is having an affair with the much younger woman.

2. You have been a rape victim, and your client discloses that she has been raped. Or your client informs you that he has raped someone.

3. You were abused as a child, and your client tells you that he has abused some of his own children.

4. You have just dealt at home with a rebellious teenage daughter, and your first client for the day is a hostile, acting-out boy.

5. You lost a grandfather, but you have never really gone through a mourning process and come to terms with his death. One of your elderly male clients is in poor health and almost dies. As he talks about his feelings, you are extremely uncomfortable and find yourself unable to respond to him. You attempt to reassure him that he will be all right.

- *"You are too much like me."* Some of your clients are bound to remind you of some of the traits that you would rather not acknowledge in yourself. Even if you do recognize certain traits, you may find it disconcerting to work with clients who talk about problems and situations that are very much like your own. A client may be a compulsive workaholic, for example, and you may see yourself as working too hard. You might find yourself spending a lot of energy getting this client to slow down and take it easy.

- *"My own reactions are getting in my way."* Sometimes your clients will express pain and show tears. This anguish may make you anxious, because it reminds you of some past or present situation in your life that you would rather avoid. You may intervene by attempting to stop the client's feelings. It is important to realize that such interventions are motivated by bringing comfort to the helper, not by doing what is in the best interest of the client.

No one is immune to countertransference. It is therefore crucial that you be alert to its subtle signs and that you not be too quick to pin the blame for your reactions on your clients. For example, you may find that certain clients evoke a parental response in you. Their behavior can bring out your own critical responses to them. Knowing this about yourself enables you to work through some of your own projections or places where you get stuck.

Among the most vulnerable to the effects of countertransference may be those caregivers who work with the seriously ill or dying. These caregivers are continually confronted with the reality of mortality. In their work they watch others around them die. Unless these caregivers are able to process their reactions, this work will take an emotional toll on them. Unless you have come to terms with your own feelings about death, loss, separation, and grief, your own unfinished business will continue to be activated as you work with clients who trigger your fears. In our experience in training students, we find that many of them have difficulty working with the terminally ill or the elderly because of the constant reminder of their own mortality. Working with the elderly can be very rewarding, but it can sometimes be anxiety-provoking and stressful as well (Brockett & Gleckman, 1991).

You will probably not be able to eliminate countertransference altogether, but you can learn to recognize it and deal nondefensively with whatever your clients evoke in you. Here are some additional signs to watch for in recognizing your own countertransference:

- You become easily irritated by certain clients.
- You feel intense anger toward a person you hardly know.
- With some clients you continually run overtime.
- You find yourself wanting to lend money to some unfortunate clients.
- You feel like adopting an abused child.
- You quickly take away pain from a grieving client.
- You regularly feel depressed after seeing a particular client.
- You feel excited knowing that a certain client is soon to arrive.
- You tend to become very bored with a certain client.
- You are aware of typically working much harder than your client.
- You get highly emotional and get lost in the client's world.
- You become aware of giving a great deal of advice and wanting to have clients do what you think they should do.
- You are quick not to accept a certain type of client, or you suggest a referral with little data.
- You find yourself lecturing or debating with certain clients.

To manage countertransference, you must have a receptive attitude and welcome self-awareness, be self-disciplined, and be willing to share your responses in a timely and therapeutic manner (Brockett & Gleckman, 1991). Accept whatever feelings you are experiencing without getting stuck in guilt and without criticizing yourself. Here are some red flags that could indicate countertransference (Brems, 2001) :

- You avoid certain topics or certain types of clients.
- You have predictable reactions to certain types of clients.
- You have sexual or romantic feelings for certain types of clients.
- You are overprotective with certain types of clients.
- You seek approval or admiration from your clients.
- You encourage client dependency.

When you begin to realize that certain topics or issues stimulate heightened feelings or specific reactions on your part, it is essential that you strive to understand what is contributing to your excessive or inappropriate responses. Self-exploration and consultation are excellent paths toward gaining this self-understanding (Brems, 2001).

Your own supervision will be a central factor in learning how to deal effectively with both transference and countertransference reactions. Your blind spots can easily hamper your ability to deal with "difficult clients" or with your own old wounds. You can become more aware of your own manifestations of countertransference by focusing on yourself in your supervision sessions. Rather than talking exclusively about a client's problem, spend some time talking about how you feel when you are in a session with a client. A good way to expand your awareness of potential countertransference is by talking with colleagues and supervisors about your feelings toward clients. This can be especially helpful if you feel stuck and do not quite know what to do with some of your clients. Part of what could be stalling you is some feeling that you are reluctant to acknowledge.

Ongoing supervision will enable you to accept responsibility for your reactions and at the same time prevent you from taking full responsibility for directions that your clients take. Self-knowledge is your most basic tool in dealing effectively with transference and countertransference. It is well to remember that helping others change will certainly also have the effect of changing you. If you are unwilling to resolve your own issues, you will not have much leverage when you challenge your clients to overcome their resistance.

Dealing With Difficult Clients

Professional helpers and students alike are concerned with how to handle difficult clients. They hope to learn techniques for making these clients less troublesome, for such clients tax them personally and professionally. There are no simple techniques, however—no tricks that you can pull out of a bag. In our workshops we help participants become aware of and understand their own reactions to resistance, and we teach them ways of constructively sharing their reactions with clients.

Kottler (1992) believes that by openly discussing those clients with whom helpers struggle the most, helpers put themselves in a better position to differentiate the dysfunctional behavior of clients from their own dynamics. Although he admits that some of his clients were extremely trying, he thinks that they have taught him more than any supervisor or instructor. Kottler has this to say about working with difficult clients:

> They force us to be more flexible, creative, and innovative than we ever thought possible. And they require us to look deep inside ourselves to examine every one of our own unresolved issues that get in the way of our being compassionate and effective—both as professionals and as human beings. (p. xi)

Attitude Questionnaire on Understanding and Working With Resistance and Difficult Clients

Take a few moments to complete this self-inventory to discover what your attitudes are toward resistance and difficult behaviors exhibited by clients. Indicate your position on each statement using the following scale: 1 = strongly agree; 2 = slightly agree; 3 = slightly disagree; 4 = strongly disagree.

_____ 1. Difficult clients force me to look deep inside myself and explore my own unresolved issues that get in the way of being an effective helper.
_____ 2. Resistance is best approached with a sense of interest.
_____ 3. Resistance on the part of clients generally leads to ineffective results in the helping process.
_____ 4. When I encounter clients' resistance, it generally gets me to thinking about my own part in contributing to this resistance.
_____ 5. Involuntary clients will rarely benefit from professional helping relationships.

_____ 6. When clients are silent, this is almost always a sign of resistance and lack of willingness to cooperate with treatment.

_____ 7. Resistance is often a sign of handling a transference relationship poorly.

_____ 8. The most effective way of dealing with resistance is to be highly confrontive with clients.

_____ 9. One way of working with difficult clients is to pay attention to my own countertransference.

_____ 10. Labeling or judging clients who exhibit difficult behavior tends to entrench the resistance.

Now look over your responses and try to identify patterns in your perceptions of resistance. At this point, how does resistance from clients generally affect you? What are some ways you can think of to deal with resistance effectively?

Handling Resistance With Understanding and Respect

Some people with whom you work will test you to determine if the relationship with you will be a safe one. It is essential that you encourage openness on the part of your clients so that they are able to express their hesitations and anxieties. Clients are likely to have mixed feelings regarding staying in a safe zone versus taking the risk of letting you know them. Both you and your clients need to understand the meaning of resistance and come to view it as something to explore in the helping relationship.

From a psychoanalytic perspective, resistance is defined as the individual's reluctance to bring into conscious awareness threatening material that has been previously repressed or denied. It can also be viewed as anything that prevents individuals from dealing with unconscious material. From a broader perspective, resistance can be viewed as behavior that keeps us from exploring personal conflicts or painful feelings. Resistance can be thought of as ways we attempt to protect ourselves from anxiety.

Clients may demonstrate a variety of resistances. Learn to respect resistance and understand its meaning. Teyber (2000) suggests that counselors must understand the client's reluctance as a behavior that at one time served a self-preservative and adaptive function. Teyber asserts that by honoring clients' resistance, clients are able to appreciate the fact that a particular coping strategy was the best possible response to a difficult situation at an earlier time in their development. By viewing clients' symptoms and resistive behaviors as survival mechanisms, both helpers and clients can recognize that some resistance is perfectly normal and makes good sense.

Resistance is not something that needs to be "gotten around quickly" or bypassed. Why should your clients automatically trust you? Chances are that many of them have had negative encounters with helpers or with a mental health agency, and as they approach you, they wonder whether you will be trustworthy. You don't get clients' respect immediately, nor do credentials on your office wall really earn genuine regard. Instead, your clients will come to trust you, and thus let down some of their defenses, if you approach their reluctance with compassion and regard. Part of respecting resistance means that you appreciate the functions these defenses serve. If clients give up their defenses, what will be the effect on them? If you succeed in helping clients to surrender many of their defenses, are you able to assist them in developing better ways of coping with life's challenges? There are times when people need their defensives in order to survive in a crisis situation. At such times, you need to be supportive rather than insist that your clients let go of their defenses.

Perhaps the key to understanding clients' various forms of defensive behavior is in paying attention to your countertransference that is evoked by this resistance. Avoid labeling your clients and thus entrenching their resistant styles. Do not assume that your client merely wants to annoy you. You cannot afford to have a fragile ego as a professional helper. Give your clients some rope, and do not respond to their resistance with resistance of your own. Be patient with your clients; remember that they are coming to you for help.

In dealing with difficult clients, monitor your responses to their behavior. If you respond in a belligerent tone, a tense situation is likely to worsen. If clients exhibit initial distrust, view this as a sign of strength and recognize ways you can utilize clients' cautiousness in the helping process. This is an example of how a perceived weakness can actually be reconceptualized as a strength. Your task is to approach difficult clients in a different way and work cooperatively with them so that they might learn new and more effective ways of coping.

Clients whom you perceive as being difficult or resistant may contribute to your own feelings of self-doubt and incompetence and bring out feelings of inadequacy and anger. If you too quickly become annoyed with difficult clients, you are likely to cut off avenues of reaching them. Avoid labeling clients as "resistant" and instead describe the behaviors you are observing. When you view clients as being scared, overwhelmed with grief, cautious, or hurt, you can reframe any pattern of resistance that your clients manifest. By simply changing the word "resistant" to more descriptive and nonjudgmental terminology, your own attitude toward clients who appear to be "difficult" may change. As you change the lens by which you perceive clients' behaviors, it will be easier for you to adopt an understanding attitude and to encourage clients to explore the meaning of their reluctance. Instead of viewing their resistance as behavior that is designed to make your work impossible, approach such behavior with a genuine sense of interest. If your client, Enrique, exhibits hostile behavior, consider reframing this experience: "It's interesting how hard Enrique is trying to get me to be angry with him. I wonder how his behavior is serving a purpose and whether he could find another way to get what he wants more directly." As another example, consider Maribel, a client who sits silent for much of each session. "Perhaps Maribel is scared or is a tentative person who is reluctant to experience her emotions. Maribel's silence during the sessions may be due to her lack of understanding of how to ask for help with her problems." Describe how you see your clients behaving toward you and how they are affecting you. After this declaration of your personal reactions, invite clients to explore alternative ways of getting what they want from you and from others.

Common Forms of Resistance

Albert Ellis (2002) has described many forms that resistance takes as counselors work with what he calls "difficult customers." Rational emotive behavior therapy

(REBT) acknowledges that some resistance is a normal reaction, because fears are attached to the process of change. Resistance is caused by a variety of factors within the client (such as irrational thinking), but the counselor's attitudes and behavior can also produce much client resistance. What follows is an adapted description of the common forms of resistance as detailed by Ellis (2002) and Ellis and MacLaren (1998):

- *Healthy resistance.* All forms of resistance are not to be considered dysfunctional, and some resistance to personality change and therapy is a normal reaction that serves some useful purposes for clients.

- *Resistance motivated by a client-helper mismatch.* At times clients and helpers are not compatible. Clients may simply not like a helper, for any number of reasons.

- *Resistance caused by counselors' relationship problems.* Counselors are not immune to relationship difficulties. They may not like some of their clients; they may have countertransference difficulties and therefore be biased against some clients; and they may be insensitive to their clients' feelings. The resistance that clients show in these cases is largely brought about by the counselors' difficulties.

- *Resistance related to counselors' moralistic attitudes.* Some counselors assume a moralistic stance, condemning both themselves and others. These helpers who condemn their clients for their behavior help their clients to berate themselves. Such clients will typically resist any attempts at helping.

- *Resistance created by fear of discomfort.* One of the most stubborn forms of resistance stems from low frustration tolerance, or what REBT calls discomfort anxiety. Some clients demand that they achieve pleasure immediately. They have irrational beliefs, which lead to discomfort anxiety: "It's *too hard* to change, and it *must* not be that hard. It's *awful* that I have to go through pain to experience therapeutic gain. I *can't tolerate* the discomfort of working hard. The world is a *horrible place* when it forces me to work so hard. Life *should be* easier." REBT shows clients ways to substitute long-range hedonism for short-range hedonism. It teaches clients that there is rarely any gain without pain.

- *Resistance due to secondary gain.* Many clients resist change because the payoffs that they get from their problems seem considerable. When clients improve, they sometimes discover hidden penalties. Some men learn to express their emotions, for example, only to be ill rewarded by society. They may then relapse into their old and familiar stoical ways.

- *Resistance stemming from feelings of hopelessness.* Some clients resist because they are convinced that they cannot change their dysfunctional behavior. Although they may make good progress, at the first sign of any regression they are likely to irrationally conclude that they are indeed hopeless.

- *Resistance motivated by fear of change or fear of success.* Some symptoms, such as shyness or fear of public speaking, protect clients against possible failure. Their shyness keeps them from being rejected, and their fear of speaking in public keeps them from making a fool of themselves in front of others. If they gave up their symptoms, they would open themselves to the chance of failure and disapproval. Some clients tell themselves that this would be so "catastrophic" or "awful" that they want to cling to their symptoms.

The foregoing description of some of the common kinds of resistance shows that although clients come to counseling for help because they are plagued with a variety of symptoms of emotional disturbance, they often stubbornly resist efforts on the helper's part. This resistance is at least partly due to what the helper does or does not do. More often, however, clients have their own reasons for resisting the help that they have sought.

Types of Difficult Clients

Ellis (2002) has written about how to deal with the resistance of your most difficult client—you. His main point is that therapists rarely function at an ideal level; rather, they are human and very fallible. Therapists, like their clients, all too often fall prey to irrational beliefs and accept assumptions that they have not questioned. When helpers encounter resistant clients, for example, they often assume that it is their own fault and that if they were the perfect counselors that they should be, their clients would be cooperative.

In many respects we agree with Ellis when he contends that dealing with your resistance (and your countertransference) is likely to be your greatest challenge as a helper. Rather than constantly paying attention to what your clients do or fail to do, occasionally focus on your reactions to your clients. See what these reactions tell you, both about yourself and about your client. You make resistance all the more difficult to deal with in clients when you demand perfection of yourself and labor under irrational beliefs about how the world must be fair.

If you want to be effective with difficult clients, you need to develop patience and give such clients room to maneuver. Regardless of which specific behavior a client exhibits, it is essential that you understand your own countertransference. Certain clients are more difficult for you because they evoke countertransference reactions. Think about which of the characteristics of difficult clients described in the following pages would provide the greatest challenge for you. Which clients might you find it easiest to work with?

Involuntary clients.   You may not have the luxury of seeing clients who freely come to you for your help. Some will be sent by the court, others will be sent by their parents, others will come in under duress with a spouse, and others will be referred by another helper. Involuntary clients are likely to have little motivation for change and to see little value in the help that you offer. For example, Herman attends a class for those found guilty of driving under the influence. His main motivation in coming to this class is to satisfy the judge's order. He figures that attending class is better than going to jail. Although he is willing to come to the sessions, he tells you that he doesn't believe that he has a problem. Rather, his intoxication was due to a series of unfortunate circumstances. He does not see much that he wants to change.

In your role as a helper, you could become either defensive or apologetic. We see it as a mistake to apologize for the fact that an involuntary client is sitting in your office. In Herman's case, he is responsible for being in his situation. It is *he* who needs to accept the consequences of his decisions and behavior. If you work harder than he does, there is little left for him to do. We see nothing wrong with your making some stipulations about how the two of you will spend your time. It helps to remember that when you have an involuntary client, you often have an involuntary helper. With some exploration of his resistance and willingness on your part to provide information about the services you offer, it is possible to melt resistance. Sometimes clients are reluctant to seek help because of their misconceptions about what the helping process entails. You can confront him with the reality that no one dragged him in to see you. Ultimately, he decided that it would be a better deal to come to see you than to accept the consequences if he did not. Together you can make a contract setting out how you are willing to spend your time with him.

Clients who are silent and withdrawn.   Clients who say very little are bound to evoke your anxiety. Imagine this client sitting in your office: He looks down at the floor much of the time, responds politely and briefly to your questions, and does not volunteer any information. For you the session drags on, and you feel as though you are a dentist pulling teeth. You might ask "Do you want to be here?" He will reply curtly "Sure, why not?" If you ask him what is going on in his life and what he wants to talk about, he will tell you that he doesn't know.

Do you feel that you need to do something to make this client talk? Are you taking his silence personally? Are you thinking of all sorts of ways to draw him out? Before your ego becomes too involved and you are unable to see his problem, it is useful to attempt to put his silence in some context. You might ask yourself, and even at times your client, what the silence means. His silence could have any one of the following meanings: He is frightened. He sees you as the expert and is waiting for you to ask a question or tell him what to do. He feels dumb; he may be rehearsing every thought and critically judging his every reaction. He is responding to past conditioning of "being seen but not heard." His culture may put a value on silence. He may have been taught to listen respectfully and merely to answer questions. Furthermore, your client may be quiet and invisible because this pattern served to protect him as a child. In other words, all forms of silence should not be interpreted as stubborn resistance and a refusal to cooperate with your attempts to help.

Silent clients in a group counseling situation can affect you and the other members in many ways. You may begin to judge yourself, thinking that if you knew the right things to say and do, your client would open up and talk fully. You could make a mistake by doing the talking for your client or by constantly drawing him out. It might be helpful to say something such as this: "I notice that you are very quiet in this group. You seem to pay attention to what other group members are saying, yet I rarely hear from you. I'd like to know more about how it is for you to be in this group. Is your silence OK with you?" If this client does not interpret his silence as a problem, maybe you will be working in vain if you try to change him. This silent group member will have many reasons for being quiet. If he sees his silence as a problem, you can explore with him the ways in which this behavior is problematic. If you assume the responsibility for bringing him out, he never has to struggle with the forces that are keeping him quiet.

Clients who talk excessively.   The opposite of the client who says nothing is the one who seems never to stop talking. Some clients tend to get lost in telling stories. They jump from one topic to another. They take great care in providing you with every detail so they won't be misunderstood. They often get lost in relating their stories, and you wonder what the point of the story is. Instead of talking about how they are affected by a particular situation, they give you much irrelevant information.

Consider the case of Bertha. When she is in your office, she goes on and on and on. Any attempt you make to stop her results in her telling you that she wants to be sure that you know what she is saying. She gets very involved in "he-said" and "she-said" monologues. Bertha's defense is to keep talking, for then she doesn't have to stay long enough to experience any feelings or insights. If she slows down and experiences some of the things she is talking about, she is likely to feel anxiety.

In working with Bertha, you might feel intimidated. Although she is talking about painful situations, she is doing so in a very detached and rehearsed style. You might have reservations about interrupting her, out of fear of cutting her off. One of your functions is to help Bertha gain awareness into how her behavior serves as a defense. Here are a few examples of some helpful comments you might make:

- I notice that when you speak of your relationship with your mother you have tears in your eyes. Yet you quickly move away from your tears when you start talking *about* her instead of how you feel when you are with her.
- I have trouble following what you're saying, and I wonder why you are telling me all of this.
- Let's stop right here, and you tell me what you are feeling at this moment.
- You are making a real effort to give me a lot of details so that I can understand you better. I'm getting lost, and I'm not understanding you. I want you to know that I do want to understand you, and I can't when you go into so many details.
- If you had to express in one sentence all that you have been trying to tell me, what would you say?

If you are having reactions to a client like Bertha who overwhelms you with words, such as noticing that you have a hard time staying with her, it could be therapeutic to deal with your own reactions. Chances are that Bertha is affecting many people in her life in much the same way as she is affecting you. This is an opportunity for her to get feedback on how she comes across and for her to determine if she wants to do anything different. If you chronically suppress your reactions and pretend that you are listening with unconditional positive regard, she will soon pick up that you are not present for her. Also, by not dealing with her, you are reinforcing her talkativeness.

Clients who overwhelm themselves.   Some of your clients have so many problems that they feel chronically overwhelmed. Not only that, they may overwhelm you as well. Disaster seems to lurk constantly around the corner. Such clients often have an endless reserve of problems, as if they thrived on having and creating problems. They come in each week and excitedly begin with "Just wait until I tell you what happened to me this week." Although some of the situations they describe are terrible, you suspect that they get some sense of excitement out of reporting these incidents. A sample of the way some clients continue to overwhelm themselves can be seen from Ruth's statements:

> I've just got to tell you everything that happened this week. I got an "F" on one of my term papers, I'm having trouble getting financial aid, and if I don't get this aid, I can't stay in college. My daughter is having all sorts of problems with her boyfriend, and she comes to me late at night and wants to talk. Of course I listen, and then I get up in the morning feeling worn out. Then I don't have the energy to get through the day. My son is having problems at school. His counselor called me to tell me that he is truant much of the time. I had to go down to the school, and I surely didn't have time for that with all the things that went wrong last week. The toilet got stopped up, and of course I was the one who had to take care of that. Oh, by the way, the garbage disposal broke again, and there was a flood in the kitchen. I feel I have to handle everything, and all by myself. When my husband comes home, all he does is plop himself in front of the TV, watch the sports, and drink beer. I just don't see how I can hold up everything. I've got to be a terrific student, the one who repairs leaks, the counselor to my kids, and on top of that I should be understanding of my husband who doesn't want any more pressure when he comes home. Oh, I don't know where to begin. Everything seems to be pulling at me at once.

Although this may seem a bit dramatic and exaggerated, some of your clients will sound like this. As you listen, you may have a hard time making an impact. If you don't intervene actively and forcefully, yet sensitively, Ruth will not only overwhelm herself but you, too, will be at your wit's end. You will not know where to begin, and you are likely to feel burdened with all of her problems and think that you must solve them.

As with other forms of resistance, you need to explore with Ruth the ways in which she contributes to her problems by overwhelming herself. It can be helpful to tell her something like this: "Ruth, I know there are many things that you feel are pressing on you today. But we have only an hour, and we realistically can't attend to everything that has gone on with you all week. Why don't you sit quietly for a moment and reflect on what it is that you most want from this session? Select the one concern that is most pressing to you at this time." By focusing her, you are a catalyst in helping her to avoid being drowned in a sea of problems.

Clients who often say "Yes, but . . ."   You will encounter clients who are exceptionally talented at inventing reasons why your interventions just won't work. As a helper faced with such clients, you quickly feel deenergized. No matter what insights or hunches you share or what suggestions you make, the end result is the same: the client quickly retorts with an objection. Some illustrations of the "yes, but" syndrome follow:

HELPER: Have you considered telling your wife some of what you've told me?
CLIENT: "Yes, but you don't know my wife." "I agree that it might help, but my wife would be very threatened." "But my wife will never change!" "I'm willing to talk to her, but I don't think it would help."
HELPER: Every time I suggest something, you come back with plenty of reasons why my suggestion wouldn't work. I wonder if you really do want to change.

CLIENT: "Yes, but you just don't understand my situation." "You expect so much of me. I try, but things just don't work out." "Of course I want to change, but there are just so many things that keep me from changing. Only God knows how hard I try!"

When you are trying to help such clients, there is a danger of becoming too easily discouraged. It doesn't take much to get irritated with them. Even though you are willing to help this client, he is determined to prove to you that he cannot be helped. Eventually you are bound to feel helpless and to be inclined to give up. When you sense that you are working harder than your client is working, it may be time to renegotiate with him what he wants.

Clients who blame others.   Some clients assume a stance of being a victim and a martyr. They chronically blame circumstances and other people for everything that happens to them. Carrie is a good illustration of a client who is quick to find fault in the universe for her unhappiness but slow to recognize her part in contributing to her misery. She views herself as having no control over her life. She seems to refuse to consider her role in creating her own unhappiness, largely because she is so attuned to finding fault outside of herself. Here are just a few of the outside factors that she sees as being responsible for her misery: her husband does not understand her; her children are selfish and inconsiderate; she always feels miserable a few days before her period; she feels terrible when there is a full moon; she has severe allergies, which keep her from doing what she wants; she really can't lose weight because she is too depressed.

As long as Carrie puts the focus of her problems outside of herself, no change is possible in her life unless others change. If you allow her to talk continually about these others "out there," you have no power as a helper, because most of what she talks about is not in the room. It is possible for you to work with her to change, but you cannot work with all of the variables apart from her. You cannot control the moon, nor can you change some of the people in her life.

It would not be surprising if Carrie were to annoy you. You might engage in a lot of argumentation with her, challenging her on all of the ways in which she makes herself a martyr. If she continually refused to look at her own role, you might be tempted to refer her. As with most of these forms of resistance, it is important to keep clear within yourself and not get lost in the attempt to sway her. You can challenge her, share your reactions with her, listen to her, and ask her what she is willing to do to get what she says she wants.

Clients who deny needing help.   Difficult clients in another category do not see that they have a problem. Such clients may come to a marital counseling session to help their spouse but be unwilling to see their part in the troubled marriage. In fact, they may well deny that a problem even exists in the marriage. You can waste much valuable time by trying to convince these clients that they indeed have a problem when they insist otherwise. The denial of these clients is serving a function, for as long as they don't admit the problem, they don't have to cope with it.

For example, if you ask Roy what he wants from you, he will probably reply: "My wife wanted me to come to counseling, and I'm here for her sake." You may be better able to get through his resistance if you take his word for it and accept his view that he is problem free. By asking him how he is being affected by his wife's problems, you may eventually get to problems that he wants to deny. Another alternative is to ask him how it is for him to come to your office. If he replies by saying "Oh, it's fine," you could respond "What were you thinking as you approached the office?" Or you could ask: "You say you're here to help your wife. What are some of the areas that you think she needs help with?" Or you could say: "You tell me that you don't have any problems and that your wife made you come here today. Could *that* be a problem for you?"

Some of the students we work with in a counseling program are quick to say how much they want to help others but not so quick to identify issues in their own lives. We have heard such students talk about their problems in the past tense. They are ready to admit that they had problems, but they maintain that they have dealt with and solved these problems. In some of your classes you have probably had opportunities for experiential and personal-growth activities. Think about how open you were to exploring any facets of your life with others. Were you willing to look at your own life in an honest fashion? How much did you resist? How motivated were you to listen to and reflect on feedback that others gave you? If you find it difficult to own up to potential problems in your life, do you think you will be able to effectively challenge clients to make an honest assessment of what troubles them?

Clients who are overly dependent on you. Client dependency comes in many forms. There are clients who don't make any move without first checking it with you; those who continuously want you to tell them what you think of them; those who would like to call you at all hours of the day and night; those who want to become your friend; and those who want you to tell them what to do, how to do it, and when to do it.

If you have many clients whom you perceive as dependent, look at your possible role in fostering and maintaining their dependence on you. You might encourage clients to call you at any time, for example, without thinking that they will take you at your word. You might encourage them to call you before a job interview or right after the interview, so they can let you know how it went. It is important that you look at the ego gratification that you get from their dependence. These clients usually fear making decisions. For them, choices represent a threat. If they make the "wrong" choice, they are stuck with the responsibility. Along with accepting that we have choices comes the anxiety of using our freedom constructively and responsibly. Many clients want to escape from their freedom by making you responsible for choosing for them. In some ways they expect you to fill their parents' shoes. They are likely to develop transference reactions toward you and to treat you as an authority. If you buy into their manipulations and nurture their dependent tendencies, you are merely reinforcing their vision of themselves as helpless. They are bound to resent you if they consistently put you "up there" and themselves "down there."

Clients who manifest passive-aggressive behavior. Certain clients have learned to defend themselves from hurt by dealing with people indirectly. They use hostility and sarcasm as a part of their style of resistance. Whenever they do or say anything, they are highly evasive. If you want to give your reactions, they are likely to retort: "Well, you really shouldn't feel this way. When I made that remark, I was just kidding. You take me too seriously."

Some common signs of clients who exhibit passive-aggressive behavior are as follows: They often arrive late. They say little. You see reactions on their faces, yet they assure you that everything is fine. They giggle when you talk. They raise eyebrows, frown, sigh, shake their head, look bored, and show other nonverbal reactions but deny that anything is going on with them. They chronically draw attention to themselves, and when they have the attention, they do little with it. They tend to be seductive in many ways.

Clients who behave in passive-aggressive ways may be hard to deal with. You may feel that you have been hit, but you won't know what hit you. It is hard to deal directly with this kind of behavior because of its elusive quality. However, you will certainly have reactions to clients who make hostile remarks, who offer much sarcasm, and who seem to engage in hit-and-run behavior. One way of cutting through this indirect behavior is to be aware of what it brings up in you and to give your reactions. What is important in dealing with this behavior is to avoid making judgments about it. You are more likely to avoid further hostility when you describe the behavior you see and tell the clients how their behavior is affecting you. It is also useful to ask them if they are aware of their behavior and to tell you what it means.

Here are some possible questions to consider: "Do certain clients who display hostility remind me of any people in my life? What do I feel like when people are not direct and I sense that there are some things they are not telling me? Is it timely and appropriate for me to give my reactions to the hostility I perceive in my clients?"

Clients who rely primarily on their intellect. Individuals who block out any feelings and present themselves in highly detached ways are another type of difficult client. Any time they get close to an emotion, they find a way to pull themselves away from feelings and into a safer cognitive zone. They constantly try to figure out why they have a problem. They are adept at self-diagnosis and theorizing abstractly about the nature of their dysfunctions. They have learned that as long as they "stay in their head" they are safe. If they allow themselves to feel jealousy, pain, depression, anger, or any other emotion, they are not safe. To avoid experiencing anxiety, they have learned to insulate themselves from feelings.

Don't attack such clients and insist that they get to a feeling level. You can let them know how it is for you to be with them when they show little affect, but it is not helpful to try to strip away their defense. When they feel ready to let go of it, they will do so. Think about the ways in which you are affected in dealing with a man who remains very cerebral. If you are successful in getting him to give up his protection, will you be able to help him? Will you be able to be present for this person when his resistance melts and he gets in touch with years of bottled-up feelings? Will you be overwhelmed with his pain and run from it? If you are not there when he expresses his fear, will this prove to him that people will let him down when he releases his emotions?

Clients who use emotions as a defense. The opposite of the client who uses his or her intellect as a defense is the client who thrives on displaying emotions.

Such people are quick to weep, have no trouble "getting into feelings," and seem to enjoy catharsis. Their behavior may put you in a bind. You may have trouble trusting their emotions. You may become annoyed, feel manipulated by them, or somehow feel that they are not sincere.

We are not suggesting that clients who genuinely express emotions are resisting. We are talking about the difficult clients who have made a defense out of getting stuck in emotional material. When you are with such clients, reflect on what they bring out in you. It is possible that some of your highly emotional clients could remind you of people in your life who manipulated you with their emotions. For example, a sister might have succeeded in making you feel guilty when she cried and stormed out of the room. Now, as you work with clients who exhibit some of these behaviors, you may feel a lack of compassion for them and, in turn, wonder whether you have a problem with empathy.

Dealing Effectively With Resistance

It will help you greatly if you can conceptualize resistance, ambivalence, and defense as providing a window to certain inner aspects of the individual. Exploring resistance in a collaborative way provides an opportunity to observe the fascinating workings of internal conflict (Teyber, 2000). Learn to listen attentively and with respect as clients express their fears, reservations, and reluctances. Think about ways you can intervene when clients seem to make helping them extremely challenging. Here are some guidelines for you to consider:

- Express your reactions to clients without insulting them.
- Avoid responding to sarcastic remarks with sarcasm or to hostile comments with hostility.
- Provide clients with necessary information so they can get the most from the helping process.
- Encourage clients to explore their fears and hesitations rather than expecting immediate trust.
- Avoid judging a client; instead, describe the behavior you are observing that tends to be self-defeating.
- Share with a client how you are personally affected in a nonblaming way.
- State observations and hunches in a tentative way as opposed to being dogmatic.
- Be sensitive to clients who are culturally different from you without stereotyping a client because of his or her culture.
- Monitor your own countertransference reactions.
- Avoid using your power to intimidate those seeking help.
- Do not take clients' reactions in an overly personal way.

When we talk about dealing with difficult client behaviors in workshops, participants are always interested in learning specific strategies for dealing with the type of client behavior they find most frustrating. In our discussion here, we have avoided suggesting simple ways to change clients. Instead, we have put the focus on you, as a person and as a helper. You cannot directly change clients who are manifesting defensive behaviors, but you can learn significant lessons about the dynamics of their behavior as well as better understanding your own defenses.

Focus on why your clients have come to you, what they hope to get, and how you can teach them better ways of fulfilling their needs. If you respond in a negative manner to clients who exhibit negative behaviors, it will hamper your effectiveness with them. If you resist the temptation to attack their defenses, and if you avoid labeling or judging them, the chances of their defenses melting increase. If you are able to retain your own centeredness and be clear within yourself about your reactions to these clients, then avenues open up as you explore with your clients the meaning of their behavior.

By Way of Review

• Effective helpers must become aware of clients' transference and of their own countertransference. Neither of these factors is to be eliminated but is to be understood and dealt with therapeutically.

• Countertransference refers to the unrealistic reactions that therapists have toward their clients, which are likely to interfere with their objectivity. One way of becoming more aware of your potential for countertransference is by experiencing your own therapy. Another way is by focusing in your supervisory sessions on yourself and your reactions to clients.

• Resistance takes many forms, and it is necessary to understand the ways in which it serves as a protection for clients. Not all resistance stems from stubbornness on the part of the client. Some is caused, or at least contributed to, by the attitudes and behaviors of helpers.

• The goal in a helping relationship is not to eliminate resistance but to understand what functions it serves and to use it as a focus for exploration.

• There are many types of difficult clients. Some of them will evoke your own countertransference reactions. It is important to avoid reducing clients to a label.

What Will You Do Now?

1. Select the most difficult client whom you can imagine working with, and reflect on the reasons this client would present problems for you. What makes this client a difficult one? What do you think you would do if you actually had this person as a client? What might you do if you felt that you could not work with him or her?

2. Reflect on the kinds of resistance that you see within yourself. How open are you to accepting your faults and your limitations? If you were a client in

counseling, what resistances do you imagine that you might develop to changing? What do you think it would be like if your clients were very much like you? Talk with a friend about this subject as a way of confirming (or contradicting) your views.

3. Look over the descriptive list of difficult client behaviors and identity specific kinds of client behaviors you would find it most difficult to deal with in a helping relationship. In your journal write down what you can learn about yourself from your reactions to certain behaviors displayed by clients.

Look again at the inventory at the beginning of the chapter that helped you identify your self-doubts and fears pertaining to your role as a helper. Select one or two of these concerns and write about them. What are some steps you might take in dealing with your greatest concerns?

Review the attitude questionnaire on working with resistance and difficult clients. Write down your ideas about how you might become more therapeutic in dealing with resistance and difficult clients.

4. For the full bibliographic entry for each of the sources listed here, consult the References and Reading List at the back of the book. See Ellis (1999, 2002) and Ellis and MacLaren (1998) for a discussion of cognitive, emotive, and behavioral approaches in dealing with resistance. For ways of confronting and dealing with resistances, see Kottler (1993), and for an excellent treatment of what makes clients difficult and how to manage difficult cases, see Kottler (1992).

InfoTrac College Edition Resources

For additional readings, explore InfoTrac College Edition, our online library. Go to http://www.infotrac.college.com/wadsworth and select these key word searches:

transference
countertransference
difficult W1 client*
difficult W1 patient*
resistance psych*
resistance couns*
rational emotive behavior therapy

Key words are listed in a form that enables the search engine to locate a wider range of articles in the online university library. Key words should be entered exactly as shown, including asterisks, "W1," "W2," "AND," and other search engine tools.

CHAPTER *7*

Values and the Helping Relationship

Focus Questions

1. Are you aware of your key values and of how they are likely to affect the way you work with clients?

2. Is it possible for you to interact with your clients without making value judgments? Do you think it is sometimes appropriate to make value judgments? If so, when?

3. Can you remain true to your own values and at the same time make allowances for the right of your clients to make their own choices, even if they differ from the ones you might make?

4. Do you have a need to push what you think is right on your friends and your family? If so, what are the implications for the way you are likely to function as a helper with your clients?

5. Are you able to make the distinction between exposing your values and imposing them?

6. Do you see it as your job to make decisions for clients, or is it your job to help your clients make their own decisions?

7. Are you able to give your clients the latitude to make their own decisions, even if you believe that they would be better served by following a different path?

8. How can you best determine whether a conflict between your values and those of a client dictates a referral to another professional?

9. When you become aware of difficulties in working with clients because of value differences, what course of action would you take?

10. Can you identify certain key values that are an essential part of effective helping? How would you communicate such values to your clients?

Aim of the Chapter

This chapter is designed to help you clarify your values and identify how they are likely to influence your work as a helper. Toward this end, we explore how values operate in the helping relationship and process. Our focus is on the critical distinction between making your values known to a client and indoctrinating him or her with a particular ethics code or philosophy of life. To assist you in clarifying your values and identifying ways in which they might interfere with effective helping, we describe practical situations about which you may find yourself perplexed.

Conflicts between clients and helpers often surface in situations involving sexual orientation, family values, gender-role behaviors, religious and spiritual values, abortion, sexuality, and end-of-life decisions. Value issues pertaining to multicultural populations are so important that we devote Chapter 8 in its entirety to this subject.

The Role of Values in Helping

Although the professional literature reveals an interest in the role values play in the helping process, no consensus has been reached on which values are essential to helping or on how values should be used in the helping relationship (Bergin, 1991). Bergin compares the helping process to what occurs with effective parenting: After trust has been established in the relationship, helpers deal with values in a respectful way and offer guidance that allows for growth. Through the helping relationship, clients learn how to clarify and test their value choices, and they experiment with new behaviors and ideas until they become more mature and autonomous. As the person receiving help becomes stronger and more independent, the helper reduces external guidance. Helpers do not do for their clients what the clients are able to do for themselves.

Values are embedded in therapeutic theory and practice. A national survey of the mental health values of practitioners (Jensen & Bergin, 1988) found a consensus that certain basic values are important for maintaining mentally healthy lifestyles and for guiding and evaluating the course of treatment. These values include assuming responsibility for one's actions; developing effective strategies for coping with stress; developing the ability to give and receive affection; being sensitive to the feelings of others; practicing self-control; having a sense of purpose for living; being open, honest, and genuine; finding satisfaction in one's work; having a sense of identity and feelings of worth; being skilled in interpersonal relationships, sensitivity, and nurturance; being committed in marriage, family, and other relationships; having deepened self-awareness and motivation for growth; and practicing good habits of physical health. These are seen as universal values on which helping relationships are based.

We suggest that you take the following self-inventory as a way of focusing your thinking on the role that your values will play in your work. As you read the following statements, decide the degree to which each most closely identifies your attitudes and beliefs about *your role as a helper*. Use this code: 3 = this statement is true for me; 2 = this statement is not true for me; 1 = I am undecided.

_____ 1. I see it as my job to challenge a client's philosophy of life.

_____ 2. I could work objectively and effectively with clients who had values that differed sharply from my own.

_____ 3. I see it as both possible and desirable for me to remain neutral with respect to values when working with clients.

_____ 4. Although I have a clear set of values for myself, I feel quite certain that I could avoid unduly influencing my clients to adopt my beliefs.

_____ 5. I think it is appropriate to express my views and expose my values, so long as I don't impose them on clients.

_____ 6. I might be inclined to subtly influence my clients to consider my values.

_____ 7. If I discovered sharp value conflicts between a client and myself, I would refer the person.

_____ 8. I have certain religious views that would influence the way I work.

_____ 9. I would not have any difficulty counseling a pregnant adolescent who wanted to explore abortion as one of her alternatives.

_____ 10. I have certain views pertaining to gender roles that might affect the way I counsel.

_____ 11. I would not have problems counseling a gay couple.

_____ 12. I see the clarification of values as the central task of the helping process.

_____ 13. My view of family life would influence the way I would counsel a couple considering divorce.

_____ 14. I would have no trouble working with a woman (man) who wanted to leave her (his) children and live alone, if this is what my client decided.

_____ 15. I have generally been willing to challenge my values, and I think I have largely chosen them for myself.

_____ 16. I would have no trouble working in individual counseling with a married client who was having an affair, even if the client was not willing to disclose the relationship to his or her spouse.

_____ 17. I feel quite certain that my values will never interfere with my capacity to remain objective.

_____ 18. I think I will work best with clients who have values similar to mine.

_____ 19. I think it is appropriate to pray with my clients during a session, if they request this of me.

_____ 20. I could work effectively with a person with AIDS who contracted the disease through IV drug use.

There are no "right" or "wrong" answers to these statements. The inventory is designed to help you think about how your values are likely to influence the way you carry out your functions as a helper. You might take some specific items that catch your attention and talk with a fellow student about your views. As you read the rest of the chapter, assume an active stance, and think about your position on the value issues we raise. A basic question is whether it is possible for helpers to keep their values out of their work.

Exposing Values Versus Imposing Them

The clients with whom you work ultimately have the responsibility of choosing what values to adopt, what values to modify or discard, and what direction their lives will take. Through the helping process, clients can learn to examine values before making choices. You can play a significant role as a catalyst for this examination if you do not either conceal your values from your clients or try to impose your values on them. When you do expose your values, it is essential that you clearly label them as your own. In this way values can be discussed in an open and noncoercive way, which can assist clients in their exploration of their own values and the behavior that stems from these values.

At times, you may not agree with the values of your clients, but it is essential that you respect the rights of your clients to hold a different set of values. Richards, Rector, and Tjeltveit (1999) do not think helpers should attempt to teach their clients specific moral rules and values because doing so violates clients' diversity and prevents clients from growing by making their own choices based on their values. In agreement with this view is Patterson (1989), who argues against indoctrinating clients or attempting to inculcate a value system or a philosophy of life in them. Patterson rightly emphasizes that because the values helpers hold cannot be kept out of their work, they should not refuse to discuss their core values. He believes it is appropriate for practitioners to make their values known when a client requests it, when they determine that it is necessary or desirable, or when they judge that the helping process will be improved by it.

Even if you think it is inappropriate to impose your values on clients, you may unintentionally influence them in subtle ways to embrace your values. Indeed, some researchers have found evidence that clients tend to change in ways that are consistent with the values of their counselors, and clients often adopt the values of their counselors (Zinnbauer & Pargament, 2000). It is now generally recognized that the therapeutic endeavor is a value-laden process and that all counselors, to some degree, communicate their values to clients (Richards & Bergin, 1997). An abundance of evidence shows that the helping process is not only value laden but that counselors and clients often share different value systems (Zinnbauer & Pargament, 2000). It will be difficult to avoid communicating your values to your clients, even if you do not explicitly share them. What you pay attention to during counseling sessions will direct what your clients choose to explore. The methods you use will provide them with clues to what you value. Your body messages give them indications of when you like or dislike what they are doing. Because your clients may feel a need to have your approval, they may respond to these clues by acting in ways that they imagine will meet with your favor instead of developing their own inner direction.

If you cannot be neutral, your client has a right to be clearly informed about this. We hope that there would be very few instances where you would have to tell clients that you could not work with them because you do not agree with their value system. Your job is not to judge your clients' values but to help them explore and clarify their beliefs and apply their values to solving their own problems. The American Counseling Association (1995) states this clearly: "Counselors are aware of their own values, attitudes, beliefs, and behaviors and how they apply in a diverse society, and avoid imposing their values on clients" (A.5.b.). Helpers do indeed have personal values that influence their professional work. From an ethical perspective, it is imperative that helpers recognize the impact their values have on their professional work and that they learn the difference between imposing and exposing values.

Our Perspective on Values in the Helping Relationship

In our view it is neither possible nor desirable for helpers to remain neutral or to keep their values separate from their professional relationships. Because values have a significant impact on the helping process, it is important to express them openly when doing so is appropriate. If you pay attention to your clients and why they are coming to see you, you will have clues to when that is.

There are certainly helpers who do not agree with our position about the role of values. On one extreme are those who see helping as very much a process of social influence. Some helpers, for example, have definite and absolute value systems, and they believe it is their proper function to influence their clients to adopt this view of the world. At the other extreme are helpers who are so concerned about unduly influencing their clients that they remain scrupulously neutral. Out of fear that their views might contaminate the client's decision, these helpers make it a practice not to expose their values. Or they err by assuming that the nonimposition of values means that they do not commit themselves to any set of values, when, in fact, some values are fundamental to the healing process.

Our position is that the helper's main task is to provide those who seek aid with the impetus needed to look at what they are doing, determine the degree to which what they are doing is consistent with their values, and consider whether their current behavior is getting them what they want. If clients conclude that their lives are not fulfilled, they can use the helping relationship to reexamine and modify their values or their actions, and they can explore a range of options that are open to them. Clients must ask themselves who and what they are, and they are the ones who will determine what they are willing to change.

Are Your Values Showing?

As a beginning helper, you may have a tendency to expect your clients to adopt your values. Even though you may not blatantly push your values onto clients, you may lead clients in subtle ways in the direction you think they should go. If you are strongly opposed to abortion, for example, you may not even consider that your client has a right to believe differently. On the basis of such convictions, you may subtly (or not so subtly) direct your client toward choices other than abortion. It is unfortunate that some well-intentioned helpers think that their job is to help people conform to acceptable and absolute value standards or to prescribe a particular direction for their clients.

Our own practice is to tell clients of some of our values that are likely to affect our work with them. These would include value orientations that are a basic part of the counseling process. To give you an idea of what we mean, we think that the examined life is better than the unexamined life. We operate on the assumption that people are not victims and that with awareness and commitment to taking action they can make substantial changes in their lives. Another bias we hold is that psychological pain is frequently a useful source to explore. If clients identify painful experiences and are willing to express them, the chances are that they will be led to significant unfinished business that is important in their life now. One of the values that we promote is self-determination, or choosing for oneself and accepting the responsibility and consequences for these choices. Although some individuals would like others to choose for them, we assume that the helping relationship is aimed at assisting people to find their own best decisions. These are but a few examples of the values that we are open about. Furthermore, if we have a difficult time with clients because it seems to us that they are behaving in ways that are inconsistent with their values, we confront them on this discrepancy.

Value Conflicts With Clients

Exposing your values can be very useful. This is especially true in situations where you discover that you and your clients have sharp value differences. If you know that you would have a difficult time working objectively with someone because of such conflicts, ethical practice dictates that you not accept the person as a client. If you find yourself struggling with an ethical dilemma over value differences, seek consultation. Supervision is often a profitable way to explore value clashes with clients. After exploring the issues in supervision, if you find that you are still not able to work effectively with this client, the ethical course of action might be to refer the client to another professional.

If you find it necessary to make a referral because of value conflicts, we are convinced that *how* the referral is discussed with the client is crucial. Make it clear to the client that it is *your* problem as the helper, not the client's. In short, if you feel a need to refer a client, the problem is likely to reside more in you than in a particular client.

Yarhouse and VanOrman (1999) contend that value conflicts in the therapeutic relationship are inevitable. Merely having a conflict of values does not necessarily imply the need for a referral, for it is possible to work through a conflict successfully. We hope that you will not be too quick to refer when there are conflicting value systems but that you will challenge yourself to determine what it is about a client that prompts you to want to make the referral. Why is it necessary for you to embrace a client's values? Or why is it a requirement that your clients accept your values in a particular area of living?

In the remainder of this chapter, we consider some value-laden issues that you are likely to encounter in your work with a range of client populations. Some of these areas include concerns of gay, lesbian, and bisexual individuals; family issues; values pertaining to gender-role identity; religious and spiritual values; abortion; sexuality; and end-of-life decisions.

Gay, Lesbian, and Bisexual Issues

Many helpers have blind spots, biases, negative attitudes, and misconceptions about lesbian, gay, and bisexual issues. If you hope to work effectively with these clients, it is absolutely essential that you begin by becoming aware of and challenging your own attitudes and assumptions about homosexuality and bisexuality. It is also essential that you identify your own biases, challenge any myths and misconceptions that you might hold, and that you be open to understanding how your values regarding sexual orientation are likely to affect your work.

Imagine yourself in a situation where you are seeing a gay man who wants to talk about his relationship with his lover and the difficulties they have in communicating with each other. As you work with him, you become aware that it is difficult for you to accept his sexual orientation. You find yourself challenging him about this, and you are not concentrating on what he says he wants to work on. Instead, you are focused on his sexual orientation, which is totally unacceptable to you, for it goes against what you think is morally right. These reactions are so much in the foreground that you and your client recognize that you are not helping him. If you were in this situation, what steps would you take in addressing the role of value differences? What would you be willing to do to explore the impact of your values on your interventions with this gay man?

Now, put yourself in the following situation and consider how your values are likely to influence the way in which you would work with Art.

The situation.   You are doing an intake interview with a gay man, age 33. Art tells you that he is coming to counseling because he often feels lonely and isolated. He has difficulty in intimate relationships, with men or women. Once people get to know him, Art feels they will not accept him and somehow won't like him. During the interview you find out that Art has a lot of pain over his father, with whom he has very little contact. He would like a closer relationship with his father, but being gay stands in the way. His father has let him know that he feels guilty that Art "turned out that way." He just cannot understand why Art is not "normal" and why he can't find a woman and get married like his brother. Art mainly wants to work on his relationship with his father, and he also wants to overcome his fear of rejection by others with whom he would like a close relationship. He tells you that he would like those he cares about to accept him as he is.

Your stance.   What are your initial reactions to Art's situation? Considering your own values, do you expect that you would have any trouble establishing a therapeutic relationship with him? In light of the fact that he lets you know that he does not want to change his sexual orientation, would you be able to respect this decision? As you think about how you would proceed with Art, reflect on your own attitudes toward gay men. Think especially whether you might be inclined to push any of your values, regardless of your stance. For example, if you have personal difficulty in accepting homosexuality on moral or other grounds, might you encourage Art to become heterosexual? You might focus on a number of issues in your counseling sessions with Art, some of which are his fear of rejection, pain with his father, desire for his father to be different, difficulty in getting close to both men and women, sexual orientation, and values. With the information you have, which of these areas are you likely to emphasize? Are there other areas you might want to explore with Art?

Discussion.   If you have a conservative value system, you may be challenged if you work with lesbian, gay, and bisexual people. Although you may tell yourself and others that you accept the right of others to live their lives as they see fit, you may have trouble when you are in an actual encounter with a client. There could be a gap between what you can intellectually accept and what you can emotionally accept. If you have negative emotional or intellectual reactions to lesbian, gay, and bisexual people, there is a danger that you could try to impose your own values if you accepted these individuals as clients.

Homosexuality and bisexuality were assumed to be a form of mental illness for over a century. Today, all major American mental health professional associations have affirmed that homosexuality is not a mental illness, and the American Psychological Association's Division 44 (2000) has developed a set of guidelines for working with lesbian, gay, and bisexual clients. But bias and misinformation about homosexuality and bisexuality continue to be widespread in society, and many lesbian, gay, and bisexual people face social stigmatization, discrimination, and violence. Oftentimes families of origin are unprepared to accept a lesbian, gay, or bisexual family member because of familial, ethnic, cultural, or religious beliefs. Families may need assistance in developing new understandings of sexual orientation (APA, 2000).

Helpers who intend to provide services for lesbian, gay, and bisexual people are ethically obligated to develop the knowledge and skills to competently deliver services to these clients. Although space restricts the full discussion this topic deserves, we present a few guidelines from APA's Division 44 (Committee on Lesbian, Gay, and Bisexual Concerns Joint Task Force on Guidelines for Psychotherapy with Lesbian, Gay, and Bisexual Clients). These guidelines address attitudes toward homosexuality and bisexuality, relationships and families, issues of diversity, and education.

- Psychologists are encouraged to recognize how their attitudes and knowledge about lesbian, gay, and bisexual issues may be relevant to assessment and treatment and seek consultation or make appropriate referrals when indicated.
- Psychologists strive to understand the particular circumstances and challenges faced by lesbian, gay, and bisexual parents.
- Psychologists are encouraged to recognize the particular life issues or challenges that are related to multiple and often conflicting cultural norms, values, and beliefs that lesbian, gay, and bisexual members of racial and ethnic minorities face.
- Psychologists strive to understand the special problems and risks that exist for lesbian, gay, and bisexual youth.

- Psychologists are encouraged to increase their knowledge and understanding of homosexuality and bisexuality through continuing education, training, supervision, and consultation.
- Psychologists make reasonable efforts to familiarize themselves with relevant mental health, educational, and community resources for lesbian, gay, and bisexual people.

If you do not have the knowledge and skill competencies to work with lesbian, gay, and bisexual clients, take advantage of continuing-education workshops in coming to a fuller understanding of these special client populations. By participating in such workshops, you can learn about referral resources as well as about specific interventions and strategies that are appropriate for gay and lesbian clients. If you do not possess knowledge and training about a specific group, ethically you would be required to seek supervision and consultation or make referrals to appropriately trained professionals. Crawford and colleagues (1999) recommend that before you offer mental health services to gay and lesbian people and their children, you should complete formal, systematic training on sexual diversity.

You might well be unaware of your client's sexual orientation until the therapeutic relationship develops. Even if you do not plan to work with a homosexual or bisexual client population, you need to have a clear idea of your own attitudes and values relative to issues associated with sexual orientation.

As a way of clarifying your values pertaining to homosexuality, take the following inventory, using this code: 3 = I agree, in most respects, with this statement; 2 = I am undecided in my opinion about this statement; 1 = I disagree, in most respects, with this statement.

_____ 1. Lesbian, gay, and bisexual clients are best served by lesbian, gay, and bisexual helpers.

_____ 2. A counselor who is homosexual or bisexual is likely to push his or her values on a heterosexual client.

_____ 3. I would have trouble working with either a gay male couple or a lesbian couple who wanted to adopt children, even if they were fit parents.

_____ 4. Homosexuality is a form of mental illness.

_____ 5. A lesbian, gay, or bisexual person can be as well adjusted (or poorly adjusted) as a heterosexual person.

_____ 6. Homosexuality and bisexuality are immoral.

_____ 7. I would have no difficulty being objective in counseling lesbian, gay, and bisexual clients.

_____ 8. I have adequate information about referral sources in the local gay community.

_____ 9. I feel a need for specialized training and knowledge before I can effectively counsel lesbian, gay, and bisexual clients.

_____ 10. I expect that I would have no difficulty conducting family therapy if the father were gay.

After you finish the inventory, look over your responses to identify any patterns. Are there any attitudes that you want to change? Are there any areas of information or skills that you are willing to acquire?

Family Issues

A situation involving a restless mother.   Veronika has lived a repressed life. She got married at 17, had four children by the age of 22, and is now going back to college at age 32. She is a good student—excited, eager to learn, and discovering all that she missed. She finds that she is attracted to a younger peer group and to professors. She is now experiencing her second adolescence, and she is getting a lot of affirmation that she did not have before. At home she has been taken for granted, and the members of her family are mostly interested in what she can do for them. At school she is special and is respected for her intellect.

Ultimately, Veronika becomes involved in an affair with a younger man. She is close to a decision to leave her husband and her four children, ages 10 to 15. She comes to see you at the university counseling center. Veronika is in turmoil over what to do, and she wants to find some way to deal with her guilt and ambivalence.

Your stance.   For a moment, consider your own value system. If Veronika were asking for your advice, what would you be inclined to say? What are your thoughts about her leaving her husband? her four children? Would you encourage her to "do her own thing"? If Veronika gave this matter considerable thought and then told you that, as painful as it would be for her own growth and well-being, she needed to leave her family, what would be your stance? Would you be inclined to encourage her to bring her entire family in for some counseling sessions? What values do you think you might push, if any? If she told you that she was leaning toward staying married and at home, even though she would be resentful, what interventions might you make? If you had been left yourself, either as a child or by a spouse, how might this trauma affect you in working with Veronika?

A situation involving a family in crisis.   A wife, husband, and three adolescent children come to your office. The family was referred by the youngest boy's child-welfare and attendance officer. The boy is acting out by stealing and is viewed as the problem person in the family.

The husband is in your office reluctantly. He appears angry and resistant, and he lets you know that he doesn't believe in this "therapy stuff." He makes excuses for the boy and says he doesn't see that there is much of a problem, either in the marriage or in the family.

The wife tells you that she and her husband fight a lot, that there is much tension in the home, and that the children are suffering. She is fearful and says that she is afraid of what might happen to her family. She has no way of supporting herself and her three children and is willing to work on the relationship.

Your stance.   How would you be affected by having this family in your office? What course of action would you take? How would your values pertaining to family life influence your interventions with this family? Would you expose your own values in this case, even if the family members did not ask you? If they asked you what you thought of their situation and what you thought they should do, what would you say?

A situation involving an affair. A couple seek your services for marital counseling. The husband has confessed to his wife that he is having an affair, and the incident has precipitated the most recent crisis in their relationship. Although the wife is highly distraught, she wants to stay married. She realizes that their marriage needs work and that there is boredom between the two of them, yet she thinks it is worth it to work on their problems. They have children, and the family is well respected and liked in the community.

The husband wants to leave and live with his newfound lover, yet he is struggling with conflicting feelings and is not sure what to do. He is very confused, for he still loves his wife and children. He is aware that he is going through a midlife crisis, and each day he comes up with a different decision. His wife is in a great deal of pain and feels desperate. She has been totally dependent on him, with no means of support.

Your stance. What are your values pertaining to affairs in a marriage? What would you want to say to the wife? to the husband? Should a helper counsel a couple to stay together or get divorced?

In thinking about the direction you might pursue with this family, consider whether you have ever been in this situation yourself in your own family. If so, how do you think this experience would affect the way you worked with the couple? If the husband said he was confused, desperately wanted an answer, and was hoping that you would point him in some direction, would you be inclined to tell him what you thought he should do?

Gender-Role Identity

The situation. Fernando and Elizabeth describe themselves as a "traditional couple." They are in marriage counseling with you to work on the strains in their relationship that arise from rearing their two adolescent sons. The couple talk a lot about their sons. Both Elizabeth and Fernando work full time outside the home. Besides working as an elementary school principal, Elizabeth has another full-time job as mother and homemaker. Fernando says he is not about to do any "women's work" around the house. Elizabeth has never really given much thought to the fact that she has a dual career. Neither Elizabeth nor Fernando shows a great deal of interest in critically examining the cultural stereotypes that they have incorporated. Each of them has a definite vision of what women and men "should be." Rather than talking about their relationship or the inequalities of the distribution of tasks at home, they focus the attention on troubles with their sons. Elizabeth wants advice on how to deal with their problems.

Your stance. If you become aware of the tension between this couple over traditional gender roles, will you call it to their attention in your counseling with them? Do you see it as your job to challenge Fernando on his traditional views? Do you see it as your job to encourage Elizabeth to want more equality in their relationship? If you were counseling this couple, what do you think you might say to each of them? How would your values influence the direction in which you might go? What bearing would your own gender-role conditioning and your own views have on what you did?

Discussion. If you will be working with couples and families, it is essential that you appreciate the fact that gender-role stereotypes serve a purpose and are not easily modified. As a helper, your role is to guide your clients in the process of examining their gender-role attitudes and behaviors, if doing so is relevant to the problem for which they are seeking your services. You must examine your own beliefs about appropriate family roles and responsibilities, child-rearing practices, multiple roles for women, and traditional and nontraditional family arrangements. Effective communication between you and your clients can be undermined by stereotypical views about how women and men think, feel, and behave. You need to be alert to the particular issues women and men struggle with and the ways their own views about gender keep them locked in traditional roles. You can offer assistance to both female and male clients in exploring and evaluating cultural messages they received about gender-role expectations. Without deciding for them what changes they should make, you can facilitate awareness on the part of your clients, which will open up new possibilities for making self-directed choices.

Margolin (1982) provides some recommendations on how to be a nonsexist family therapist and to confront negative expectations and stereotyped roles in the family. One suggestion is that helpers should examine their own behavior and attitudes that would imply sex-differentiated roles and status. For example, helpers can show their bias in subtle ways by looking at the husband when talking about making decisions and looking at the wife when talking about home matters and rearing children. Margolin also contends that practitioners are especially vulnerable to the following biases: (1) assuming that remaining married would be the best choice for a woman, (2) demonstrating less interest in a woman's career than in a man's career, (3) encouraging couples to accept the belief that child rearing is solely the responsibility of the mother, (4) showing a different reaction to a wife's affair than to a husband's, and (5) giving more importance to satisfying the husband's needs than to satisfying the wife's needs. Margolin raises two critical questions for those who work with couples and families:

- How does the counselor respond when members of the family seem to agree that they want to work toward goals that (from the counselor's vantage point) are sexist in nature?
- To what extent does the helper accept the family's definition of gender-role identities rather than trying to challenge and eventually change these attitudes?

Religious and Spiritual Values

Contrary to the myth that helping professionals have little interest in spiritual matters, Elkins (1994) suggests that the majority of clinicians are now paying more attention to the spiritual dimensions of the human being. Many clients are hungry for therapeutic experiences that offer them help with the spiritual and existential issues of life. Elkins calls for a "soulful psychology" and concludes that psychotherapy ought to be considered a journey of the soul in search of its own healing.

Miranti and Burke (1995) state that helpers must be prepared to deal with spiritual issues that lie at the very core and essence of the client's being. For many clients who are in crisis, the spiritual domain offers solace and comfort and is a major sustaining power that keeps them going when all else seems to fail. According to Miranti and Burke, the guilt, anger, and sadness that clients experience often result from a misinterpretation of the spiritual and religious realm, which can lead to depression and a sense of worthlessness. It is essential that helpers be open and nonjudgmental to their clients who may be going through some life transition, for their spiritual beliefs can be a major source of strength as they make crucial life decisions. Miranti and Burke remind us: "For counselors, the challenge is not whether the issue of spirituality should be addressed, but how it can best be addressed by well-prepared and sensitive professionals" (p. 3).

The situation.   Your client has a fundamentalist background. Peter has definite ideas about right and wrong, sin, guilt, and damnation, and he has accepted the teachings of his church without question. When he encountered difficulties and problems in the past, he was able to pray and find comfort in his relationship with his God. Lately, however, he has been suffering from chronic depression, an inability to sleep, extreme feelings of guilt, and an overwhelming sense of doom that God is going to punish him for his transgressions. He consulted his physician and asked for medication to help him sleep better. The physician, as well as his minister, both suggested that he seek counseling. At first Peter resisted this idea, for he strongly felt that he should find comfort in his religion. With the continuation of his bouts of depression and sleeplessness, he hesitantly comes to you for advice.

He requests that you open the session with a prayer so that he can get into a proper spiritual frame of mind. He also quotes you a verse from the Bible that has special meaning to him. He tells you about his doubts about seeing you for counseling, and he is concerned that you will not accept his religious convictions, which he sees as being at the center of his life. He inquires about your religious beliefs.

Your stance.   Would you have any trouble counseling Peter? He is struggling with trusting you and with seeing the value in counseling. What are your reactions to some of his specific views, especially those pertaining to his fear of punishment? Do you have reactions to his strong fundamentalist beliefs? If you have definite disagreements with his beliefs, could you be accepting of him? Would you challenge him to think for himself and do what he thinks is right? Would you encourage him to question his religion?

Assume that you have a religious orientation, yet you believe in a God of love whereas Peter believes in a God of fear. You let him know that you have differences in the way the two of you perceive religion. Yet you also say that you want to explore with him how well his religious beliefs are serving him in his life and also examine possible connections between some of his beliefs and how they are contributing to his symptoms. With these assumptions, do you think you could be helpful to Peter? Would you accept him as a client?

Now assume that you don't share any of Peter's religious values, that you are intolerant of fundamentalist beliefs, and that you see such beliefs as doing far more harm than good for people. Given these values, would you accept a client like Peter? Would you be able to work with him objectively, or would you try to find ways to sway him to give up his view of the world?

Discussion. Research reveals that approximately 96% of Americans believe in God and 75% of the American population view religious faith as being a very important part of their lives. At the same time, only 33% of psychologists believe that religious faith is important in their own lives (Plante, 1999). It is essential that helpers seek clarity about their own spiritual and religious beliefs if they hope to gain an in-depth appreciation of the beliefs and worldviews of their clients (Faiver, Ingersoll, O'Brien, & McNally, 2001). Ethical practice requires that you avoid indoctrinating clients with a particular set of spiritual or religious values. You have an ethical responsibility to be aware of how your beliefs affect your work and to make sure you do not unduly influence your clients.

Even if spiritual and religious issues are not the focus of a client's concern, these values may enter into the sessions indirectly as the client explores moral conflicts or grapples with questions of meaning in life. Can you keep your spiritual and religious values out of these sessions? How do you think they will influence the way you counsel? If you have little belief in spirituality or are hostile to organized religions, can you be nonjudgmental? Can you empathize with clients who view themselves as being deeply spiritual or who feel committed to the teachings of a particular church?

As you formulate your own position on the place of spiritual and religious values in the helping relationship, reflect on these questions:

- Is it appropriate to deal with religious issues in an open and forthright manner as clients' needs arise in the helping process?
- Do clients have the right to explore their religious concerns in the context of the helping process?
- If you have no religious or spiritual commitment, how might this hinder or help you in working with diverse clients?
- Are you willing to refer a client to a rabbi, minister, or priest if it appears that clients have questions that you are not qualified to answer?

The situation. Guiza is a student intern who feels deeply committed to spirituality and also claims that her religious faith guides her in finding meaning in life. While she does not want to impose her values on her clients, she does feel it is essential to at least make a general assessment of clients' spiritual/religious beliefs and experiences during the intake session. One of her clients, Alejandro, tells Guiza that he is depressed most of the time and feels a sense of emptiness. He wonders what is the meaning of his life. In Guiza's assessment of Alejandro, she finds that he grew up without any kind of spiritual or religious guidance in his home, and he states that he is agnostic. He never has explored either religion or spirituality, for these ideas seem too abstract to help with the practical problems of everyday living. Guiza becomes aware that she is strongly inclined to suggest to Alejandro that he open up to spiritual ways of thinking, especially because of his stated problem with finding meaning in his life. Guiza is tempted to suggest that Alejandro at least go to a few church services to see if he might find any meaning in doing so. She brings her struggle to her supervisor.

Your stance.   It is very likely that you will experience conflicts in values with your clients in the spiritual realm. If you hold a definite system of religious values, you may have a tendency to want your clients to adopt these values. Without blatantly pushing your values, you might subtly persuade clients to your religious beliefs or lead them in a direction you hope they will take. Conversely, if you do not place a high priority on spirituality and do not view religion as a salient force in your life, you may not be open to assessing your client's religious and spiritual beliefs. Consider Guiza's situation as you reflect on how your values might influence your approach with clients. When, if ever, would you recommend to your client that he or she talk to a minister, priest, or rabbi? If you sought consultation from your supervisor, what key issues would you most want to explore and clarify? Could you maintain your objectivity? When would you consider suggesting a referral because of conflicts between you and your client with respect to spiritual/religious beliefs and values?

Discussion.   Faiver and O'Brien (1993) have devised a form to assess the religious beliefs of clients for diagnostic, treatment, and referral purposes. They suggest that the assessment process can include questions pertaining to spiritual and religious issues as they are relevant to a client's presenting problems, questions about the roles religion and spirituality have played or currently play in a client's life, and questions about how spiritual/religious beliefs might be related to the client's cognitive, affective, and behavioral processes. Kelly (1995b) is in agreement with Faiver and O'Brien that a first step is to include the spiritual and religious dimensions as a regular part of the intake procedure and the early phase of the counseling process. Including questions pertaining to the client's spirituality and religion serves three purposes: (a) obtaining a preliminary indication of the relevance of spirituality and religion for each client, (b) gathering information that the helper might refer to at a later point in the helping process, and (c) indicating to the client that it is acceptable to talk about religious and spiritual concerns.

There are many paths toward fulfilling spiritual needs, and it is not the helper's task to prescribe any particular pathway. However, we think that it is the helper's responsibility to be aware that spirituality is a significant force for many of their clients. It is especially important for a practitioner to pursue spiritual concerns if the client initiates them. As part of the assessment process, it is good practice to ask about a client's spiritual and religious beliefs and values. If clients indicate that they are concerned about any of their beliefs or practices, this is a useful focal point for exploration. The key here is that the practitioner remain finely tuned to the client's story and to the purpose for which he or she sought professional assistance.

In clarifying your values pertaining to religion and counseling, consider these questions: Does an exploration of religion belong in formal helping relationships? Is the helping process complete without a spiritual dimension? If a client's religious needs arise in the therapeutic relationship, is it appropriate to deal with them? Are helpers pushing their values on their clients when they decide what topics can and cannot be discussed in counseling? Do you have to hold the same religious beliefs to work effectively with clients who have religious struggles?

Abortion

The situation.   Connie, a 19-year-old college student, seeks your assistance because she is contemplating having an abortion. A part of her wants to have the abortion, while another part of her wants to have the child. Connie is thinking about telling her parents, but is concerned because they would have a definite idea of what she should do. She is also considering the option of having her child and giving it up for adoption. She is unable to sleep and feels guilty for having gotten herself into this situation. She has talked to her friends and solicited their advice. She has gotten many contradictory recommendations. Connie lets you know that she is not at all sure about what to do and asks you for advice.

Your stance.   With the information you have, what are some things you would say to Connie? Think about your values pertaining to abortion. Would you dissuade her from having an abortion and suggest other options? To what extent do you think you could keep your values out of this session?

Sometimes we hear students say that they would refer a pregnant client who was considering an abortion to another professional because of their values. They would not like to sway the woman, and they fear that they could not remain objective. Does this apply to you? What would you do if a client of yours happened to get pregnant while she was in treatment with you? Would you refer her at this point? What if she felt that you were abandoning her?

Sexuality

Situation involving a sex-education program.   You are working in a facility for adolescents and are doing a good deal of individual and group counseling. You discover that many young teenagers are sexually active and that a number of them have gotten pregnant. Abortion is common. Many of these young women keep their babies, whether or not they get married. The agency director asks you to design a comprehensive education program for preventing unwanted pregnancy.

Your stance.   In thinking about the kind of program you would suggest, consider these questions: What are your values with respect to teenagers' being sexually active? What are your attitudes about providing detailed birth-control information to children and adolescents? How would your own values influence the design of your program?

Situation involving sex in a nursing home.   You are working in a nursing home. You discover that several of the unmarried elderly residents have sexual relationships. At a staff meeting several other workers begin to complain that supervision is not tight enough and that sex between unmarried residents should not be permitted. What input would you want to have in this staff meeting? What are your thoughts about unmarried elderly people engaging in sex? How would your own values affect your recommendations to the staff?

Assessing your sexual values. Consider your values with respect to sexuality, as well as where you acquired them. How comfortable are you in discussing sexual issues with clients? Are you aware of any barriers that could prevent you from working with clients on sexual issues? How would your experiences in sexual relationships (or the lack of them) influence your work with clients in this area? Would you promote your sexual values? For example, if a teenage client was promiscuous and this behavior was in large part a form of rebellion against her parents, would you be inclined to challenge her behavior? Or if a teenage client took no birth-control precautions yet was sexually active with many partners, would you urge him or her to use birth control? Or would you encourage abstinence? Or would you recommend that he or she be more selective in choosing sexual partners?

Although you may say that you are open-minded and that you can accept sexual attitudes and values that differ from your own, it may be the case that you are inclined to try to change clients who you believed were involved in self-destructive practices. Assess your attitudes toward casual sex, premarital sex, teen sexuality, and extramarital sex. What are your attitudes toward monogamy? What do you consider to be the physical and psychological hazards of sex with more than one partner? How would your views on this issue influence the direction you would take with clients in exploring sexual concerns?

When you have made this assessment, ask yourself whether you would be able to work objectively with a person who had sexual values sharply divergent from yours. If you have very conservative views about sexual behavior, for example, will you be able to accept the liberal views of some of your clients? If you think their moral values are contributing to the difficulties they are experiencing in their lives, will you be inclined to persuade them to adopt your conservative values?

From another perspective, if you see yourself as having liberal sexual attitudes, how do you think you would react to a person with traditional values? Assume your unmarried client says that he would like to have more sexual experiences but that his religious upbringing has instilled in him the belief that premarital sex is a sin. Whenever he has come close to having sexual experiences, he has been burdened with guilt. He would like to learn to enjoy sex without feeling guilty, yet he does not want to betray his values. What do you think you would say to him? Could you help him explore his own value conflict without contributing to his dilemma by imposing your own?

End-of-Life Decisions

Studies of attitudes toward suicide reveal sharp divisions of opinion regarding the meaning of the decision to end one's life. Some regard this as a basic personal right, and others consider it a sign of moral evil or personal pathology (Neimeyer, 2000). As a helper, you need to be willing to discuss end-of-life decisions when clients bring such concerns to you. If you are closed to any personal examination of this issue, you may interrupt these dialogues, cut off your clients' exploration of their feelings, or attempt to provide your clients with your own solutions based on your values and beliefs. It is your responsibility to clarify your own beliefs and values pertaining to end-of-life decisions so you can assist your clients in making decisions within the framework of their own belief and value systems. Once you understand your own perspectives on end-of-life decisions, you can focus on the needs of your clients.

Your stance.   Imagine yourself in a rest home, growing more and more confused and demented. You are unable to read, to carry on meaningful conversation, or to go places, and you are partially paralyzed by a series of strokes. Do you think you would be able to find meaning through suffering in an extreme circumstance? Would you want to be kept alive at all costs, or might you want to end your life? Would you feel justified in doing so? What might stop you?

Now apply this line of thought to other situations in life. If you accept the premise that your life is yours to do with as you choose, do you believe it is permissible to commit suicide at *any* period in your life? Suppose you felt like ending your life even after trying various ways of making your life meaningful. Imagine that you felt as if nothing worked and that nothing will change. What would you do? Would you continue to live until natural causes took over? Would you feel justified in ending your own life if your active search had failed to bring you peace? Put yourself in the following case as Walfred's counselor.

The situation.   A man in his 30s, Walfred discovers that he has tested HIV-positive. He says that he wants to participate in a physician-assisted suicide before he gets to an intolerable state. Too many of his friends have died from AIDS and he vowed to himself that he would take active measures to be sure that he would not die in the same way. Because he is rational and knows what he wants, he believes that taking this action is reasonable and in accord with his basic human rights. He has been your client for several months and has been successfully exploring other issues in his life. When he suddenly learned of his HIV status, it got him to wondering what was the point in living with a bleak future. He does want your help in making a decision, but he is clearly leaning in the direction of ending his life before he is faced with extreme suffering.

Your stance.   What would you want to say to Walfred? Because Walfred is rational and able to make decisions that affect his life, should he be allowed to take measures to end his life far before he becomes terminally ill? Because he is not yet seriously ill, should he be prevented from ending his life, even if it means taking away his freedom of choice? Given the fact that you have been working with Walfred for some time, would you respect his self-determination, or would you influence him to search for alternatives to suicide at this stage in his life? As a mental health worker, if there were no legal mandates to report his intentions, would you feel justified in attempting to persuade Walfred to change his mind?

Discussion.   What is the role of mental health professionals in working with people who are considering some form of hastened dying or end-of-life decision? Is the proper role of the helper to steer the client in a particular direction? Should the helper's personal values enter the picture? What is the ethical course to follow when there is a conflict between the therapist's and the client's values on this matter? Are you legally obliged to report a client who is seriously considering hastening the process of dying?

The situation.   Esmeralda, who is in her early 40s, is suffering from advanced rheumatoid arthritis. She is in constant pain, and many of the pain medications have resulted in serious side effects. This is a debilitating disease, and she sees no hope of any improvement. She has lost her will to live and has expressed her desire to end her life, but her parents cling to hope. They deeply believe that it is always wrong to take your own life.

Your stance.   Think about how your values might influence your interventions in this case. If her parents were coming to you for counseling, what might you say to them? To what degree can you empathize with Esmeralda's desire to end her life? What role would your beliefs play in your counseling? How might your values affect the things you say to the family?

Now assume that Esmeralda herself comes to you, her therapist of long standing, and says: "I am in too much pain, and I don't want to suffer anymore. I don't want to involve you in it, but as my counselor, I would like you to know my last wishes." She tells you of her plan to take an overdose of pills, an action she sees as more humane than continuing to endure her suffering. What legal implications are involved here? Do you see any conflict between ethics and the law in this case? Do you have an ethical and legal responsibility to prevent Esmeralda from carrying out her intended course of action? If you were in full agreement with her wishes, how might this feeling influence your intervention? What do you consider to be the ethical course of action?

Discussion.   Werth and Holdwick (2000) suggest that mental health professionals whose values preclude consideration of hastened death should not be obligated to provide professional services to clients who want to explore this issue. However, for helpers who do counsel these clients, Werth and Holdwick provide some guidelines for dealing with end-of-life issues:

- Assess your personal values and professional beliefs regarding the acceptability of rational suicide.
- As a part of the informed consent process, give prospective clients information about the limitations of confidentiality as it applies to assisted death, if applicable.
- Make full use of consultation throughout the process.
- Keep risk-management-oriented notes.
- Assess your clients' capacity to make reasoned decisions about their health care.
- Review clients' understanding of their condition, prognosis, and treatment options.
- Strive to include clients' significant others in the counseling process.
- Assess the impact of external coercion on clients' decision making.
- Determine the degree to which clients' decisions are congruent with their cultural and spiritual values.

Your stance.   Where do you stand with respect to key questions on end-of-life decisions? What is your position on an individual's right to decide about matters pertaining to living and dying? What religious, ethical, and moral beliefs do you hold that might enable you to support a client's decision about ending his or her life under certain circumstances? If your personal or professional value system is not accepting of an individual ending his or her own life, is it ethical for you to work with clients who may be contemplating some form of hastened death? How might your beliefs get in the way of assisting your client in making his or her own decision? Are you aware of the laws of your state and the ethical standards of your professional organization concerning an individual's freedom to make end-of-life decisions?

By Way of Review

- Ethical practice dictates that helpers seriously consider the impact of their values on their clients and the conflicts that might arise if values are sharply different.

- Ultimately, it is the responsibility of clients to choose in which direction they will go, what values they will adopt, and what values they will modify or discard.

- It is neither possible nor desirable for helpers to remain neutral or to keep their values separate from their professional relationships.

- It is not the helper's role to indoctrinate clients or to push them to adopt the value system of the helper.

- At times, it can be useful for helpers to expose their values to their clients, yet it is counterproductive to impose these values on them.

- Simply because you do not embrace a client's values does not mean that you cannot work effectively with the person. The key is that you be objective and respect your client's right to autonomy.

- There are numerous areas in which your values can potentially conflict with the values of your clients. You may have to refer some clients because of such differences.

What Will You Do Now?

1. Spend some time reflecting on the role you expect your values to play as you work with a range of clients. How might your values work for you? against you? Reflect also on the source of your values. Are you clear where you stand on

the value issues raised in this chapter? In your journal, write some of your thoughts to these questions. Under what circumstances might you be inclined to share and perhaps explore your values and beliefs with your clients? Can you think of situations in which it might be counterproductive for you to do so?

2. Consider a personal value that could get in the way of your being objective in working with a client. Take a value that you hold strongly, and challenge it. Do this by going to a source that holds values opposite to your own. If you are strongly convinced that abortion is immoral, for instance, consider going to an abortion clinic and talking with someone there. If you are uncomfortable with homosexuality because of your own values, go to a gay organization on campus or in your community and talk with people there. If you think you may have difficulty with religious values of clients, find out more about a group that holds religious views different from yours.

3. For the full bibliographic entry for each of the sources listed here, consult the References and Reading List at the back of the book. For books dealing with the role of spiritual values in the helping process, see Burke and Miranti (1995), Faiver, Ingersoll, O'Brien, and McNally (2001), Faiver and O'Brien (1993), Kelly (1995b), Miller (1999), Miller and Thoresen (1999), and Richards and Bergin (1997, 2000).

Ethics in Action CD-ROM Exercises

4. For supplemental activities that accompany this chapter, see Part Two [Values and the Helping Relationship] of the *Ethics in Action* CD-ROM. Before viewing role-play segments 4, 5, 6, and 7, complete the self-inventory provided in Part Two and bring your completed responses to class for discussion.

5. Complete the exercises and follow-up discussion questions after each of the role-play segments dealing with value conflicts in Part Two. To derive the maximum benefit, after viewing each role-play segment write out your reactions to the situation portrayed.

6. In role-play segment 4, The Divorce, it is clear that the counselor has an agenda for the client when she says that she has decided to leave her husband and get a divorce. The counselor's line of inquiry is about who will look after the welfare of her children. The client feels misunderstood and does not think the counselor is of help to her. Have one student role-play the counselor, using a different approach from the one that Gary used with this client. Have another student play the role of the client. After the role play, explore the issues you see being played out. What are some other alternatives helpers could employ when dealing with a value conflict?

7. In role-play segment 5, Doing It My Way, Sally is attempting to influence her client to think about the effect of her behavior on her parents. The client (Charlae) is seeking increased independence and wants to break away from her

parents and be "free." Her father wants her to stay at home, but she wants to live at college in the dorms. Sally suggests that Charlae talk with her parents about this, but she just wants to move out, without any discussion with her parents. Sally is concerned about what Charlae's parents' reaction might be if she moves out without involving her parents in this decision. Charlae says, "I could really care less what they think." Sally wants Charlae to think about the consequences and the effect on her parents and the fact that they have made sacrifices for her. Have one student role-play Sally and another Sally's supervisor. Demonstrate how you might approach the counselor as her supervisor. What would you most want Sally to consider?

8. In role-play segment 6, The Promiscuous One, the client (Suzanne) is having indiscriminate sexual encounters. Richard expresses concern for his client, who reports meeting a guy in a bar and having sex with him, which she says is the best she has had in a week. He asks if she is protecting herself from pregnancy and/or HIV. She claims she has the greatest life as it is. Suzanne says, "I'm not going to get HIV. People are blowing it totally out of proportion." She says she doesn't know why he is so worried about it, for after all, it's her life. Richard then focuses on how Suzanne's behavior plays out the recurring theme of abandonment by her father. She thinks there is no connection.

If you were Suzanne's counselor, how would you deal with the situation as she presents it? Is it ethically appropriate for you to strongly influence your client to engage in safe sex practices? Demonstrate how you would approach Suzanne through role playing.

9. In role-play segment 7, The Affair, the client (Natalie) shares with her counselor that she is having a long-term affair. Natalie is struggling with her marriage and the fact that she is having a long-term affair. She feels alive, youthful, and beautiful when she is with this other person. At home she feels depressed and sees her purpose as being just to serve her husband. For years she has been there for others, but now she has to think about herself. The counselor (Janice) says, "Having an affair is not a good answer for someone—it just hurts everyone. I just don't think it is a good idea."

What are your values as they pertain to this issue, and how would your values influence your interventions? In a role play, show how you might work with Natalie.

InfoTrac College Edition Resources

For additional readings, explore InfoTrac College Edition, our online library. Go to http://www.infotrac.college.com/wadsworth and select these key word searches:

    values couns*
    values therap*
    values psych*

spiritual W1 values psych*
religious W1 values psych*
end-of-life decisions
rational W1 suicide
gay W1 relationship*
homosexuality
heterosexuality

Key words are listed in a form that enables the search engine to locate a wider range of articles in the online university library. Key words should be entered exactly as shown, including asterisks, "W1," "W2," "AND," and other search engine tools.

CHAPTER 8

Cultural Diversity in the Helping Professions

Focus Questions

1. How much thought have you given to your own cultural background and the assumptions that you have developed? To what degree are you open to expanding your vision of reality?

2. How prepared are you to work with client populations that differ from you significantly in a number of dimensions (age, gender, culture, ethnicity, sexual orientation, socioeconomic status, and educational background)? What life experiences can you draw from to bridge any gap of differences between you and your clients?

3. What ethical issues are involved in failing to take cultural factors into account in the helping relationship?

4. What problems and pitfalls are associated with a multicultural perspective?

5. What values do you hold that could make it difficult for you to work with clients who have a different worldview or a different cultural background? For example, if you value self-determination and this is not a central value in your client's culture, could this pose problems?

6. What might you do if a client who sought your help wondered if you would be able to help him or her despite differences in worldview or culture?

7. In your college program, how much attention is given to developing awareness of your cultural assumptions, knowledge about diverse cultural groups, and skills for working in a pluralistic society?

8. What can you do to increase your ability to make contact with clients who are different from you? How can you move toward becoming a culturally skilled helper?

Aim of the Chapter

In most places where you might work, it will be necessary for you to relate effectively to a wide variety of clients. At this point in your development as a helper, it is essential that you be open to considering how to establish contact with clients who differ from you in age, gender, ethnicity, race, culture, socioeconomic status, sexual orientation, lifestyle, life circumstances, or basic values.

You do not need to be the same as your client or to have experienced the same life circumstances to form a therapeutic alliance. But it is necessary that you have a range of experiences upon which to draw to understand the human condition. Universal human themes link people in spite of their differences. What is crucial is your openness to learn from the lessons that life has presented to you, your respect for contrasting perspectives, your interest in understanding the diverse worldviews of the clients you will meet, and your capacity for breaking out of the narrow grooves that filter reality. If you have grown up in a monocultural world, it is not impossible for you to understand people with a different worldview, but it will demand a good deal of challenging and changing of your attitudes and views.

In Chapter 7 we focused on the influence your values have on the interventions you make as a helper. This theme continues as we examine the basic role that cultural values play in every helping relationship. Both you and the person seeking your help bring attitudes, behaviors, and life perspectives into the relationship. If these values are in conflict, there is little chance for a helping relationship to form. To function effectively as a helper, you need to remain aware of clients' cultural attributes and to realize how cultural values operate in the helping process. You need to know about specific cultural differences and realize how certain cultural values affect your work. It is crucial that all helpers seriously consider these issues, regardless of their racial, ethnic, and cultural background.

This chapter will not teach you all you need to know to understand diversity. Our intention is to offer a perspective on learning how to appreciate and work with diversity in the helping relationship. We stress coming to an understanding of the ways in which your own cultural background has contributed to who and what you are and honestly examining your basic views about diversity. You will probably take a course in cultural diversity, which is likely to cover gender concerns, ageism, racism, multicultural issues, physical disabilities, and issues pertaining to sexual orientation. We hope that you do not view such a course merely as a "requirement" to get through but rather view it as a challenging and awakening experience that can broaden your vision of the world. A good course in cultural diversity is a necessity in helping you formulate alternative perspectives and in giving you tools for working with all client populations.

Self-Assessment:
Cultural Diversity and Gender Equity

Understanding cultural pluralism begins with self-analysis. D. W. Sue (1996) contends that becoming multiculturally competent is best conceptualized as a lifelong developmental process that requires continual education and training. Sue admits that realistically it is not possible to acquire an in-depth understanding of all the different cultural groups. Part of multicultural competence entails recognizing our limitations and is manifested in our willingness to (a) seek consultation, (b) seek continuing education, and (c) make referrals to a professional who is competent to work with a particular client population.

Before delving into the issues related to a multicultural and diversity perspective in the helping process, we think it makes sense to identify your present attitudes and beliefs about cultural diversity and gender equity issues. Complete the Quick Discrimination Index on pages 194–195. This survey is designed to assess sensitivity, awareness, and receptivity to cultural diversity and gender equity. Respond to each item as honestly as possible. This inventory is designed to assess subtle racial and gender bias. You can use this inventory to become more aware of your attitudes and beliefs pertaining to these issues.

A Multicultural Perspective on Helping

Multicultural counseling refers to practices that integrate culture-specific awareness, knowledge, and skills in the helping process. The United States is a pluralistic or multicultural society that includes individuals from different ethnic, racial, and cultural backgrounds (Arredondo, et al., 1996). When you become a helper, you will encounter many individuals from cultures different from your own. In many instances, your first step toward helping these clients will be coming to an understanding of their cultural values.

Culture can be defined narrowly or broadly. Lee (1997a) contends that the term *culture* should be limited to categories of race or ethnicity and focus on the mental health issues and developmental needs of those racial and ethnic groups in the United States that do not have European roots. Pedersen (2000) looks at culture from a broader perspective, defining cultural groups by *ethnographic* variables (nationality, ethnicity, language, and religion), *demographic* variables (age, gender, and place of residence), *status* variables (educational and socioeconomic background), and formal and informal *affiliations*. According to Pedersen, the multicultural perspective provides a conceptual framework that both recognizes the complex diversity of a pluralistic society and suggests bridges of shared concern that link all people, regardless of their differences. This perspective looks both at the unique dimensions of a person and at how this person shares common themes with those who are different.

Arredondo and her colleagues (1996) make a distinction between multiculturalism and diversity. Multiculturalism puts the focus on ethnicity, race, and culture. In the context of training helpers, the term *multicultural* refers to five major cultural groups in the United States and its territories: African/black, Asian, European/white, Hispanic/Latino, and Native American. *Diversity* refers to other individual differences and characteristics by which persons may self-define. This includes but is not limited to an individual's age, gender, sexual orientation, religion or spiritual identification, physical ability/disability, social and economic class background, and residential location.

Ethical Dimensions in Multicultural Practice

Becoming an ethical and effective helper in a multicultural society is a continuing process, not a destination that we reach once and for all. Sue (1996) suggests that ethical and effective multicultural counseling evolves from three primary practices. First, helpers must be aware of their own assumptions, biases, and values about human behavior, and of their own worldview as well. Second, helpers need to become increasingly aware of the cultural values, biases, and assumptions of diverse groups in our society, and come to an understanding of the worldview of culturally different clients in nonjudgmental ways. Third, with this knowledge helpers will begin to develop culturally appropriate, relevant, and sensitive strategies for intervening with individuals and with systems.

Recognizing diversity in our society and embracing a multicultural approach in the helping relationship are fundamental tenets of professional codes of ethics. Respecting diversity implies a commitment to acquiring the knowledge, skills, and personal awareness that are essential to working effectively with a wide variety of client groups. The ACA (1995) ethics code explains this requirement: "Counselors will actively attempt to understand the diverse cultural backgrounds of the clients with whom they work. This includes, but is not limited to, learning how the counselor's own cultural/racial identity impacts her or his values and beliefs about the counseling process."

The *Ethical Standards of Human Service Professionals* (NOHSE, 2000) contain six principles aimed at the human service professional's responsibility to the community and society, with a specific emphasis on ethics and human diversity. Human service professionals must adhere to these standards:

- Advocate for the rights of all members of society, particularly those who are members of minorities and groups at which discriminatory practices have been directed.
- Provide services without discrimination or preference based on age, ethnicity, culture, race, disability, gender, religion, sexual orientation, or socioeconomic status.
- Become knowledgeable about the cultures and communities within which they practice.
- Become aware of their own cultural backgrounds, beliefs, and values, recognizing the potential impact these values may have on their relationships with others.
- Become aware of sociopolitical issues that differently affect clients from diverse backgrounds.
- Seek the training, education, experience, and supervision necessary to ensure their effectiveness in working with culturally diverse client populations.

Quick Discrimination Index*

Directions: Remember there are no right or wrong answers. Please circle the appropriate number to the right.

	Strongly Disagree	Disagree	Not Sure	Agree	Strongly Agree
1. I do think it is more appropriate for the mother of a newborn baby, rather than the father, to stay home with the baby (not work) during the first year.	1	2	3	4	5
2. It is as easy for women to succeed in business as it is for men.	1	2	3	4	5
3. I really think affirmative-action programs on college campuses constitute reverse discrimination.	1	2	3	4	5
4. I feel I could develop an intimate relationship with someone from a different race.	1	2	3	4	5
5. All Americans should learn to speak two languages.	1	2	3	4	5
6. It upsets (or angers) me that a woman has never been president of the United States.	1	2	3	4	5
7. Generally speaking, men work harder than women.	1	2	3	4	5
8. My friendship network is very racially mixed.	1	2	3	4	5
9. I am against affirmative-action programs in business.	1	2	3	4	5
10. Generally, men seem less concerned with building relationships than women.	1	2	3	4	5
11. I would feel OK about my son or daughter dating someone from a different race.	1	2	3	4	5
12. It upsets (or angers) me that a racial minority person has never been president of the United States.	1	2	3	4	5
13. In the past few years, too much attention has been directed toward multicultural or minority issues in education.	1	2	3	4	5
14. I think feminist perspectives should be an integral part of the higher education curriculum.	1	2	3	4	5
15. Most of my close friends are from my own racial group.	1	2	3	4	5
16. I feel somewhat more secure that a man rather than a woman is currently president of the United States.	1	2	3	4	5
17. I think that it is (or would be) important for my children to attend schools that are racially mixed.	1	2	3	4	5

	Strongly Disagree	Disagree	Not Sure	Agree	Strongly Agree
18. In the past few years too much attention has been directed toward multicultural or minority issues in business.	1	2	3	4	5
19. Overall, I think racial minorities in America complain too much about racial discrimination.	1	2	3	4	5
20. I feel (or would feel) very comfortable having a woman as my primary physician.	1	2	3	4	5
21. I think the president of the United States should make a concerted effort to appoint more women and racial minorities to the country's Supreme Court.	1	2	3	4	5
22. I think white people's racism toward racial-minority groups still constitutes a major problem in America.	1	2	3	4	5
23. I think the school system, from elementary school through college, should encourage minority and immigrant children to learn and fully adopt traditional American values.	1	2	3	4	5
24. If I were to adopt a child, I would be happy to adopt a child of any race.	1	2	3	4	5
25. I think there is as much female physical violence toward men as there is male physical violence toward women.	1	2	3	4	5
26. I think the school system, from elementary school through college, should promote values representative of diverse cultures.	1	2	3	4	5
27. I believe that reading the autobiography of Malcolm X would be of value.	1	2	3	4	5
28. I would enjoy living in a neighborhood consisting of a racially diverse population (Asian, blacks, Latinos, whites).	1	2	3	4	5
29. I think it is better if people marry within their own race.	1	2	3	4	5
30. Women make too big a deal out of sexual-harassment issues in the workplace.	1	2	3	4	5

The total score measures overall sensitivity, awareness, and receptivity to cultural diversity and gender equality. Of the 30 items on the QDI, 15 are worded and scored in a positive direction (high scores indicate high sensitivity to multicultural/gender issues), and 15 are worded and scored in a negative direction (where low scores are indicative of high sensitivity). Naturally, when tallying the total score response, these latter 15 items need to be *reverse-scored*. Reverse scoring simply means that if a respondent circles a "1" he or she should get five points, a "2" four points, a "3" three points, a "4" two points, and a "5" one point.

The following QDI items need to be *reverse-scored*: 1, 2, 3, 7, 9, 10, 13, 15, 16, 18, 19, 23, 25, 29, 30.

Score range = 30 to 150, with high scores indicating more awareness, sensitivity, and receptivity to racial diversity and gender equality.

Cultural diversity is a fact of life in today's world, and ethical practice demands that helpers pay attention to the issues involved in working with culturally diverse populations. Helpers may misunderstand clients of a different gender, race, age, religion, social class, educational level, or sexual orientation. If practitioners fail to integrate these diversity factors into their practice, they are infringing on the client's cultural autonomy and basic human rights, which will reduce the chance of establishing an effective helping relationship. For some clients religious values may be important. Other clients may focus on gender or age discrimination. By paying attention to what a client is saying, helpers can discover which factors are salient for this person at this time.

The Need for a Multicultural Emphasis

In the past decade we have seen an increased awareness on the part of the helping professions to address the special issues involved in working with people of various cultures. D. W. Sue (1996) cites United States Census figures indicating that sometime between the years 2030 and 2050 racial and ethnic minorities will become the majority population. Because of these changes in demographics, it is important for human service professionals to embrace a broad multicultural perspective if they hope to understand the behavior of culturally diverse client populations.

Pedersen (2000) maintains that human service workers have two choices—to ignore the influence of culture or to attend to it. Whatever choice is made, culture will continue to influence the behavior of both the client and the helper. Adopting a multicultural perspective enables us to think about diversity without polarizing issues into "right" or "wrong." When two people argue from culturally different assumptions, they can disagree without one being right and the other being wrong. Depending on the cultural perspective from which a problem is considered, there can be several appropriate solutions. In some cases, a similar problem may have very different solutions depending on one's culture. For example, helpers may encourage some clients to express feelings of hurt to parents but encourage other clients to practice restraint in self-expression so as not to offend their elders.

A multicultural perspective respects the needs and strengths of diverse client populations, and it recognizes the experiences of these clients. However, do not fall into the trap of perceiving individuals as simply belonging to a group. Remember that the differences between individuals within the same group are often greater than the differences between groups. Pedersen (2000) indicates that individuals who share the same ethnic and cultural background are likely to have sharp differences. Not all Native Americans have the same experience, nor do all African Americans, all Asian Americans, all women, all old people, or all people who are physically challenged. Helpers must be prepared to deal with the complex differences among individuals from every cultural group. Sue, Arredondo, and McDavis (1992) point out that although all of us are racial, ethnic, and cultural beings belonging to a particular group, we are not innately endowed with the competencies and skills necessary to be multiculturally skilled helpers.

We hope that you will not view the tapestry of culture that is woven into the fabric of all helping relationships as a barrier to break through. Try to approach cultural diversity in a positive way. As Pedersen (2000) reminds us, multiculturalism can make your job as a helper easier and more fun; it can also increase rather than decrease the quality of your life. Adopting a perspective that cultural differences are positive attributes that add richness to relationships will expand your ability to work with diverse client groups.

Overcoming Cultural Tunnel Vision

Our work with students in a human services training program has shown us that many of them have cultural "tunnel vision." Many students are unaware of the difficulty of dealing with clients who have a cultural background different from their own. They have limited cultural experiences, and in some cases they see it as their role to transmit their values to their clients. Some students have made inappropriate generalizations about a particular group of clients. For example, helpers often assert that minorities are unresponsive to psychological intervention because of a lack of motivation to change or a "resistance" to seeking professional help.

In a sense, all helping relationships are multicultural. Both those providing help and those receiving help bring to their relationship attitudes, values, and behaviors that can vary widely. One mistake is to deny the importance of these cultural variables; another mistake is to overemphasize such cultural differences to the extent that helpers lose their spontaneity and thus fail to be present for their clients. You need to understand and accept clients who have a different set of assumptions about life, and you need to be alert to the likelihood of imposing your own worldview. Honestly examine your own expectations, attitudes, and assumptions about working with various cultural and ethnic groups. In working with clients with different cultural experiences, it is important that you resist making value judgments for them.

The *culturally encapsulated counselor,* a concept introduced by Wrenn (1962, 1985), identifies the characteristics common to cultural tunnel vision. Think about how broad your own vision is as you consider these traits of culturally encapsulated counselors:

- Defines reality according to one set of cultural assumptions.
- Shows insensitivity to cultural variations among individuals.
- Accepts unreasoned assumptions without proof or ignores proof because that might disconfirm one's assumptions.
- Fails to evaluate other viewpoints and makes little attempt to accommodate the behavior of others.
- Is trapped in one way of thinking that resists adaptation and rejects alternatives.

Years after first identifying the concept, Wrenn (1985) maintained that cultural encapsulation continues to be a problem for mental health professionals.

Encapsulation is a potential trap that all helpers must be wary of falling into. If you accept the idea that certain cultural values are necessarily supreme, you become limited by refusing to consider alternatives. If you possess cultural tunnel vision, you are likely to misinterpret patterns of behavior displayed by clients who are culturally different from you. Unless you understand the values of other cultures, you are likely to misunderstand these clients. Because of this lack of understanding, you may label certain client behavior as resistant, you may make an inaccurate diagnosis of a particular behavior as maladaptive, and you may impose your own value system on the client. For example, many Hispanic women might resist changing what you view as dependency on their husband. If you work with Hispanic women, you need to appreciate that they are likely to live by the value of remaining with their husband, even if he is unfaithful. Hispanic tradition tells these women that no matter what, it is not appropriate to leave one's husband. If you are unaware of this traditional value, you could make the mistake of pushing such women to take an action that will violate their belief system.

It is important that helpers respect the cultural heritage of their clients and that they avoid encouraging clients to "give up" this culture so that they can "make it" in the dominant culture. Certainly, clients need to consider the consequences of not accepting certain values of the society in which they live, but they should not be pressured to accept wholesale a set of values that may be alien to them. Although clients who inhabit more than one culture are likely to struggle in finding ways to integrate what is best for them from both cultures, the synthesis is bound to be richer with possibilities.

Helpers from all cultural groups need to honestly examine their expectations and attitudes about the helping process. Realize that there is no sanctuary from cultural bias. We tend to carry our bias around with us, yet we often do not recognize this fact. It takes a concerted effort and vigilance to monitor our biases and value systems so that they do not interfere with establishing and maintaining successful helping relationships.

Western and Eastern Values

The theories and practices of the helping process that you have learned are grounded in Western assumptions, yet most of the world differs from mainstream U.S. culture. Hogan-Garcia (1999) points out that the mainstream culture in the United States derives from the Anglo-Saxon culture of the English who colonized America. She summarizes the underlying value orientations of the mainstream culture as characterized by an emphasis on a patriarchal nuclear family; "getting things done" and keeping busy; measurable and visible accomplishments; individual choice, responsibility, and achievement; self-reliance and self-motivation; the pragmatic notion of "If an idea works, use it"; change and novel ideas; and equality, informality, and fair play. The degree to which these values fit culturally diverse client groups needs to be carefully considered by human service practitioners.

Some writers in the multicultural field are critical of the strong individualistic bias of contemporary theories and the lack of emphasis on broader social contexts such as families, groups, and communities (Ivey, D'Andrea, Ivey, & Simik-Morgan, 2002; Sue, Ivey, & Pedersen, 1996). The Western model of helping does have certain limitations when applied to minority groups such as Asian Americans, Hispanics, Native Americans, and African Americans. Seeking professional help is not typical for many of these groups. In most non-Western cultures, in fact, informal groups of friends and relatives provide a supportive network. Many of the clients with whom you will work have a cultural heritage associated with non-Western values. Some of the interventions you have learned will be of questionable relevance if you do not modify your techniques.

Eastern and Western are not just geographic terms but also represent philosophical, social, political, and cultural orientations. It is typical to examine individualism and collectivism through comparisons between the cultures of the West, which reflect individualism, and those of the East, which reflect collectivism (Sampson, 2000). Ho (1985) states that a comparison of Western and Eastern systems shows some striking differences in value orientations. Western culture places a prime value on choice, the uniqueness of the individual, self-assertion, and strengthening the ego. By contrast, the Eastern view stresses interdependence, downplays individuality, and emphasizes losing oneself in the totality of the cosmos. From the Western perspective, the primary values are the primacy of the individual, youth, independence, nonconformity, competition, conflict, and freedom. The guiding principles for action (individualism) are found in the fulfillment of individual needs and individual responsibility. From the Eastern perspective, the primary values are the primacy of relationships, maturity, compliance, conformity, cooperation, harmony, and security. The guiding principles for action (collectivism) are found in the achievement of collective goals and collective responsibility.

Behavioral orientations also differ. The Western view encourages expression of feelings and striving for self-actualization, whereas the Eastern view encourages control of feelings and striving for collective actualization. Western approaches emphasize outcomes such as improving the environment, changing one's coping behavior, learning to manage stress, and changing objective reality in other ways to improve one's way of life. Eastern approaches emphasize acceptance of one's environment and inner enlightenment.

Sampson (2000) maintains that individualism and collectivism have become increasingly important cultural variables that have significant effects on an individual's experiences and behavior. He contends that it is not necessary to pit individualism against collectivism. Recognizing both individualism *and* collectivism, independence *and* interdependence, as aspects of a total process can encourage clients to move toward a synthesis of these characteristics.

Patterson (1996) believes that Western approaches can be useful despite cultural differences. He contends that focusing on the universal factors that link all humanity can help East and West move toward each other. For Patterson, the overemphasis on cultural diversity and training in specific techniques for various cultural groups "ignores the fact that we are rapidly becoming one world, with rapid communication and increasing interrelations among persons from varying cultures, leading to increasing homogeneity and a worldview representing the common humanity that binds all humans together as one species" (p. 230).

Some time ago we presented a series of workshops in Hong Kong for human service professionals. This gave us the opportunity to rethink the challenges of applying Western approaches to working with non-Western clients. Almost all the participants in these workshops were Chinese, but some of them had obtained their graduate training in social work or counseling in the United States. These professionals were challenged with retaining the values that were basic to their Chinese heritage while integrating a Western counseling viewpoint.

In talking with these practitioners, we learned that their focus is on the individual in the context of the social system. In their interventions they pay more attention to the family than to individuals' interests. They are learning how to balance a stress on personal growth with what is in the best interest of the family and society. They are able to respect the values of their clients, who are also mostly Chinese, yet at the same time challenge them to think of some ways to change. Many of the helping professionals in Hong Kong told us that they had to demonstrate patience and understanding with their clients. They saw it as essential to form a trusting relationship before engaging in confrontation. Although this necessity applies to counseling in general, it seems especially important for non-Western clients.

   Case example.   A student is seeing you because he continues to get "B" and "C" grades, which is a source of embarrassment to his family. He is in great difficulty because he feels that he is letting his family down and actually bringing shame to them by what he considers his "academic failure." If you were working with this student, how would you help him deal with his feelings of guilt and failure and at the same time be cognizant of his cultural values? Would you challenge your client? Would you try to change his reactions to his family? Would you help him become more self-accepting? Would you tend to focus on the issue of what constitutes academic success, or would your focus be on what constitutes "bringing shame to the family"?

Challenging Your Cultural Assumptions

Culturally learned basic assumptions deeply influence the ways in which we perceive and think about reality and how we act. A willingness to examine such assumptions opens doors to seeing others from their vantage point rather than from a preconceived perspective. Helpers often make cultural assumptions that they are unaware of. By reflecting on how your assumptions could interfere with effective helping in multicultural situations, you can begin to see ways to challenge your assumptions as you work with any client.

   Assumptions about self-disclosure.   Self-disclosure is highly valued in traditional counseling. Most helpers assume that no effective helping can occur unless clients reveal themselves in the helping relationship. Patterson (1996) asserts that the inability to self-disclose is something to be overcome, not accepted. He writes: "The only way in which the counselor can enter the world of the client is with the permission of the client, who communicates the nature of his or her world to the counselor through self-disclosure. Thus, client self-disclosure is the *sine qua non* for counseling. Counselor respect and genuineness facilitate client self-disclosure" (p. 230). According to Patterson, unless clients are willing to verbalize and communicate their thoughts, feelings, attitudes, and perceptions, there is no basis for empathic understanding by the helper.

   Some would contend that this assumption ignores the fact that in some cultures self-disclosure is taboo and that some European ethnic groups stress keeping problems "in the family." This assumption does not address the fact that self-disclosure is foreign to the values of some cultural groups.

Related to this issue of client self-disclosure is helper self-disclosure. One way to facilitate meaningful disclosure on the part of clients is for helpers to model appropriate self-disclosure. Ivey and Ivey (1999) comment that helper self-disclosure can increase client self-disclosure, create trust between counselor and client, and establish a more equal relationship in the interview. However, some writers have reservations about the value of helper self-disclosure, contending that the helping process can work quite well without this kind of sharing.

Both Ivey and Ivey (1999) and Patterson (1996) make points worth considering. Unless clients challenge the obstacles to some level of disclosure, they are not likely to be able to participate in the helping relationship. However, you can recognize and appreciate that some of your clients will struggle in letting you know the nature of their problems. This struggle in itself is a useful focus for exploration. Rather than expecting such clients to disclose freely, you can demonstrate respect for their values and at the same time ask them what they want from you. With your support and encouragement, clients can sort through their values and conditioning pertaining to self-disclosure and decide the degree to which they want to change.

Other forms of helping place less stress on verbal disclosure. These can include music therapy, occupational and recreational therapy, and other forms of activity therapy. Helpers can also assume an advocacy role for the client in the system, can help clients build on their natural sources of support, or can teach clients to use the resources within the community. As you will see in Chapter 11, a number of community-based interventions may be more appropriate for some clients than traditional approaches to helping.

Assumptions about family values. D. Sue (1997) has written about some traditional Chinese family values. Filial piety is a significant value in Chinese American families, emphasizing obedience to parents and respect and honor for them. They value family bonds and unity more than self-determination and independence. Family communication patterns are based on cultural tradition and emphasize appropriate roles and status. Academic achievement is prized. Helpers who fail to understand and appreciate these values are likely to err by pushing Chinese American clients to change in directions that are not consistent with their values.

In one of his multicultural workshops, Paul Pedersen related that many Asian students with whom he worked reflected values from their family when they were confronted with a problem. They first tended to reflect inward for some answer. If they did not find an answer within themselves, they tended to go to someone in the family. If neither of these routes worked, they were likely to seek a teacher, a friend, or someone with wisdom for guidance. If none of these avenues resulted in a satisfactory solution, they might then consult a professional helper.

Assumptions about nonverbal behavior. Clients can disclose themselves in many nonverbal ways, but cultural expressions are subject to misinterpretation. Personal space requirements, eye contact, handshaking, dress, formality of greeting, perspective on time, and so forth all vary among cultural groups. Mainstream Americans often feel uncomfortable with silence and tend to fill in quiet gaps with words. In some cultures, in contrast, silence indicates a sign of respect and politeness. You could misinterpret a quiet client's behavior if you did not realize that the client might be waiting for you to ask questions. It is good to keep in mind that there are no universal meanings of nonverbal behaviors.

You may have been systematically trained in a range of microskills: attending skills, open communication, observational skills, hearing clients accurately, noting and reflecting feelings, selecting and structuring skills, to mention a few (Ivey & Ivey, 1999). Although these behaviors are aimed at creating a positive therapeutic relationship, individuals from certain ethnic groups may have difficulty responding positively or understanding the intent of the counselor's attitudes and behavior. The helper whose confrontational style involves direct eye contact, physical gestures, and probing personal questions may be seen as offensively intrusive by clients from some other cultures.

In European North American middle-class culture, direct eye contact is usually considered a sign of interest and presence, and a lack thereof is interpreted as being evasive. It is common for individuals to maintain more eye contact while listening and less while talking. Some research indicates that African Americans may reverse this pattern by looking more when talking and slightly less when listening. Among some Native American and Hispanic groups, eye contact by the young is a sign of disrespect. Some cultural groups generally avoid eye contact when talking about serious subjects (Ivey & Ivey, 1999). Clearly, helpers who interpret a client's lack of eye contact as "resistive" or "pathological" may not be understanding or respecting important cultural differences. Helpers need to acquire sensitivity to cultural differences to reduce the probability of miscommunication, misdiagnosis, and misinterpretation of nonverbal behaviors.

Assumptions about trusting relationships.   Many Americans of European background tend to form quick relationships and to talk easily about their personal life. This characteristic is often reflected in their helping style. Thus, the helper expects that the client will approach their relationship in an open and trusting manner. Doing this is very difficult for some clients, however, especially given that they are expected to talk about themselves in personal ways to a stranger. Among many cultures it takes a long time to develop meaningful relationships. What is more, you will have to *earn* the trust of these clients before they will confide in you.

Assumptions about self-actualization.   Helping professionals commonly assume that it is important for the individual to become a fully self-actualized person. But some clients are more concerned about how their problems or changes are likely to affect others in their life. You will recall that in the Eastern orientation one of the guiding principles is achievement of collective goals. Likewise, Native Americans judge their worth primarily in relation to how their behavior contributes to the harmonious functioning of their tribe. Native Americans have a value system that is fundamentally different from that of the dominant culture, determining their self-worth in reference to the betterment of the tribe rather than their own gain (Anderson & Ellis, 1988).

Assumptions about directness and assertiveness.   Although the Western orientation prizes directness, some cultures see it as a sign of rudeness and as something to be avoided. If you are not aware of this cultural difference, you could make the mistake of interpreting a lack of directness as a sign of being unassertive rather than as a sign of respect. Although getting to the point immediately is a prized value in Western culture, clients from other cultures may prefer to delay dealing with their problems or to cope with them in indirect ways. If you are operating from a Western orientation, you are likely to assume that your clients are better off if they can behave in assertive ways, such as telling people what they think, feel, and want. Some training programs teach participants coping skills that involve taking an active stance toward life.

You could offend certain clients by automatically assuming that they would be better off if they became more assertive. For example, assume that you are working with a woman who seems very unassertive to you. She rarely asks for what she wants, she allows others to decide her priorities, and she almost never denies a request or demand from anyone in her family. If you worked hard at helping her become an assertive woman, it could very well create conflicts within her family system. If she changed her role, she might no longer fit in her family or in her culture. Therefore, it is crucial that both you and your clients consider the consequences of making changes that challenge their cultural values.

One way to respect your clients is to ask them to tell you about themselves and listen to their underlying values. Ask your clients what behaviors are and are not working in their lives. If clients tell you that being indirect or unassertive is problematic for them, then this is certainly to be explored. However, if such behaviors are not posing difficulty for them, you need to monitor how your biases may be operating if you attempt to change clients in directions that they are not interested in moving toward. Asking your clients what they want from you is a way of decreasing the chances that you will impose your cultural values on them.

Review the basic cultural assumptions that influence helping practices, and determine where you stand with regard to them. What forces have shaped your basic assumptions? Are you open to considering the relevance of such assumptions in working with a variety of clients?

Challenging Your Stereotypical Beliefs

Although you may think you are without bias, stereotypical beliefs could well affect your practice. Stereotyping involves assuming that the behavior of an individual will reflect or be typical of that of most members of his or her cultural group. This assumption leads to statements such as these: "Asian American clients are emotionally repressed." "African American clients are suspicious by nature and will not trust professional helpers." "White people are arrogant." "Native Americans have very low motivation."

Helpers who view themselves as being without any stereotypes, biases, and prejudices are underestimating the impact of their socialization. Such helpers can be even more dangerous than those who are more open about their biases and prejudices. According to Pedersen (2000), this form of racism emerges unintentionally from well-meaning and caring professionals who are no more nor less culturally biased than segments of the general public. He believes that unintentional racists must be challenged either to become intentional racists or to modify their attitudes and behaviors. The key to changing the unintentional racist lies in examining basic underlying assumptions, such as those we described earlier.

Besides cultural stereotypes, there are stereotypes associated with other special populations, such as people with disabilities, the elderly, and the homeless. Statements that lump together individuals within a group reflect a myth of uniformity. In your professional work you need to realize that there are variations within cultural groups and that such differences may be at least as important as those among different groups. In your attempt to be culturally sensitive, be careful to avoid further stereotyping of certain groups.

Although cultural differences both among and within groups are obvious, we think that it is important not to go to the extreme of focusing exclusively on the differences that can separate us. In working with mental health professionals in foreign countries, we have become even more convinced that there are some basic similarities among the peoples of the world. Universal experiences can bind people together. Although personal circumstances differ, most people experience the pain of making decisions and attempting to live with integrity in their world. It is essential to be respectful of the real cultural differences that exist, and it is equally critical that we not forget the common denominators of all people.

Effective Multicultural Helpers

Increasingly, helpers will come into contact with culturally diverse client populations who may not share their worldview of what constitutes normality and abnormality. Because the helping professions continue to emphasize a monocultural approach to training and practice, many helpers are ill prepared to deal effectively with cultural diversity (Sue, Arredondo, & McDavis, 1992). Although referral is sometimes an appropriate course of action, it should not be viewed as a solution to the problem of inadequately trained practitioners. With the increasing number of culturally diverse clients seeking professional help, and with the decreasing number of resources to meet these needs, helpers may not have the luxury of referral. Given this reality, we recommend that students in the human service professions, regardless of their racial or ethnic background, receive training in multicultural helping.

Working with culturally diverse client populations requires that helpers possess the awareness, knowledge, and skills to effectively deal with the concerns of the people with whom they work. Although it is unrealistic to expect that you will have an in-depth knowledge of all cultural backgrounds, it is feasible for you to have a comprehensive grasp of general principles for working successfully amid cultural diversity. If you are open to the values inherent in a diversity perspective, you will find ways to avoid getting trapped in provincialism, and you will be able to challenge the degree to which you may be culturally encapsulated (see Wrenn, 1985).

Sue and his colleagues (1992, 1998) developed a conceptual framework for multicultural counseling competencies and standards in three areas. The first area deals with the helper's beliefs and attitudes about race, culture, gender, and sexual orientation. The second dimension involves knowledge and understanding of the worldview of the helper and specific knowledge of the diverse groups with whom he or she works. The third area deals with skills and intervention strategies needed to serve diverse client groups. Arredondo and her colleagues (1996) developed a revised set of multicultural competency standards that clarify and define these three domains. A brief version of the multicultural competencies and standards identified by Sue and his colleagues (1992, 1998) and by Arredondo and her colleagues (1996) follows. You can use this checklist to identify areas of competence you now possess as well as areas in which you need to acquire skills.

Beliefs and Attitudes of Culturally Skilled Helpers

Put a check mark in the box before each of the beliefs and attitudes in this section that you think you already hold or each area of awareness that you already possess. *With respect to beliefs and attitudes, culturally skilled helpers . . .*

❑ recognize and understand their own stereotypes and preconceived notions that they may hold toward other racial and ethnic minority groups.

❑ do not allow their personal biases, values, or problems to interfere with their ability to work with clients who are culturally different from them.

❑ believe that cultural self-awareness and sensitivity to one's own cultural heritage are essential for any form of helping.

❑ are aware of their negative and positive emotional reactions toward other racial and ethnic groups that may prove detrimental to establishing collaborative helping relationships.

❑ are aware of how their own cultural background and experiences have influenced attitudes, values, and biases about what constitutes psychologically healthy individuals.

❑ have moved from being culturally unaware to knowing their cultural heritage.

❑ are able to recognize the limits of their multicultural competence and expertise.

❑ seek to examine and understand the world from the vantage point of their clients.

❑ respect clients' religious and spiritual beliefs and values.

❑ recognize their sources of discomfort with differences that exist between themselves and others in terms of race, ethnicity, culture, and beliefs.

❑ welcome diverse value orientations and diverse assumptions about human behavior and, thus, have a basis for sharing the worldview of their clients as opposed to being culturally encapsulated.

❑ rather than maintaining that their cultural heritage is superior, are able to accept and value cultural diversity.

❑ are able to identify and understand the central cultural constructs of their clients and to avoid applying their own cultural constructs inappropriately to people with whom they work.

❑ respect indigenous helping practices and respect help-giving networks within the community.

❑ monitor their functioning through consultation, supervision, and further training or education.

❑ realize that traditional concepts and helping strategies may not be appropriate for all clients or for all problems.

Knowledge of Culturally Skilled Helpers

Put a check mark in the box before each type of knowledge in this section that you think you already possess.

With respect to knowledge areas, culturally skilled helpers . . .

❏ possess knowledge about their own racial and cultural heritage and how it affects them personally and in their work.

❏ possess knowledge and understanding about how oppression, racism, discrimination, and stereotyping affect them personally and professionally.

❏ acknowledge their own racist attitudes, beliefs, and feelings.

❏ do not impose their values and expectations on their clients from differing cultural backgrounds and avoid stereotyping clients.

❏ understand the worldview of their clients and attempt to learn about their clients' cultural backgrounds.

❏ understand the basic values underlying the helping process and know how these values may clash with the cultural values of various minority groups.

❏ are aware of the institutional barriers that prevent minorities from utilizing the mental health services available in their communities.

❏ have knowledge of the potential bias in assessment instruments and use procedures and interpret findings keeping in mind the cultural and linguistic characteristics of clients.

❏ possess specific knowledge and information about the particular individuals with whom they are working.

❏ are aware of the values, life experiences, cultural heritage, and historical background of their culturally different clients.

❏ possess knowledge about their social impact on others.

❏ are knowledgeable about communication style differences and how their style may clash with or foster the helping process with persons from different cultural groups.

❏ are knowledgeable about the community characteristics and the resources in the community as well as those in the family.

❏ have knowledge about sociopolitical influences that impinge upon the lives of ethnic and racial minorities, including immigration issues, poverty, racism, stereotyping, and powerlessness.

❏ view diversity in a positive light, which enables them to meet and resolve the challenges that arise in their work with a wide range of client populations.

❏ know how to help clients make use of indigenous support systems. In areas where they are lacking in knowledge, they seek resources to assist them.

Skills and Intervention Strategies of Culturally Skilled Helpers

Put a check mark in the box before each of the skill areas in this section that you think you already possess.

With respect to specific skills, culturally skilled helpers . . .

❑ take responsibility for educating their clients to the way the helping process works, including matters such as goals, expectations, legal rights, and the helper's orientation.

❑ familiarize themselves with relevant research and the latest findings regarding mental health and mental disorders that affect diverse client populations.

❑ are willing to seek out educational, consultative, and training experiences to enhance their ability to work with culturally diverse client populations.

❑ are open to seeking consultation with traditional healers or religious and spiritual leaders to better serve culturally different clients, when appropriate.

❑ use methods and strategies and define goals consistent with the life experiences and cultural values of their clients and modify and adapt their interventions to accommodate cultural differences.

❑ are not limited to only one approach in helping but recognize that helping strategies may be culture bound.

❑ are able to send and receive both verbal and nonverbal messages accurately and appropriately.

❑ are able to exercise institutional intervention skills on behalf of their clients.

❑ become actively involved with minority individuals outside of the office (community events, celebrations, and neighborhood groups) to the extent possible.

❑ are committed to understanding themselves as racial and cultural beings and are actively seeking a nonracist identity.

❑ actively pursue and engage in professional and personal-growth activities to address their limitations.

❑ consult regularly with other professionals regarding issues of culture to determine whether or where referral may be necessary.

Reflection Questions

Now that you have completed the checklist, summarize and think about the implications of your current level of awareness, knowledge, and skills. Reflect on the following questions:

- Are you familiar with how your own culture has a present influence on the way you think, feel, and act? What steps could you take to broaden your base of understanding, both of your own culture and of other cultures?
- Are you able to identify your basic assumptions, especially as they apply to diversity in culture, ethnicity, race, gender, class, religion, and sexual orientation? To what degree are you clear about how your assumptions are likely to affect your practice as a helper?
- How open are you to being flexible in applying the techniques you use with clients?
- How prepared are you to understand and work with clients of different cultural backgrounds?
- To what degree are you now able to accurately compare your own cultural perspective with that of a person from another culture?

- Is your academic program preparing you to gain the awareness, knowledge, and skills you will need to work with diverse client populations?
- What kinds of life experiences have you had that will better enable you to understand and counsel people who have a different worldview?
- Can you identify any areas of cultural bias that could inhibit your ability to work effectively with people who are different from you? If so, what steps might you take to challenge your biases?

Recognizing Your Own Limitations

As a culturally skilled helper, you are able to recognize the limits of your multicultural competency and expertise. When necessary, you will refer clients to more qualified individuals or resources. Furthermore, it is not realistic to expect that you will know everything about the cultural background of people with whom you will work. There is much to be said for letting your clients teach you about relevant aspects of their culture. Ask clients to provide you with the information you will need to work effectively with them. In working with culturally diverse individuals, it helps to assess the degree of acculturation and identity development that has taken place. This is especially true for individuals who have had the experience of living in another culture. They often have allegiance to their own home culture but find certain characteristics of their new culture attractive. They may experience conflicts when integrating the values from the two cultures in which they live. These core struggles can be productively explored in the context of a collaborative helping relationship.

We encourage you to accept your limitations and to be patient with yourself as you expand your vision of how your culture continues to influence the person you are today. It is not helpful to overwhelm yourself with all that you do not know or to feel guilty over your limitations or parochial views. You will not become a more effective and culturally skilled helper by expecting to be completely knowledgeable about the cultural backgrounds of all your clients, by thinking that you should have a complete repertoire of skills, or by demanding perfection. Instead, recognize and appreciate your efforts toward becoming a more multiculturally competent helper.

The first step is to become more comfortable in accepting diversity as a value and in taking actions to increase your ability to work with a range of clients. You can also recognize when referral is in the best interest of your client. It is important to make a commitment to lifelong learning and to take the steps necessary to continually upgrade your knowledge and skills to better serve diverse client populations (NOHSE, 2000). This kind of continuing education extends throughout your professional career.

Multicultural Training

Helpers must be able to adapt their interventions to meet not just the developmental needs of clients but also their cultural dimensions (Sue, 1992). To enable helpers to utilize a multicultural perspective in their work, we support specialized training through formal courses and supervised field experiences with diverse client populations. We believe that a self-exploratory class should be required for helpers so that they can better identify their cultural and ethnic blind spots. In addition to enabling students to learn about cultures other than their own, such a course could offer opportunities for trainees to learn more about their own race, ethnicity, and culture.

A good program should include at least one course dealing exclusively with multicultural issues and minority groups, but a multicultural perspective should be integrated throughout the curriculum. For example, a fieldwork or internship seminar can introduce ways that helping strategies can be adapted to the special needs of diverse client populations and show how some techniques may be quite inappropriate for culturally different clients. The integration of multiculturalism and gender awareness can certainly be a thread running through relevant formal courses. In addition, there could be at least one required field placement or internship in which trainees have multicultural experiences. Ideally, the supervisor at this agency will be well versed in the cultural variables of that particular setting and also be skilled in cross-cultural understanding. Further, trainees should have access to both individual and group supervision on campus from a faculty member.

Supervised experience, along with opportunities for trainees to discuss what they are learning, is the core of a good program. We encourage you to select supervised field placements and internships that will challenge you to work on gender issues, cultural concerns, developmental issues, and lifestyle differences. You will not learn to become an effective multicultural counselor by working exclusively with clients with whom you are comfortable and who are "like you." Lee (1997b) maintains that although courses and workshops are valuable sources of learning about cultural diversity, more can be learned by going out into the community and interacting with diverse groups of people who face a myriad of problems. Through well-selected internship experiences, you will not only expand your own consciousness but increase your knowledge of diverse groups. This will provide a basis for acquiring intervention skills.

Pedersen (2000) has identified the basic components of an effective multicultural training program as including the components of awareness, knowledge, skill development, and experiential interaction, all of which are integrated in actual practice. As you have seen, awareness of personal attitudes and of attitudes toward diverse client populations is integral to becoming an effective helper. From a knowledge perspective, helpers need to understand what makes a diverse population special. They need to know what is acceptable behavior within the diverse population and how this behavior differs from that of other groups. Skill development is a necessary but not sufficient component of learning to work with diverse populations. The skills themselves are not unique, but the ways in which these skills are applied to particular clients should be the focus of training. Effective training will pay sufficient attention to each of these domains. If any of them are neglected, helpers are at a disadvantage.

Arredondo and her colleagues (1996) offer a number of suggestions that we think are well worth considering as a way to gain and maintain competence when working from a multicultural perspective.

- Read materials regarding identity development. Not only is it a good idea to read about your own cultural and ethnic identity development, but it is important to read about others' identity development processes.
- Attend annual conferences and workshops that deal with multicultural concerns.
- Read newspapers and other periodicals targeting specific populations different from your own.
- Engage a mentor from your own culture who you see as working toward becoming a culturally competent counselor and who is making the kind of strides that you would like to be making.
- Engage a mentor or two from cultures different from your own who are willing to provide you with honest feedback regarding your attitudes, beliefs, and behavior.
- Enroll in an ethnic studies course at a community college or university that focuses on cultures different from your own.
- Spend time in communities different from your own (such as shopping in grocery stores, attending churches, and walking in marches).
- Take part in activities and celebrations within communities different from your own.
- Accept that it is your responsibility to learn about other cultures and the implications for counseling, and do not expect or rely on individuals from those cultures to teach you.
- Seek out and engage in consultation with professionals from cultures relevant to the clients with whom you work.
- Language barriers may be one of your biggest problems in working with certain cultural groups. Make attempts to learn the language and the culture of the major group with whom you will be working.
- Spend some time in a civil service office, and observe the service orientation toward people of color. Contrast that with the service orientation toward white individuals. Also observe any differences in service orientation that may be based on class issues.
- Become familiar with some of the more recent immigrant populations that are changing the face of practice in many areas in the country. The Internet and local resettlement agencies and public schools teaching English as a second language are resources for learning about new cultural groups and special issues affecting resettlement.
- Actively communicate to your organization the need for multicultural training.

Training programs have come a long way in the past decade, but they still have some way to go if they are to meet the challenges of equipping helpers to acquire the knowledge and develop the skills required to meet the needs of diverse clients. As a student, you can begin to meet this challenge by taking some small, yet significant, steps toward recognizing and examining the impact of your own cultural background and learning about cultures different from your own. Deciding to act upon even a few of the suggestions listed here is one way to move in the direction of becoming a culturally skilled helper.

By Way of Review

- Multiculturalism can be considered as the fourth force in the helping professions. This perspective recognizes and values diversity in helping relationships and calls on helpers to develop strategies that are culturally appropriate.

- A multicultural perspective on the helping process takes into consideration specific values, beliefs, and actions related to race, ethnicity, gender, age, ability, religion, socioeconomic status, sexual orientation, political views, and geographic region.

- To function effectively with clients of various cultures, you need to know and respect specific cultural differences and realize how cultural values operate in the helping process.

- Be aware of any tendencies toward cultural tunnel vision. If you have limited cultural experiences, you may have difficulties relating to clients who have a different view of the world. You are likely to misinterpret many patterns of behavior displayed by such clients.

- It is important to pay attention to ways in which you can express unintentional racism through your attitudes and behaviors. One way to change this form of racism is by making your assumptions explicit.

- There are some striking differences in value orientations between Western and Eastern cultures. A main difference is the Western emphasis on individualism and the Eastern emphasis on collectivism. Individualism and collectivism are not necessarily oppositional concepts, for they are both elements of a total system. These value orientations have important implications for the process of helping.

- In working with people from other cultures, avoid stereotyping and challenge your assumptions about the use of self-disclosure, nonverbal behavior, trusting relationships, self-actualization, and directness and assertiveness.

- Effective multicultural helpers have been identified in terms of the specific knowledge, beliefs and attitudes, and skills they possess.

- Helpers who view differences as positive attributes will be most likely to meet and resolve the challenges that arise in multicultural helping situations.

- Rather than thinking of cultural differences as barriers to effective helping relationships, learn to welcome diversity as something positive. Recognize that consciously dealing with cultural variables in helping can make your job easier, not more difficult.

What Will You Do Now?

1. If your program does not require a course on cultural diversity, consider taking such a course as an elective. You might also ask if you can sit in on some class sessions in various courses that deal with special populations. For example, in one university these are a few of the courses offered: The Black Family, The Chicano Family, American Indian Women, The African Experience, The Chicano and Contemporary Issues, Afro-American Music Appreciation, The White Ethnic in America, Women and American Society, The Chicano Child, and Barrio Studies.

2. On your campus you will probably find a number of student organizations for particular cultural groups. Approach some members of one of these organizations for information about the group. See if you can attend one of their functions to get a better perspective on their culture.

3. Challenge yourself to broaden your cultural horizons. Go to a restaurant, social event, church service, concert, play, or movie with a person from a cultural background that is different from your own. Ask this person to teach you about salient aspects of his or her culture.

4. If your grandparents originally came from another country, interview them about their experiences growing up in their culture. If they are bicultural, ask them about any experiences with combining both cultures. What have been their experiences in assimilation? Do they retain their original cultural identity? What do they most value in both cultures? Do what you can to discover the ways in which your cultural roots have some influence on your thinking and behavior today. In Chapter 3 you were introduced to the importance of discovering how your family of origin continues to influence you. This exercise can help you develop a richer appreciation of your cultural heritage.

5. Take a few minutes to look at the results of the self-assessment inventory (QDI) pertaining to awareness and receptivity to cultural diversity and equity that is found in the early part of this chapter. After reading this chapter, are you more aware of your attitudes and beliefs pertaining to cultural diversity? In your journal, write about strengths that you see in yourself that will assist you in becoming a culturally competent helper. Write also about any of your beliefs, values, and assumptions that could inhibit your ability to make good contact with individuals who are culturally different from you. Then review the checklist of knowledge, skills, and awareness competencies that appeared later in this chapter and determine your current level of proficiency in these competencies. List some steps you can take to either acquire or refine your knowledge and skills.

6. For the full bibliographic entry for each of the sources listed here, consult the References and Reading List at the back of the book. For a state-of-the-art book on multicultural perspectives on supervision and training, practice, and research and on models of racial and ethnic identity development, see Ponterotto, Casas, Suzuki, and Alexander (1995). For a good overview of counseling strategies and issues for various ethnic and racial groups, consult Atkinson, Morten, and Sue (1998). Pedersen (2000) deals extensively with the topic of developing multi-

cultural awareness, knowledge, and skills. For a discussion of unintentional racism in counseling, see Ridley (1995). Sue, Ivey, and Pedersen (1996) deal in a comprehensive manner with multicultural counseling from the perspectives of theory, practice, and research. Sue and Sue (1999) have written a comprehensive text on helping diverse client populations. Consult W. Lee (1999) for an introductory overview of multicultural counseling; and for additional information consult Axelson (1999), Hwang (2000), Okun, Fried, and Okun (1999), and Wehrly (1995). For a framework for developing cultural competency in the areas of cultural awareness, knowledge acquisition, and skill development, see Lum (1999); and for a useful treatment of culturally diverse social work practice, see Lum (2000).

Ethics in Action CD-ROM Exercises

7. Review role-play segment 12 in Part Three on the CD-ROM. How would you respond if your client presented you with a gift and told you that in his culture this was a way to express appreciation? How might the cultural context make a difference in deciding to accept or not accept a gift?

8. Put yourself into role-play segment 3, Culture Clash, in Part Two [Values and Helping Professions] on the CD-ROM. You are the counselor, and your client directly questions you about your background, wondering if you are able to understand her life experience and thus help her. When you consider the range of differences between yourself and a given client, what specific differences concern you the most? Role-play a situation where a clash between you and a client might develop (such as a difference in age, race, sexual orientation, or culture).

9. Refer to the CD-ROM section entitled "Becoming an Effective Multicultural Practitioner," which is found in Part Two immediately following role-play 3. Complete the self-examination of multicultural counseling competencies. Bring your answers into class and explore in small discussion groups what you need to learn to become competent as a counselor of clients whose cultural backgrounds differ from yours.

InfoTrac College Edition Resources

For additional readings, explore InfoTrac College Edition, our online library. Go to http://www.infotrac.college.com/wadsworth and select these key word searches:

    cultural W1 diversity therap*
    gender W1 equity
    effective multicult*

Key words are listed in a form that enables the search engine to locate a wider range of articles in the online university library. Key words should be entered exactly as shown, including asterisks, "W1," "W2," "AND," and other search engine tools.

CHAPTER 9

Ethical and Legal Issues Facing Helpers

Focus Questions

1. What ethical issues most concern you at this stage in your professional development?

2. When you are faced with an ethical dilemma, what route do you take in attempting to resolve the conflicts involved, and how do you make an ethical decision? What specific steps would you take in dealing with an ethical dilemma?

3. When would you be inclined to refer a client? On what grounds might you make the referral, and how would you go about it?

4. There are limits to confidentiality in any helping relationship. What would you want your clients to know about the purposes and limitations of confidentiality?

5. What is the role of ethics codes in guiding professionals to practice ethically? What value do you find in ethics codes?

6. What are your concerns, if any, about the prospects of being involved in a malpractice suit? What steps can you take to lessen the chances of such an action being taken against you?

7. What are some of the ways a client's privacy can be violated through the inappropriate use of various forms of technology (voice mail, pagers, faxes, cellular phones, and e-mail)?

8. What are some of the key ethical issues that need to be considered in a managed care context?

9. What do you consider to be the most essential components of informed consent?

10. How are you likely to secure informed consent from your clients?

Aim of the Chapter

Regardless of what helping profession you decide on, you will be faced with ethical dilemmas. Part of becoming a professional involves being able to apply codes of ethics to practical situations. In this chapter we introduce you to an array of ethical and legal concerns that helpers encounter.

There has been an increased interest in ethics in the mental health profession in recent years. Articles pertaining to ethical and legal issues in the helping field are common in professional journals, and a number of books have been written in the field of professional ethics. Many undergraduate and graduate programs include a discussion of these topics in various courses, with separate courses in ethical, legal, and professional issues now required in most graduate programs. Although we don't want to be cynical about the motivations for the rising interest in ethics, we suspect that some of this trend is a response to the rising tide of malpractice actions against those in the helping professions. How to lessen the chances of a malpractice suit is one topic of this chapter. In addition to the realities of legal constraints, we hope you will become increasingly sensitive to the ethical dimensions of your professional practice by focusing on what is best for your clients.

The chapter will not provide you with an in-depth knowledge of ethical issues, but we hope it will stimulate you to read some of the books listed at the end of the chapter. We encourage you to take an ethics course or, at the very least, to attend professional conferences and workshops dealing with ethical, legal, and professional concerns.

Inventory of Ethical Issues

What are some of your major concerns about ethical practices? Perhaps at this point you have not even raised this question. We hope you will broaden your awareness of the significant ethical issues that you may face. For each statement in this inventory, indicate the response that most closely identifies your beliefs and attitudes. Use the following code:

> 5 = I *strongly agree* with this statement.
> 4 = I *agree* with this statement.
> 3 = I am *undecided* about this statement.
> 2 = I *disagree* with this statement.
> 1 = I *strongly disagree* with this statement.

_____ 1. When an ethical concern arises, the best way to deal with it is to refer to the code of ethics.

_____ 2. If I were faced with an ethical dilemma in one of my cases, I would take the initiative in seeking guidance from one of my professors or supervisors.

_____ 3. It would be hard for me to refer a client to another professional, even if I felt this was in the client's best interest.

    4. If I felt that I lacked the competency to work with a certain client, but he or she refused to accept a referral to another professional, I would continue seeing this person.

    5. It would be difficult for me to decide when I had to break confidentiality.

    6. If I were uncertain about keeping a client's confidence, I would want to discuss this with my client.

    7. I would have trouble terminating a client even if it were clear that the client was no longer benefiting.

    8. I am uncertain about how to go about resolving many ethical dilemmas.

    9. I often doubt whether I know enough or possess the skills needed to effectively help others.

    10. I am not at all certain what I might do if I felt that one of my clients posed a danger either to self or to others.

    11. I am likely to promote dependency on the part of my clients by being too ready to offer advice or too quick to find solutions to their problems.

    12. The obligation to warn and protect others is an area where I am uncertain about taking the appropriate action.

    13. What constitutes ethical practice is very much a concern of mine.

    14. I know the steps I am likely to take in cases where I become aware of unethical behavior on the part of my colleagues.

    15. I am concerned about the possibility of becoming involved in a malpractice suit as a result of something I do or don't do as a helper.

Once you have finished this inventory, spend a few minutes reflecting on any ethical concerns you have at this time. This reflection can help you read the chapter more actively and formulate ethical questions. Identify a few of the areas where you are uncertain about your position, and bring this ambiguity up in class discussions.

Ethical Decision Making

Ethical practice involves far more than merely knowing and following a professional code of ethics. In dealing with ethical dilemmas, you will rarely find clear-cut answers. Most of the problems are complex and defy simple solution. Making ethical decisions involves acquiring a tolerance for dealing with gray areas and for coping with ambiguity. Although knowing the ethical standards of your profession is important, this knowledge alone is not sufficient. Ethics codes are not dogma but provide guidance in assisting you in making the best possible decisions for the benefit of your clients and yourself. Standards vary among agencies. It is essential that you become aware of the specific policies and practices of the agency in which you are working.

In our teaching we find that students often begin an ethics course with the expectation of getting concrete answers to some of the questions raised in their fieldwork. They do not expect to have to engage in personal and professional self-exploration to find the best course of action. At times, readers of our ethics book (G. Corey, M. Corey, & Callanan, 2003) comment that it raises many more questions than it answers. We tell them that the book's purpose is to challenge them to develop the resources to deal intelligently with ethical dilemmas.

Consider the example of Gerlinde, who became aware of unethical practices in a community agency where she was an intern. She and other interns were expected to take on some difficult clients. She realized that doing so would mean that she was clearly practicing beyond the boundaries of her competence. To make the situation worse, supervision at the agency left much to be desired. Her superior was not willing to offer regular supervision and was often "too busy" to keep appointments to talk about her cases. In her fieldwork seminar on campus she learned that supervisors are ethically and legally responsible for what interns do. Gerlinde had some trouble deciding what to do. She did not want to change placements in the middle of the semester, yet she was struggling with the appropriateness of confronting her supervisor about the situation. Unclear about how to proceed, she made an appointment with her fieldwork professor on campus, who shared responsibility with the agency supervisor.

In consultation with her professor, Gerlinde explored a number of alternatives. She might approach her agency supervisor herself and be more assertive in getting an appointment. Another option could be a meeting with Gerlinde, her agency supervisor, and her professor to explore the situation. It might be decided that this particular agency was inappropriate for students. What was important was that Gerlinde knew she could get help in dealing with her problem. Sometimes students who are in similar predicaments arrive too quickly at the conclusion that they will merely tolerate things as they are rather than challenge an uncomfortable situation.

At the beginning of the course, Gerlinde thought that clear answers were available for the variety of situations that would surface. By the end of the semester, she was learning to appreciate that ethics codes are not laws; they are standards that provide guidance in dealing with a range of ethical dilemmas. She had also learned the value of initiating the consultation process in ethical decision making.

Another example involves interpreting the ethical standard that the client's welfare should be the primary consideration in the therapeutic relationship. Consider the case of a client who is talking about his struggles in an alcoholic family. As the therapist listens, his own pain over having alcoholic parents is triggered. He wonders whether he should tell his client about his personal reactions. Will his disclosure meet his own needs or the needs of the client? How is the therapist to judge whether the disclosure will help or hinder the client in working through places where he is stuck?

Ethical issues in counseling are often complex and multifaceted, and they defy simplistic solutions. There are many gray areas that require decision-making skills. This process entails not only learning information about ethical standards but also learning how to define and work through a variety of difficult situations. Thinking about ethical issues and learning to make wise decisions is an evolutionary process that requires an open mind.

Law and Ethics

Most professional organizations affirm that practitioners should be aware of the prevailing community standards and of the possible impact on their practice of deviation from these standards. Ethical and legal issues are frequently intertwined, which makes it imperative not only that practitioners follow the ethics codes of their profession but also that they know their state's laws and their legal boundaries and responsibilities.

Laws and ethics codes provide guidelines, yet neither offers clear-cut answers to situational problems. *Law* defines the minimum standards society will tolerate; these standards are enforced by government. All of the codes of ethics state that practitioners must act in accordance with relevant federal and state statutes and governmental regulations. But counselors often have doubts about whether they have a legal problem, or what to do with this legal issue once it has been identified (Remley & Herlihy, 2001). It is essential that practitioners be able to identify legal problems as they arise in their work; many of the situations helpers encounter that involve ethical and professional judgment will also have legal implications.

Helpers who work with minors and certain involuntary populations are especially advised to learn the laws restricting their practices. Areas that may be governed by law include confidentiality, parental consent, informed consent, protection of client welfare, and civil rights of institutionalized persons. Because most helpers do not possess detailed legal knowledge, it is a good idea for helpers to obtain legal advice about the procedures they use in their practice. Awareness of legal rights and responsibilities as they pertain to helping relationships protects not only the clients but also practitioners from needless lawsuits arising from negligence or ignorance.

Crawford (1999) points out that counselors do not have to be lawyers to practice with a lawful perspective. As is the case with dealing with ethical dilemmas, Crawford tells us not to expect to find simple solutions to every legal problem. Lacking a definitive answer to what the legal path to follow entails, some professionals increasingly limit their options of ways to work with clients out of fear of a possible lawsuit. This raises a potential ethical issue of delivering less than effective services, especially if this narrowing of available options to clients is not clearly expressed during the initial interview.

Unlike law, *ethics* represents aspirational goals, or the maximum or ideal standards set by the profession. Ethical standards are enforced by professional associations, national certification boards, and government boards that regulate professions (Remley, 1996). Codes of ethics are conceptually broad in nature and generally subject to interpretation by practitioners.

Laws and ethics codes, by their very nature, tend to be reactive, emerging from what has occurred rather than anticipating what may occur. We hope that you will not limit your behavior to obeying statutes and following ethical standards but will develop a sensitivity to doing what is best for your clients by working toward the best standards of practice. It is very important that you acquire this ethical sense at the beginning of your professional program. Remember that the basic purpose of practicing ethically is to further the welfare of your clients.

Professional Codes and Ethical Decision Making

Various professional organizations have established codes of ethics that provide broad guidelines for professional helpers. These codes are not static; they are revised as new concerns arise. Some of the professional mental health organizations that have formulated codes of ethics are the National Association of Social Workers ([NASW], 1999), the American Psychological Association ([APA], 1992), the American Counseling Association ([ACA], 1995), the American Association for Marriage and Family Therapy ([AAMFT], 2001), and the National Organization for Human Service Education ([NOHSE], 2000). Herlihy and Corey (1997b) identify several purposes that codes of ethics serve:

- Codes of ethics educate helpers about sound ethical practice. The application of these codes to particular situations demands a keen ethical sensitivity.
- Codes of ethics provide a mechanism for professional accountability. The ultimate end of a code of ethics is to protect the consumers of mental health services.
- Codes of ethics serve as catalysts for improving practice. Codes can get us to critically examine both the letter and the spirit of ethical principles.

Ethics codes are necessary, but not sufficient, for the exercise of ethical responsibility. Although you have or will become familiar with the ethics codes of your specialization, you must still develop your own personal ethical stance that will govern your practice. You have the ongoing challenge of examining your own practices to determine whether you are acting as ethically as you might. Ethics codes do not convey ultimate truth, nor do they provide ready-made answers for the ethical dilemmas that you will face. Although ethics codes offer guidance, they do not make decisions for you. You will be challenged to grapple with the gray areas, raise questions, discuss your ethical concerns with colleagues, and monitor your own behavior (Herlihy & Corey, 1996a). When dealing with the uniqueness of each client, it is up to you to apply ethics codes to specific situations and to engage in a process of ethical decision making in determining the best course of action.

According to Frame (1999), most ethics codes are punitive rather than preventative, reactive rather than proactive. Codes of ethics are largely designed to protect the client by describing parameters within which the helper should operate so that clients are not harmed. In addition, codes are partially designed to protect practitioners in cases of malpractice. If you conscientiously practice in accordance with accepted professional codes, you have some measure of protection in case of litigation. Compliance with or violation of ethics codes of conduct may be admissible as evidence in some legal proceedings. In a lawsuit, your conduct would probably be judged in comparison with that of other professionals with similar qualifications and duties.

The NASW *Code of Ethics* (1999) states that an ethics code cannot guarantee ethical behavior, nor can it resolve all ethical issues or disputes, nor can it capture the complexity involved in making responsible choices within a moral community. Instead, the code identifies ethical principles and standards to which professionals should aspire and by which their actions can be judged. Indeed, the NASW document reinforces the idea that ethical decision making is a process:

> Reasonable differences of opinion can and do exist among social workers with respect to the ways in which values, ethical principles, and ethical standards should be rank-ordered when they conflict. Ethical decision making in a given situation must apply the informed judgment of the individual social worker and should also consider how the issues would be judged in a peer review process where the ethical standards of the profession would be applied.
>
> Ethical decision making is a process. There are many instances in social work where simple answers are not available to resolve complex ethical issues. Social workers should take into consideration all the values, principles, and standards in this *Code* that are relevant to any situation in which ethical judgment is warranted. Social workers' decisions and actions should be consistent with the spirit as well as the letter of this *Code*.

We suggest that you devote some time to reviewing the codes of ethics of one or more of the professional organizations. Examine the assets and limitations of these codes. As you think about these codes of ethics, identify any areas of possible disagreement that you might have with a particular standard. If your practice goes against a specific ethics code, be aware that you must have a rationale for your course of action. Realize also that there are consequences for violating the codes of your profession.

Must you follow all the ethics codes of your profession to be considered an ethical practitioner? If you agree with and follow all the ethics codes of your profession, does this necessarily mean that you are an ethical professional? Practical application of codes is often difficult. The complex issues you will encounter as a helper will require not only an understanding of the codes for your profession but also knowledgeable interpretations of these codes to the real-life situations you face.

Recognizing Unethical Behavior in Yourself

It is easier to see the shortcomings of others and to judge their behavior than to develop an attitude of honest self-examination. You can control your own professional behavior far more easily than you can that of your colleagues, so the proper focus is to look honestly at what you are doing. There is a tendency to think in terms of gross ethical violations while overlooking more subtle ways of being unethical. Consider for a moment these two scenarios, and ask yourself the degree to which you could picture yourself in each situation:

- A client calls you frequently and pleads that he is in great need of your direction. He is afraid to make decisions lest "I mess up my life even more than it is." Might you be flattered by being needed? Could you see yourself fostering his dependency out of your need to be needed?
- A client who is in private therapy with you is ambivalent about continuing counseling sessions. She wonders whether it is time to terminate and "try it alone." Things are rather tight financially for you right now, and several

other clients have recently terminated. Would you be inclined to support her decision? Might you be inclined to encourage her to continue, partly for financial reasons?

Unethical Behavior by Colleagues

You may occasionally encounter colleagues who are behaving in unethical and unprofessional ways. Professional codes of conduct generally state that in such cases the most prudent action is to approach the colleague and share your concerns directly in an attempt to rectify the situation. If this step fails, you are then expected to make use of procedures established by your professional organization, such as reporting the colleague.

Reflect for a few minutes on being in each of the following situations. What would you do in each case?

- A colleague frequently talks about his clients in inappropriate ways in places where others are able to hear him. The colleague says that joking about his clients is his way of "letting off steam" and preventing himself from taking life too seriously.
- A couple of female clients have told you that they were sexually seduced by another counselor at the agency where you work. In their counseling sessions with you, they are dealing with their anger over having been taken advantage of by this counselor.
- A colleague has several times initiated social contacts with her clients. She thinks that this practice is acceptable because she sees her clients as consenting adults. Furthermore, she contends that time spent socializing with these clients gives her insights into issues with which she can productively work in the therapy sessions.
- You see that one of your colleagues is practicing beyond what you think is the scope of his competence and training. This person is unwilling to seek additional training and is also not receiving adequate supervision. He maintains that the best way to learn to work with unfamiliar problems that clients present is simply to "jump in and learn by doing."

The ethics codes generally address the matter of how to respond to unethical behavior of colleagues. For example, NOHSE (2000) provides this standard:

> Human service professionals respond appropriately to unethical behavior of colleagues. Usually this means initially talking directly with the colleague and, if no resolution is forthcoming, reporting the colleague's behavior to supervisory or administrative staff and/or to the professional organization(s) to which the colleague belongs.

Certainly, dealing with the unethical behavior of colleagues demands a measure of courage. If these people are in a position of power, you are obviously vulnerable. Even in the case of peers, confrontations usually are difficult. The other person may react defensively and tell you to mind your own business.

An Ethical Decision-Making Model

Having a systematic way of examining difficult ethical dilemmas increases your chances of making sound ethical decisions. We cannot overemphasize the importance of seeking consultation when deciding on the best course of action. It is a good idea to consult with more than one colleague or supervisor; doing so can help you see various dimensions of a problem. Responsible and ethical practice requires that you do the following things:

- Base your actions on informed, sound, and responsible judgment.
- Consult with colleagues or seek supervision.
- Keep your knowledge and skills current.
- Engage in a continual process of self-examination.
- Remain open.

As much as possible, and when appropriate, include your client in the ethical decision-making process. Make ethical decisions *with* clients, not simply *for* them. Respecting the autonomy of your clients implies that you do not decide for them, nor do you foster dependent attitudes and behaviors. Cottone (2001) describes a social constructivism model of ethical decision making that is collaborative in nature. This approach involves negotiating, consensualizing, and when necessary, arbitrating. In dealing with an ethical dilemma or concern, Cottone recommends following these steps:

> [T]he ethically sensitive professional operating from a social contructivism mode would take several steps: (a) obtain information from those involved, (b) assess the nature of the relationships operating at that moment in time, (c) consult valued colleagues and professional expert opinion (including ethics codes and literature), (d) negotiate when there is a disagreement, and (e) respond in a way that allows for a reasonable consensus as to what should happen or what really occurred. Every relationship involved must be examined for potential linkage to another (possibly adversarial) system of thought. In addition, every relationship must be assessed for a potential conflict of opinion over what should or did happen. If consensus is not possible, further negotiation, interactive reflection, or arbitration may be necessary. (p. 43)

The ethical decision-making model we present here involves the inclusion of the clients as collaborators whenever possible. The procedural steps we describe below should not be thought of as a simplified and linear way to reach a resolution on ethical matters. It has been our experience that the application of these steps generally stimulates self-reflection and encourages discussion. Following these systematic steps will help you think through ethical problems.

1. Identify the problem or dilemma. Gather as much information as you can to clarify the situation you are facing. You might ask yourself these questions: "Is this an ethical, legal, professional, or clinical problem? Is it a combination of more than one of these?" If there are legal dimensions to the problem, seek legal consultation. Remember that many ethical dilemmas are complex, which means that it is best to examine the problem from various perspectives and to avoid looking for a simplistic solution. Ethical dilemmas do not have "right" or "wrong" answers, so you will be challenged to deal with ambiguity. It may be helpful to seek consultation to determine whether there actually is an ethical concern—or to identify the exact nature of the problem. Including the client begins at this initial step and continues throughout the process of working through an ethical problem, as does the process of documenting your decisions and actions.

2. Identify the potential issues involved. After the information is collected, list and describe the critical issues and discard the irrelevant ones. Evaluate the rights, responsibilities, and welfare of all those who are affected by the situation. Good reasons can be presented that support various sides of a given issue, and different ethical principles may indicate different courses of action. Ask yourself these questions: "How can I best promote client independence and self-determination? What actions have the least chance of bringing harm to a client? What decision will best safeguard the welfare of the client? How can I create a trusting and therapeutic climate where clients can find their own solutions?"

3. Apply the ethics code. Once you have a clearer picture of the nature of the problem, review the code of ethics to see if the issue is addressed. If there are specific and clear guidelines, following them may resolve the problem. However, if the problem is more complex and a resolution is not apparent, you may need to employ additional steps to resolve the problem. Ask yourself whether the standards of your professional organization offer a possible solution to the problem. Consider whether your own values and ethics are consistent with or in conflict with the relevant codes. If you are in disagreement with a particular standard, do you have a rationale to support your position? Your state or national professional association may be able to provide you with guidance in resolving a dilemma. Such associations often make legal counsel available to their members.

4. Know the applicable laws and regulations. It is essential for you to keep up to date on relevant state and federal laws. This is especially critical in matters of keeping or divulging confidentiality, reporting child or elder abuse, dealing with issues pertaining to danger to self or others, parental rights, record keeping, testing and assessment, and diagnosis. In addition, be sure you understand the current rules and regulations of the agency or organization where you work.

5. Obtain consultation. At this point, it is generally helpful to consult with a colleague or colleagues to obtain a different perspective on the problem. Consider consulting with more than one professional, and do not limit the individuals with whom you will consult to those who share your orientation. If there is a legal question, seek legal counsel. After you present your assessment of the situation and your ideas of how you might proceed, ask the person for feedback on your analysis. Reflect on questions such as these:

- What kinds of questions do you want to ask of those with whom you consult?
- How can you use the consultation process as an opportunity to test the justification of a course of action you are inclined to take?

- Are you considering all of the ethical, clinical, and legal issues involved in the case?

Consultation can help you think about information or circumstances that you may have overlooked. It is wise to document the nature of your consultation, including the suggestions provided by those with whom you consulted.

6. Consider possible and probable courses of action. Brainstorm as many possible courses of action as you can. In doing so, ask colleagues to help you generate possible courses of action. By listing a wide variety of courses of action, you may identify a possibility that seems most useful to you. Evaluate each option with reference to the potential consequences for all parties involved. Eliminate those options that do not promise to give the desired results or that may have problematic consequences. As you think about the many possibilities for action, discuss these options with your client, if or when appropriate, as well as with other professionals. Care needs to be taken to ensure that the client does not become the "helper" in cases where they are included in these discussions. Determine which of the remaining options or combination of options is best suited to the situation. A good guideline in choosing your course of action would be the degree to which you would feel comfortable knowing your actions would be published in the newspaper or as a part of the news on radio or television. If your answer is "no," you have reason to reconsider your selected course of action.

7. Explore the consequences of various decisions. Ponder the implications of each course of action for the client, for others who are related to the client, and for you as the counselor. Again, a discussion with your client about consequences for him or her can be most important, when appropriate. Review the consequences of key decisions to determine if any new ethical problems might arise. If so, go back to the beginning and reevaluate each step of the process.

8. Decide on the best course of action. In making the best decision, carefully consider the information you have received from various sources. The more obvious the dilemma, the clearer is the course of action; the more subtle the dilemma, the more difficult the decision will be. In carrying out your plan, realize that other professionals might choose different courses of action in the same situation. However, you can only act in accordance with the best information you have. After you carry out your course of action, it is wise to follow up on the situation to evaluate whether your actions had the anticipated effect and consequences. Determine the outcomes and see if any further action is needed. Reflecting on your assessment of the situation and the actions you took is essential if you are to learn from your experience. This is where reviewing your notes can be particularly helpful in assessing the process. To obtain the most accurate picture, involve your client in this process, when appropriate.

Even if you follow a systematic model such as the one we have described, you may still experience some anxiety about whether you made the best decision possible in a given case. Rarely is ethical thinking a clear-cut matter. Many ethical issues are controversial, and some involve blending ethics and the law. An important sign of your good faith is your willingness to share concerns or struggles with colleagues, supervisors, and fellow students. It is essential that you keep informed about laws that affect your practice, maintain awareness of new developments in your field, reflect on ways that your values will influence your practice, and be willing to engage in an ongoing process of self-reflection. Developing a sense of professional and ethical responsibility is a task never completely finished.

Recognizing Competence and Learning to Refer

As a beginning helper, you are not alone if you have doubts about your general level of competence. In fact, it is not at all unusual for even highly experienced mental health practitioners to wonder seriously at times whether they have the personal and professional abilities needed to work with some of their clients. It is more troubling to think of helpers who rarely question their competence. In thinking about the matter, you may range from one extreme to the other, at times being plagued with self-doubts and at other times feeling overly confident, thinking that you can tackle any problem a client presents.

Virtually all of the professional codes spell out that you should not practice beyond the limits of your competence. Here are two examples from these codes.

American Psychological Association (1992)
Psychologists provide services, teach, and conduct research only within the boundaries of their competence, based on their education, training, supervised experience, or appropriate professional experience.

American Counseling Association (1995)
Counselors practice only within the boundaries of their competence, based on their education, training, supervised experience, state and national professional credentials, and appropriate professional experience. Counselors will demonstrate a commitment to gain knowledge, personal awareness, sensitivity, and skills pertinent to working with a diverse client population.

Assessing competence is not an easy task. Many people who complete a doctoral program lack the skills or knowledge needed to carry out certain therapeutic tasks. Obviously, a degree alone does not guarantee competence for any and all psychological services. Practitioners must also assess how far they can safely go with clients and when to refer them to other professionals. Similarly, it is important to learn when to consult another professional if the counselor has not had extensive experience working with a particular problem.

Knowing When and How to Make Referrals

The ethics codes of most professional organizations stipulate that making referrals is one of the main responsibilities of the professional helper. For example, the National Association of Social Workers (1999) provides this guideline:

Social workers should refer clients to other professionals when other professionals' specialized knowledge or expertise is needed to serve clients fully or when social workers believe they are not being effective or making reasonable progress with clients and additional service is required. (2.06.a.)

How do you know when and how to refer? Why would you want to refer? What kind of referral might be the most appropriate? What if few referral resources are available? It is crucial for you to refer clients to other resources when working with them is beyond your ability or when personal factors are likely to interfere with a productive working relationship. A client's failure to make progress with you is another reason to consider a referral. Other circumstances may also lead you to wonder if a referral is in order. You and a client may decide that because of value conflicts or for some other reason your relationship is not productive, but the client may want to continue working with another helper. For these and other reasons you will need to develop a framework for evaluating when to refer a client, and you will need to learn how to make this referral in such a manner that your client will be open to accepting your suggestion rather than be harmed by it.

We would hope that you would not see referring a client with whom you have difficulty as the best solution to the problem. Clients can be negatively affected when you too quickly refer them. If you follow the practice of referring all clients with whom you have difficulty, you might soon have very few clients left! It is a good idea to think about the reasons you would be inclined to suggest a referral. If you recognize a pattern of frequent referrals, then you may need to examine your reasons for doing so.

In cases where you have limited experience, it is especially important to be open to consulting another professional as a way to acquire or upgrade your skills. We hope that you will always be willing to say to a client "I don't know what to do, but I know where we can get some help." Beginning helpers sometimes believe that they must have all the answers, and they hesitate to let their clients know that they might not be sure how best to proceed. Although we do not expect you to know everything, we certainly expect that you can learn much under supervision. You can also learn new skills by going to conferences and conventions, by taking additional courses in areas you do not know well and in theories that you are not necessarily drawn to, and by participating in workshops that combine didactic work with supervised practice. The feedback you receive can give you an additional resource for evaluating your readiness to undertake certain therapeutic tasks.

Referral resources are sometimes limited. This is particularly true in some less-populated areas where mental health facilities are scant. One helper told us: "I realize that I may not be much to some of my clients, but then again, I'm all they have! The nearest referral agency is over a hundred miles away, so what are they to do?" To make good referrals, first you must know of the possibilities that might be available for your clients.

Imagine that you are an intern at a community mental health center. This is your first experience in this type of setting. One of your first clients presents himself with much confusion about his sexual identity. He is unclear about how to proceed. Should he follow through on his homosexual inclinations or remain in his marriage? You feel overwhelmed, you are very uncomfortable with his choice, and you don't know quite how to handle this situation. What might you say or do? Here are some possible approaches:

- You could deny your discomfort and not express any of your feelings or reactions.
- You could share your negative reactions about homosexuality and attempt to persuade the client to remain in his marriage.
- You might let your client know that you feel both uncomfortable and overwhelmed but that you would like to challenge yourself by working with him. You could also tell him that you will seek supervision to help you avoid imposing your values on him.
- You could tell this client that you are very new in this work, that you are uncertain about how to proceed, and that you would like to refer him.

What are your thoughts about this situation and how might you proceed?

Deciding Whether to Terminate

Ethical standards usually state that it is improper to continue a professional relationship if it is clear that a client is not benefiting. The tricky problem is to assess whether the client is really being helped. What if you are convinced that a client is not making significant gains, yet she assures you that she is growing from the experience? Consider the issues in the following case example, and think about what you would do if you were confronted with a similar situation.

You have been seeing a client for some time. She is very consistent, yet she typically reports that she really has nothing to discuss. You have confronted her on her unwillingness to invest much of herself in the counseling sessions. The client agrees yet continues to return. Finally, you suggest termination because, in your opinion, she is not benefiting from the relationship. The client is reluctant to follow your suggestion, despite her lack of involvement in the sessions. How would you handle this situation?

Respecting the Client's Autonomy

Perhaps one of the most basic rights of clients is to have their autonomy safeguarded by the helper. Helpers can foster clients' dependent attitudes and behaviors in many subtle ways. Instead of helping clients find their own direction, helpers sometimes do too much for them, which results in clients assuming too little responsibility for action and change. Most professional codes warn about creating a dependent relationship with clients. Although your clients may temporarily become dependent on you, an ethical issue arises if you foster their dependency and actually prevent their growth. You might ask yourself these questions as a way of determining the degree to which you encourage either dependent or independent behavior:

- Do I have a hard time terminating a case? Do I have trouble "losing" a client? Am I concerned about a reduction in my income?
- Might I need some clients more than they need me? Do I have a need to be needed? On some level do I feel a sense of power when clients express dependency on me?
- Do I challenge clients to do for themselves what they are able to do? Am I unwilling to provide clients with quick resolutions or easy answers, even when they press me for such solutions?
- To what degree do I encourage clients to look within themselves for potential resources to find their own answers?

Some helpers foster dependence in their clients as a way of feeling important. They convince themselves that they are all-wise and that they can direct their clients' life. These helpers may feed off the dependent needs of clients to derive a sense of significance. When clients play a helpless role and beg for answers, these helpers respond all too quickly with problem-solving solutions. Such actions may not be helpful in the long run, for clients are being reinforced for their lack of willingness to support themselves. Your main job as a helper is to eventually put yourself out of business, which is done by encouraging clients to rely on their own resources rather than on yours. By reinforcing the dependency of your clients, you are telling them that you do not trust that they can help themselves or that they can function independently from you.

Informed Consent

For most clients, asking for formal or professional help is a new experience. They are often unclear about what is expected of them and what they should expect from the helper. The ethics codes of most professional organizations require that clients be given adequate information to make informed choices about entering and continuing in the therapeutic relationship. The National Association of Social Workers (1999) provides this requirement about informed consent:

> Social workers should provide services to clients only in the context of a professional relationship based, when appropriate, on valid informed consent. Social workers should use clear and understandable language to inform clients of the purpose of the service, risks related to the service, limits to service because of the requirements of a third-party payor, relevant costs, reasonable alternatives, clients' right to refuse or withdraw consent, and the time frame covered by the consent. Social workers should provide clients with an opportunity to ask questions. (1.03.a.)

The American Counseling Association (1995) has a similar code regarding informed consent:

> When counseling is initiated, and throughout the counseling process as necessary, counselors inform clients of the purposes, goals, techniques, procedures, limitations, potential risks, and benefits of services to be performed, and other pertinent information. Counselors take steps to ensure that clients understand

the implications of diagnosis, the intended use of tests and reports, fees, and billing arrangements. Clients have a right to expect confidentiality and to be provided with an explanation of its limitations, including supervision and/or treatment team professionals; to obtain clear information about their case records; to participate in the ongoing counseling plans; and to refuse any recommended services and be advised of the consequences of such refusal. (A.3.a.)

Perhaps the best way to safeguard the rights of clients is to develop procedures to help them make informed choices. Informed consent involves the right of clients to be informed about what their relationship with you will entail and to make autonomous decisions pertaining to it. How can you teach your clients about their rights and responsibilities from the outset of the helping relationship? This process begins with the intake interview and continues for the duration of the relationship. Getting informed consent involves a delicate balance between telling clients too little and overwhelming them with too much information too soon.

According to Bednar, Bednar, Lambert, and Waite (1991), informed consent is a legal doctrine that is rooted in the law's recognition of the importance of self-determination. Bednar and his colleagues write that the informed consent process is a standard part of ethical and legal practice. Although most professionals agree on the ethical duty to provide clients with relevant information about the helping process, there is not much consensus about what should be revealed and in what manner. In deciding what you would most want to tell a client, consider these questions:

- What are the goals of the helping relationship?
- What services are you willing to provide?
- What do you expect of your client? What can your client expect of you?
- What are the risks and benefits of helping strategies that are likely to be employed?
- What do you want to tell your client about yourself?
- What are the qualifications of the provider of the services?
- What are the financial considerations?
- What is the estimated duration of the professional relationship? How will termination be handled?
- What are the limitations of confidentiality? When does the law require mandatory reporting?
- Under what circumstances are you likely to consult with a supervisor or other colleagues about the case?
- Are there any alternatives to the approaches you might suggest?

If you are part of a managed behavioral health care program, you will also need to explain to your clients the number of sessions allowed, the limitations of confidentiality, and the narrower scope of short-term interventions.

Although some mental health workers use written informed consent procedures, you will need to decide which approach works best for you and your clients. We suggest that you develop a comprehensive written statement to give to clients at the first session so that they can take the materials home and read them before the next session. In this way clients have a basis for asking questions and valuable time is saved. It is important to have this client sign the document indicating an understanding of the policies and procedures.

When clients finally make an appointment, they are often anxious to get help on some pressing problem. Talking about the process in great detail can dampen the client's inclination to return for further sessions. Yet it is a mistake to withhold important information that clients need if they are to make wise choices. *What* and *how much* to tell clients is determined in part by the client. It is a good practice for helpers to employ an educational approach, encouraging clients' questions about evaluation or treatment and offering useful feedback as the helping process progresses. By providing your clients with adequate information, you are increasing the chances that they will become active participants and carry their share of the responsibilities in the helping relationship.

Confidentiality and Privacy

The helping relationship is built on a foundation of trust. If clients do not trust their helper, they will be unlikely to engage in significant self-disclosure and self-exploration. Trust is largely measured by the degree to which clients feel assured that what they share will be kept confidential. Mental health professionals have a dual ethical and legal responsibility to safeguard clients from unauthorized disclosures of information given in the context of the helping relationship. Helpers must not disclose this information except when required by law or authorized by the client to do so.

Although your clients have every right to expect that their relationship with you will remain confidential, your obligation to safeguard client disclosures is not absolute. You need to develop the legal knowledge and an ethical sense for when you must break confidentiality. The number one concern of counselors is confidentiality and its limits (Welfel, 2002). This matter should be spelled out for clients in their informed consent. According to Herlihy and Corey (1996b), it is a good idea to discuss the following points with your clients:

- The helping relationship will be kept confidential, except in certain circumstances. At times it is permissible to share information with others in the interest of providing the best possible services to the client.
- Confidential information may also be shared with other helping professionals when the client requests it or gives permission.
- Confidentiality is not an absolute, and other obligations may override the helper's pledge. For example, it is required that confidentiality be breached to protect someone who is in danger.
- Confidentiality cannot be guaranteed when the client is a minor or when counseling couples, families, or groups.
- Confidentiality can be compromised if a client's records are subpoenaed.

State law specifies the circumstances under which confidentiality must be compromised. You may have to reveal information when there is clear and imminent danger that clients will bring harm to others or to themselves. Know the laws in your state as there may be options other than breaking confidentiality available to you. Not all states have the same laws, but all states have mandatory reporting laws for incest and child abuse and several states have mandatory reporting laws for elder abuse. You have an ethical and legal obligation to report suspected child and elder abuse and neglect, so it is essential that you know how to assess signs of abuse. All states require reporting child abuse or neglect if it results in physical injury. In addition, you are expected to take action when clients are likely to harm themselves or others. If a client is suicidal, you cannot merely ignore this situation, even if your client asks you not to report it.

Human services professionals are vulnerable to lawsuits if they improperly handle confidentiality issues, so it behooves you to know the laws, to follow them, and to be aware of the ethical standards of your profession. Seek help from your professional organization when dealing with thorny ethical dilemmas.

As a way to sharpen your thinking about issues surrounding confidentiality, think about what you would do in these cases:

1. Child abuse. Two young girls are brought to a community agency by their aunt, who has gained custody of them in the last few months. One girl, age 11, is quite verbal, but the other, 13, is not. As they begin to talk and you ask about their history, they tell you of aunts and uncles who attempted to touch one of them and of an aunt who severely beat them. The 11-year-old tells of a suicide attempt by her sister after one such beating. If you were working with these girls, what action would you take, and why? Would you have available the telephone number of the Child Protective Service for the area in which you are working?

2. Runaway plan. A student intern works with pupils in an elementary school. She says to the children in a group "Everything you say in here will stay in here." Then a boy reveals a detailed plan to run away from home. The counselor, who has not talked about the exceptions to confidentiality with the children, does not know what to do. If she reports the boy, he may feel betrayed. If she does not report him, she may face a malpractice action for having failed to notify the parents. What might you suggest to her if she came to you for advice in this situation?

3. Students' violation of confidentiality. You are a counselor intern in a local agency. You are part of a training group of students that meets weekly to discuss cases. One day, while you are having lunch in a restaurant with some of the students, they begin to discuss their cases in detail, mentioning names and details of the clients loudly enough for others in the restaurant to overhear. What would you do in this situation?

It is tempting to talk about your clients and their stories, especially as others are usually curious about what you do. It may give you a sense of importance to be able to tell interesting anecdotes. You may talk more than you should when you feel overwhelmed by your clients and need to unburden yourself. As a professional helper, you must learn how to talk about clients and how to report without breaking confidentiality. Clients should know that confidentiality cannot be guaranteed absolutely, but they should have your sincere assurance that you will avoid talking about them except when the law requires you to disclose information or it is professionally necessary to do so.

Confidentiality in Couples and Family Therapy

Generally speaking, from a *legal* perspective, confidentiality does not apply to couples counseling, couples and family therapy, group counseling, and counseling minors. However, from an *ethical* perspective, confidentiality is of the utmost importance and must be discussed so all parties are aware of what confidentiality involves in these forms of counseling. If you are working with couples or families, confidentiality takes on a special meaning. Some helpers contend that whatever information they get from one family member should never be divulged to the other members. By contrast, other helpers have a policy of refusing to keep any information private within the family. Their assumption is that secrets are counterproductive in the attempt to help family members be open with one another. These helpers encourage bringing all secrets out into the open. It is essential that you be clear in your own mind about how you will deal with disclosures obtained from family members and that you let your clients know your policy before they enter into a relationship with you.

Case example.   Owen is involved in individual therapy and later has his wife, Flora, attend some of the sessions so they can receive marriage counseling. Owen discloses to the therapist that he became involved in a gay relationship a few months previously. He doesn't want his wife to know for fear that she will divorce him. In a later session in which the therapist is seeing the couple, Flora complains that she feels neglected and wonders if her husband is really committed to working on their marriage. She says that she is willing to continue marital counseling as long as she is sure that he wants to stay in the marriage and devote his efforts to working through their difficulties. The therapist knows about this gay relationship that is causing Owen a great deal of difficulty. She decides to say nothing about it in the joint session and maintains that it is the husband's decision whether to mention it.

- What do you think of the therapist's ethical decision in this situation?
- If you were involved in a somewhat similar situation, what might you do differently?
- Suppose Owen confided that he was concerned that he had contracted AIDS and was very worried. What action might you take? Are you concerned about the ethics of his withholding this information from Flora? Can a case be made for the duty to warn and protect an innocent party? (This is a topic we take up later in this chapter.)

Confidentiality in Group Counseling

If you ever lead a group, you will have to consider some special ethical, legal, and professional aspects of confidentiality. In a group setting, as is true for individual counseling, you must disclose the limitations of confidentiality. Because so many more people are privy to information shared in the group, you must also make it clear that you cannot guarantee confidentiality. Even if you continually emphasize to the members how essential it is to maintain confidentiality, there is still the possibility that some of them will talk inappropriately to others about what has been shared in the group. Leaders need to encourage members to bring up any of their reservations about possible breaches of confidentiality. If members see it as their responsibility to talk about these concerns, this topic can be openly explored in the group.

Assume that members of a group you were co-leading brought up their reluctance to participate because they were concerned about the need for a firm commitment to keep in the group whatever was discussed. How would you deal with their concerns?

Confidentiality in School Counseling

In the context of school counseling, protection of confidentiality and privacy is a major concern. Children and adolescent clients have a right to know what information will and will not be kept confidential from their first contact with a school counselor. In cases involving minors who are unable to give informed consent, the parents or guardians will need to provide this informed consent and may need to be included in the counseling process. Parents and guardians have some legal right to request information about counseling sessions, as do school personnel, but this should be done in a manner that will minimize intrusion of the child or adolescent's privacy and in a way that demonstrates respect for the student. It is essential that school counselors clearly inform the students they see of the limitations of confidentiality and how and when confidential information may be shared.

When minor clients pose a danger to themselves or to others, school counselors must breach confidentiality. From both an ethical and legal perspective, any threat of suicide or of violence to others must be taken very seriously. Even if the risk of the student actually committing suicide is remote, the possibility may be enough to establish a duty to contact the parents and inform them of the potential for suicidal behavior. Courts have found that the burden involved in making a telephone call is minor considering the risk of harm to a student who is suicidal. In short, school personnel are advised to take every precaution to protect the student. The same is true in all cases where there is a potential for violent acts.

This is an area where continuing education is of the utmost importance, as is the willingness to seek appropriate consultation when you become aware of students who are at risk. You can be held legally accountable only for judgment that is clearly negligent in light of the standard of care of other similar professionals with similar education and experience. As long as you act in an ethical and reasonable manner, you should not be overly concerned about legal sanctions related to student suicide or harm to others (Remley & Sparkman, 1993).

Confidentiality and Privacy in a Technological World

There are a host of ways to violate a client's privacy through the inappropriate use of various forms of technology. The use of the telephone, answering machines, voice mail, pagers, faxes, cellular phones, and e-mail can pose a number of potential ethical problems regarding the protection of privacy of clients. Mental health practitioners need to exercise caution in discussing confidential information with anyone over the telephone. Remley and Herlihy (2001, pp. 124–125) offer these guidelines for counselors using the telephone or leaving a message for clients:

- Do not acknowledge that clients are receiving services or give out information regarding clients to unknown callers.
- Verify that you are actually talking to the intended person when you make or receive calls in which confidential information will be discussed.
- Avoid making any comments that you would not want your client to hear or that you would not want to repeat in a legal proceeding.
- Do not allow unauthorized persons to hear answering machine messages in your office, as they are being left or retrieved.
- Personal messages should not be left on an answering machine unless this is prearranged with your client as another family member may retrieve the message left for your client.
- If you are talking to a client by cellular phone, assume that he or she is not in a private place. Your conversation may also be intercepted by an unauthorized person.
- If you use a pager, exercise caution when retrieving messages. In sending a pager message to a client, be mindful of ensuring your client's privacy by exercising the same caution you would if you were sending answering machine or voice mail messages.

Using fax machines to send confidential material is another source of potential invasion of a client's privacy. It is the helper's responsibility to make sure fax transmissions arrive in a secured environment in such a way as to protect confidential information. Before sending a confidential fax, it is a good idea to make a telephone call to assure the appropriate person will be able to receive this information in a safe and sensitive manner (Cottone & Tarvydas, 1998).

Communication by way of electronic mail is fraught with potential privacy problems. Because e-mail messages can be easily accessed by people other than their intended recipients, you cannot count on privacy. Since there is no reasonable expectation of confidentiality for e-mail, clients need to have input regarding how they want communication to be handled so that their privacy is protected.

This discussion of privacy may appear to be mere common sense. However, we have become so accustomed to relying on technology that careful thought is not always given to subtle ways that privacy can be violated. We emphasize the importance of using caution and paying attention to ways that you could unintentionally breach the privacy of your clients. As a part of the informed consent process, it is wise to discuss with your clients the potential problems of privacy regarding a wide range of technology and to take preventive measures so that both you and your clients have an understanding and agreement about these important concerns.

Privacy in a Small Community

I [Marianne] practiced for many years as a marriage and family therapist in a small community. This situation presented a set of ethical considerations involving safeguarding the privacy of clients. First, it was important that I choose an office that afforded privacy to clients as they entered and left. I considered leasing space in a small professional building in the center of town, but I quickly discovered that people would be uncomfortable making themselves that visible when seeking psychological help. A home office, which was remote from the center of the village, worked out well. However, I had to carefully schedule clients, allowing ample time between sessions so clients who might know each other would not meet in the office. When an office is located within a home, it is essential that a professional atmosphere be provided. Clients have a right to expect privacy and should not have to deal with intrusions by the therapist's family members.

I discussed with my clients the unique variables pertaining to confidentiality in a small community. I informed them that I would not discuss professional concerns with them should we meet at the grocery store or the post office, and I respected their preferences regarding interactions away from the office. Knowing that they were aware that I saw many people from the town, I reassured them that I would not talk with anyone about who my clients were. Another example of protecting my clients' privacy pertained to the manner of depositing checks at the local bank. Because the bank employees knew my profession, it would have been easy for them to identify my clients. Again, I talked with my clients about their preferences. If they had any discomfort about my depositing their checks in the local bank, I arranged to have them deposited elsewhere.

Your Obligation to Warn and Protect

Courts have created an exception to confidentiality when the mental health professional has a reasonable basis for believing that clients pose a danger either to themselves or to others. Despite your ethical duty to maintain your client's confidentiality, you are legally bound to breach confidentiality when it becomes necessary to protect your client or others.

Put yourself in this situation: A new client visits you at a college counseling center. He says he was severely abused by his father as a child and is now extremely angry. He is making threats to kill his father and tells you he has a gun. How do you proceed?

How do you decide whether a particular client is dangerous? Although practitioners are generally not held legally liable for their failure to predict violent behavior of a client, an inadequate assessment of client dangerousness can result in liability for the therapist, harm to third parties, and inappropriate breaches of client confidentiality. Helping professionals faced with potentially dangerous clients should take specific steps designed to protect the public and to minimize their own liability. They should take careful histories, advise clients of the limits of confidentiality, keep accurate notes of threats and other client statements, seek consultation, and record steps they have taken to protect others.

It is extremely difficult to decide when breaching confidentiality to protect potential victims is justified. Most states either permit or require therapists to breach confidentiality to warn or protect victims. In light of a number of court cases, mental health professionals have become increasingly conscious of a double duty—to protect other people from potentially dangerous clients and to protect clients from themselves. The responsibility to protect the public from potentially violent clients entails liability for civil damages when professionals neglect this duty by failing to diagnose or predict dangerousness, failing to warn potential victims of violent behavior, failing to commit dangerous individuals, and prematurely discharging dangerous clients from a hospital. Practitioners are advised to consult with a supervisor or an attorney because they may be subject to liability for either failing to warn those entitled to warnings or warning those who are not entitled.

HIV issues. One of the more controversial ethical dilemmas pertaining to a helper's duty to warn and protect others involves working with HIV-positive clients. As a helper, you may need to balance your client's right to confidentiality against the right of a third party to know about your client's HIV status. The ACA's *Code of Ethics* (1995) has a standard pertaining to the helper's role in dealing with contagious, fatal diseases:

> A counselor who receives information confirming that a client has a disease commonly known to be both communicable and fatal is justified in disclosing information to an identifiable third party, who by his or her relationship with the client is at a high risk of contracting the disease. Prior to making a disclosure the counselor should ascertain that the client has not already informed the third party about his or her disease and that the client is not intending to inform the third party in the immediate future. (B.1.d.)

At this time, there is no *legal* duty to warn, and it will take a court decision to resolve the legal obligation. In the meantime, practitioners who work with HIV-positive clients will have to wrestle with what they think is the moral and *ethical* course of action to take in certain situations. It is difficult to identify who in particular is at risk and to assess the degree to which individuals who have intimate relationships with persons with HIV are in imminent danger. Disclosure requires a careful decision and should be made only when the client has not informed the third party and has no intentions of doing so in the immediate future. Although the ACA's standard for contagious, fatal diseases gives practitioners *permission* to breach confidentiality, it does not state that they have a *duty* to warn, for such a provision would make them vulnerable to a malpractice suit (Herlihy & Corey, 1996b). This example illustrates a situation that could represent a conflict for the helper regarding following a legal versus an ethical course of action.

Case example. One of your male clients discloses to you that he is HIV-positive, but he says nothing about his sexual practices with a partner or partners. At a later session he discloses that he is not monogamous and that one of his partners is unaware of his condition. Since he has been engaging in unprotected sex with this person for some time, he sees no point in either disclosing his condition or changing his sexual practices.

What might you do in this case? How useful is the ACA guideline in determining your course of action? Would you initially address possible disclosure of information with others as part of the informed consent process? Why or why not? What do you see as your ethical and legal duty? How might you resolve potential conflicts between ethical and legal actions? How would you go about making the best decision?

Harm-to-self issues.   In addition to the duty to warn and to protect others from harm, helpers have a duty to protect clients who are likely to harm themselves. Many therapists inform their clients that they have an ethical and legal responsibility to break confidentiality when they have good reason to suspect suicidal behavior. Even if clients take the position that they are free to do with their lives what they want, therapists have a legal duty to protect them. The problem is to determine when a client is serious about committing suicide.

Cases have been made both for and against suicide prevention. Fujimura, Weis, and Cochran (1985) contend that most suicides can be prevented if those who work with suicidal clients learn to recognize, evaluate, and intervene effectively in crisis situations. Many clients who are in crisis may feel temporary hopelessness, yet if they are given help in learning to cope with the immediate problem, their potential for suicide can be greatly reduced. It is generally held that once mental health professionals determine that a significant risk does exist, appropriate action is necessary. Practitioners who fail to act to prevent suicide can be held liable.

Szasz (1986) argues the case against suicide prevention. He presents the thesis that suicide is an act of a moral agent who is ultimately responsible. Therefore, he opposes coercive methods of preventing suicide such as forced hospitalization. He further contends that by attempting to prevent suicide practitioners basically ally themselves with the police power of the state and resort to coercion. Clients are thus deprived of assuming responsibility for their own actions. Szasz agrees that helpers have an ethical and legal obligation to provide help to those clients who seek professional assistance for their suicidal tendencies. But for clients who do not ask for this help or who actively reject it, professionals have a duty either to persuade them to accept help or to leave them alone.

Although some have argued in favor of the right of clients to decide when and in what manner to end their lives, the codes of ethics of professional associations are in agreement that helpers must actively attempt to prevent suicide. In his article on working with suicidal clients, Wubbolding (1996) contends that counselors need to know how to handle suicide threats. They need practical skills that represent the highest level of ethical practice. He raises the following six questions as a way to assess the lethality of a threat and to determine whether further intervention is necessary:

1. Are you thinking about killing yourself?
2. Have you attempted suicide in the past?
3. Do you have a plan?
4. Do you have the means available to you?
5. Will you make a unilateral no-suicide agreement to stay alive—that is, to not kill yourself accidentally or on purpose—for a specified amount of time?
6. Is there anyone close to you who could prevent you from killing yourself and to whom you could speak when you feel the need to commit suicide?

Wubbolding (1996) contends that if clients say they are not seriously considering suicide, have not made prior suicide attempts, have neither a plan nor the means available, and are willing to make a no-suicide contract, the lethality of the threat is lessened and further intervention may not be necessary. If clients refuse to make plans to stay alive for a specified amount of time, then it is the helper's ethical responsibility to take action outside the session. Possible interventions might include informing the parents, spouse, physician, or another significant person in the client's life.

Case example.   A client is depressed and talks about putting an end to everything. He tells you that he is bringing this topic up only because he trusts you, and he insists that you not mention the conversation to anyone. He wants to talk about how desperate he feels, and he wants you to understand him and ultimately to accept whatever decision he makes. What would you say to him? How would you proceed?

Ethical Issues in a Managed Care Environment

A transformation has occurred in the delivery of helping services in the private sector. As Cummings (1995) points out, there is a shift in values and a fundamental redefinition of the role of mental health practitioners in the transition from the traditional fee-for-service model to the managed care model that is characterized by time-limited interventions, cost-effective methods, careful monitoring of services, and preventive strategies more than curative strategies.

Challenges of Managed Care

Rapidly escalating costs, especially in inpatient care, and associated concerns for quality and client outcome have led third-party payors and employers to demand more effective cost and quality controls (see Acuff et al., 1999; Cooper & Gottlieb, 2000; Cummings, 1995; Foos, Ottens, & Hill, 1991; Glosoff, Garcia, Herlihy, & Remley, 1999; Haas & Cummings, 1991; Hering, 2000; Hersch, 1995; Karon, 1995; Newman & Bricklin, 1991). In large measure, failure within the professional ranks to control rising costs has contributed to external control by the managed care industry. One of the major goals of managed care is to provide services that are as brief as possible to ameliorate presenting problems.

Although managed health care was once a reasoned response to real problems, Karon (1995) asserts that current managed care practice is more interested in reducing costs than in providing quality service. He contends that owners and managers of the managed care system are primarily interested in cost containment as a route to profitability and are concerned only secondarily with consumer needs and preferences. It is true that the costs of health care have soared, but is managed care the appropriate solution to a problem of escalating costs and restricted availability? Does managed care introduce a new set of problems that need to be solved? The debate on how to best deliver human services will continue, yet be assured that this new system will certainly have a profound influence on how you work with your clients. Overall, experts agree that managed care is here to stay (Cooper & Gottlieb, 2000).

In a managed care environment the emphasis is on making relatively quick assessments of clients' problems and designing brief interventions geared more to relief of problematic symptoms than to intensive self-exploration aimed at personal growth. This change in the focus of helping will have an impact on your role as a helper. In addition to short-term interventions aimed at a variety of client problems, you are likely to be expected to participate in prevention programs such as assertiveness training, stress management, parent education, vocational counseling, couples counseling, and a host of wellness programs that teach healthy lifestyle patterns.

Key Ethical Issues

Helpers in a managed care system clearly have divided loyalties between doing what is best for the client and keeping their commitment to a system that demands cost containment through a reliance on short-term interventions. Many times clients need more than the very brief interventions that are available. Karon (1995) reminds us that competent and ethical therapists are primarily concerned with the well-being of their clients, which is an entirely different criterion from cost-effectiveness. It is important that the welfare of the client does not get put on the back burner in the interests of preserving the financial integrity of the system. Managed care demands that practitioners adopt a set of values congruent with limited interventions that mainly treat symptoms. This could raise ethical issues for practitioners who value growth and actualization more than remedial, short-term, solution-focused strategies.

In their discussion of ethical issues in managed care, MacCluskie and Ingersoll (2001) point out that there are new challenges for delivering services in a sensitive and ethical manner. According to MacCluskie and Ingersoll, in the context of managed care, the motives for decision making are primarily economic. This factor itself does not necessarily constitute unethical behavior, unless it sacrifices the quality of care of clients in the process. Those who work in a managed care context face a number of ethical issues that revolve around these concerns:(1) informed consent, (2) confidentiality, (3) abandonment, (4) utilization review, and (5) competence.

Informed consent.   Informed consent is an ongoing process that assumes particular importance under a managed care system. Prior to entering into a professional relationship with you, your clients have a right to know that a managed care company may request a diagnosis, results on any tests given, a wide range of clinical information, treatment plans, and perhaps even the entire clinical record. From an ethical perspective, clients have a right to know that the focus on cost containment may have an adverse impact on the quality of care available to them.

Acuff and her colleagues (1999) point out that some managed care organizations make it a practice to not provide full, complete, and accurate information to their subscribers, and many of your clients will not be fully aware of how the complexities of managed care arrangements affect their benefits and rights. Do not assume that your clients have complete information regarding how the managed care system affects their specific benefit package; be sure your informed consent procedures are very clear (Cooper & Gottlieb, 2000).

Clients have a right to know that there may be other forms of treatment, possibly ones that may be more helpful, that are being denied to them solely because of cost-containment reasons. They have a right to know if you are versed in brief therapy, that an outside person is likely to judge what kind of treatment will be given and how many sessions will be allowed, the specific limitations of the plan they are participating in, and who decides the time of termination of therapy.

Confidentiality.   Although confidentiality has traditionally been considered to be an ethical and legal duty imposed on helping professionals to protect client disclosures, managed care has redefined the scope of confidentiality. Davis and Meier (2001) assert: "While maintaining confidentiality has always been a cornerstone of counseling and psychotherapy, for some managed care companies it is unfamiliar terrain" (p. 42). Because managed care providers take an active role in treatment planning, client confidentiality is compromised. Treatment is monitored by the third-party payor, who may influence decisions pertaining to interventions used, access to assessments, and access to outcomes of treatment. Managed care shifts the traditional basis for limits on confidentiality to matters pertaining to cost containment (Cooper & Gottlieb, 2000).

In exploring confidentiality in managed care, Acuff and her colleagues (1999) contend that without the assurance of confidentiality, it is reasonable to assume that many people will not seek treatment, and clients in therapy may withhold crucial information. Although there have always been exceptions to confidentiality, the demand for client information inherent in a managed care framework far exceeds previous limitations to confidentiality to the extent that the confidential nature of the therapist-client relationship is threatened. Potentially, the quality of client care is reduced. At the very least, clients should be aware that the managed care plan may require practitioners to reveal sensitive client information to a third party who is in a position to authorize initial or additional treatment. Practitioners can no longer assure their clients of confidential treatment at any level, for they have no control over confidential information once it leaves their offices. Because of these restrictions on confidentiality, helpers have an obligation to inform clients from the outset of the therapeutic process about the relevant limits of confidentiality under their managed care policy (Acuff, et al., 1999; Cooper & Gottlieb, 2000). If clients want to protect their confidentiality, they may decide to seek treatment that does not involve third-party reimbursement.

Abandonment.   The codes of ethics of the various professional organizations state that mental health practitioners do not abandon clients. Traditionally, the matter of termination of therapy is a collaborative effort involving both the client and the helper. Under managed care programs, termination generally does not come out of a collaborative process but from company policy. Clients may have a sense of abandonment if their treatment ends abruptly. It is a helper's responsibility to inform clients that the request for additional sessions may or may not be granted by the managed care company. It is essential to apply for additional sessions well in advance of the last authorized visit (Cooper & Gottlieb, 2000). Delivering mental health services under a managed care framework compels helpers to work in a restricted environment. Managed care guidelines often limit treatment to a specific number of sessions annually with lifetime cost caps. Clients may be denied the care they need if it extends beyond their benefits and they are unable to pay for additional care. For example, even though a client's policy may allow for up to 20 therapy sessions, the client may be authorized for only 6 sessions. Karon (1995) contends that ethical therapists are bound to encounter dilemmas in working in a system where the median number of sessions is 5 or 6, no matter what services are offered. He adds that medication is often relied on in managed care systems to obviate the need to provide more than 6 sessions. Although time limitations may make financial sense, this situation can become ethically problematic, forcing the practitioner to refer a client if continued therapy is needed.

It is clear that managed care presents both ethical and legal issues for professional practice. Ethically, professional helpers must not abandon their clients, and they have a responsibility to render competent services. But under managed care, many critical decisions are made for the client and the practitioner by the program. The number of sessions, the types of interventions to be used, and the content of treatment are all determined by the program. What if the practitioner is clearly aware that these external decisions are not therapeutically sound? What options do a practitioner and a client have under such a plan? What if the agency policy is not in the best interests of the client?

Utilization review. Under managed care programs, all treatment is monitored. Utilization review refers to the use of predefined criteria to evaluate treatment necessity, appropriateness of therapeutic intervention, and therapy effectiveness. This process can take place before, during, and after treatment (Cooper & Gottlieb, 2000). Acuff and her colleagues (1999) state that utilization management and review involves making decisions regarding types of treatment, setting, and the duration of treatment. They point out that ideally the needs of the client should remain paramount, yet these needs should be met in a cost-effective manner. Utilization review of clients is generally done by way of a written document that is periodically sent to the company. One disadvantage of this form of review is the possibility of the loss of confidentiality as paper reviews are sent by mail or electronic means. The disadvantage of telephone reviews is finding the time to make the call and to actually make the connection (Davis & Meier, 2001). One more potential problem pertaining to utilization review is the competence of the person doing the reviewing, who is often a technician, not a mental health professional.

Competence. A helper who works in a managed care system needs to have special knowledge and skills competencies to deliver a variety of brief services in a flexible and holistic manner with a diverse range of client populations and client problems. This requires helpers to acquire an eclectic or integrative theoretical orientation. Mental health practitioners are forced to become more proficient in time-limited and effective treatment approaches. Treatment plans need to be formulated rapidly, goals must be limited in scope, and the emphasis must be on attaining results. If helpers are not trained in brief treatment methods, and if clients will not be well served by a limited number of sessions, then helpers need to have skills in making appropriate referrals.

Legal Aspects of Managed Care

The policies of certain managed care companies are vulnerable to legal action. A landmark lawsuit in New Jersey against MCC, one of the largest managed behavioral health care providers in the United States, is believed to be the first of its kind. The 1996 lawsuit alleged that the company terminated therapists, purportedly without cause, when therapists requested more sessions for their clients than the managed care company was willing to provide In their lawsuit, the plaintiffs claimed that in limiting the number of sessions provided, the managed care company was substituting its judgment for the therapist's professional judgment, contrary to client welfare and public policy, and that these policies unlawfully prevented psychologists from exercising appropriate standards of care and clinical judgment (Jones & Higuchi, 1996). In 1996 the American Psychological Association and the New Jersey Psychological Association announced settlement of a lawsuit filed against CIGNA Behavioral Health, Incorporated. The ruling by a federal court sent a clear message that if managed care companies treat clients and practitioners inappropriately and disregard fairness, practitioners can file suit and get redress (Nessman & Herndon, 2000).

It is anticipated that more consumers of mental health services will file both ethical and legal complaints against therapists because of their willingness to terminate therapy due to decisions made by a managed care organization (Glosoff et al., 1999). Practitioners are ultimately responsible to their clients, even if the decisions are made by the managed care system. Legally, practitioners employed by managed care units are not exempt from malpractice suits if clients claim that they did not receive the standard of care they required. Professionals cannot use the limitations of the managed care plan as a shield for failing to render crisis intervention services, make appropriate referrals, or request additional services from the plan. Regardless of the structure underlying the delivery of services, ethical practice requires that you put the best interests of your client first. Consider how you can maximize short-term strategies that teach clients problem-solving skills that they can apply to their current and future problems. Ask yourself how you can best balance quality care with cost-containment requirements in the workplace.

Malpractice in the Helping Professions

Malpractice is generally defined as the failure to render proper service, through ignorance or negligence, resulting in injury or loss to the client. Professional negligence consists of departing from the usual standard of practice or not exercising due care in fulfilling one's responsibilities. For a malpractice suit to be filed against you, these three conditions must be present: (1) you must have a duty to the client, (2) you must have acted in a negligent or improper manner, and (3) there must be a causal relationship between that negligence and the damage claimed by the client.

Grounds for Malpractice Actions

The two areas that have probably received the greatest attention in the literature as grounds for malpractice are violations of confidentiality and sexual misconduct. A review of articles dealing with frequent causes of malpractice actions against people in the helping professions reveals some other key factors leading to a suit:

- Failure to obtain or document informed consent
- Abandoning a client
- Marked departures from established therapeutic practices
- Practicing beyond the scope of competency
- Improper diagnosis and utilization of assessment techniques
- Failure to respect the client's integrity and privacy
- Failure to have exercised reasonable care in cases of suicide
- Failure to protect others from a dangerous client
- Failure to supervise properly
- Failure to refer a client when the case warrants it
- Improper methods of collecting fees
- Misrepresenting one's professional training and skills
- Breaching a contract with a client

Other grounds for malpractice charges also exist; this list simply describes actions that often lead to malpractice suits.

As a student, you may think that you have no worries about being sued for malpractice. Unfortunately, student practitioners are vulnerable to such action. At this time in your professional development you might well give serious consideration to ways in which you can lessen your chances of being sued for failing to practice in a professional manner. The reality of today is that even if you abide by the ethics codes of your profession and even if you practice within the boundaries of the law, you can still be sued. No matter how careful you are, you can still be accused of wrongdoing. The best defense against becoming embroiled in a malpractice action is to practice quality client care.

Case example.   One of your teenage clients commits suicide, despite how prudent your interventions have been. The child's parents fault you for not having known more and done more to prevent this final action.

Although you do not have to prove that you are a superior or perfect being, you do have to demonstrate that you possess and exercised the knowledge and skill required for the services you provided. Ask yourself these questions: "Do I have to be able to predict a possible suicide? Assuming that I am able to spot a suicidal client, will I always know the best course of action to take?" You must be able to demonstrate that you acted in good faith, that you have been willing to seek supervision and consultation when needed, and that you have practiced within your competence. It is also essential that you can produce documentation to support your claims.

Ways to Prevent Malpractice Suits

We hope it is becoming clear that you would be wise to know your limitations in working with clients, to accept them, and to act only within the scope of your competence. Never hesitate to seek consultation, regardless of your professional experience. Consultation with colleagues often sheds light on a subject by providing a new and different perspective. Even if you are able to make wise decisions, it is validating to get support for your position from other professionals. If you are involved in litigation, it will be helpful to be able to demonstrate that your interventions were in accord with the standard of care exercised by other practitioners. If you employ unusual therapeutic techniques with little rationale behind them, you are likely to find yourself the loser in a civil action. Contending that you were following your instincts and doing what "felt right" is not likely to get you very far if you are asked to defend your therapeutic practices.

If you want a guarantee that you will not be sued for professional negligence, you probably should think about another career. There are no absolute protections in the mental health professions, but there are some practical ways to protect yourself from malpractice suits. In addition to the ways we have mentioned, here are some further guidelines:

- Make use of informed consent procedures. Do not attempt to mystify the helping process; professional honesty and openness with clients will go a long way in establishing genuine trust.
- Consider ways to define contracts with your clients that clearly structure the helping relationship. What are your clients coming to you for? How can you best help them obtain their goals?
- Because you can be sued for abandonment, take steps to provide coverage for emergencies when you are going away.
- Restrict your practice to client populations for which you are prepared by virtue of your education, training, and experience.
- Take steps to maintain your competence.
- At the outset of therapy, clearly define issues pertaining to fees.
- Carefully document a client's treatment plan.
- Keep up-to-date and accurate records of clients.
- Become aware of local and state laws that limit your practice, as well as the policies of the agency you work for. Keep abreast of legal and ethical changes by becoming involved in professional organizations.
- Be aware of the limits of confidentiality, and clearly communicate these to your clients. Attempt to obtain written consent whenever disclosure becomes necessary.
- Report any case of suspected child abuse as required by law.
- If you make a professional determination that a client is a danger to self or others, take the necessary steps to protect the client or others from harm.
- Treat your clients with respect by attending carefully to your language and your behavior. This practice generally leads to good relationships.

- Obtain written parental consent when working with minors. This is generally a good practice, even if not required by state law.
- Develop a diagnostic profile, and keep relevant notes on each client.
- When you are in doubt, always consult.
- Make it a practice to consult with colleagues or clinical supervisors whenever there is a potential ethical or legal concern. Find sources of ongoing supervision.
- Have a clear rationale for the techniques you use. Be able to intelligently and concisely discuss the theoretical underpinnings of your procedures.
- Have a clear standard of care that can be applied to your services, and communicate this standard to your clients.
- Do not promise clients anything that you cannot deliver. Help them realize that their effort and commitment will be key factors in determining the outcomes of the helping process.
- If you work for an agency or institution, have a contract that specifies the employer's legal liability for your professional functioning.
- Abide by the policies of the institution that employs you. If you disagree with certain policies, first attempt to find out the reasons for them. Then see if it is possible to work within the framework of institutional policies. Realize that you do not always have to agree with such policies to be able to work effectively.
- Adhere to billing regulations and paperwork requirements as prescribed.
- Make it a practice to assess the progress your clients are making, and teach them how to evaluate their progress toward their goals.
- Carry malpractice insurance. Students are not protected against malpractice suits.

These guidelines will lessen the chances of a malpractice suit, but we encourage you to continually assess your practices and keep up to date on legal, ethical, and community standards affecting your work setting and client populations.

A Word of Caution

Students sometimes burden themselves with the unrealistic expectation that they should have ready-made answers for the ethical issues we raise in this chapter. Quite the contrary is true. Indeed, seasoned professionals are aware that the complex nature of their work with people defies neat and absolute answers. They have an appreciation of the necessity for continuing learning, for ongoing consultation and supervision, and for remaining humble.

Our intention has not been to overwhelm you but to stimulate you to develop habits of thinking and acting that will enhance your ability to base your practice on ethical and professional principles. Working in the helping professions is a risky as well as a rewarding venture. You are bound to make mistakes from time to time. Be willing to acknowledge those mistakes and learn from them. Make full use of supervision; you will not only learn from what may seem like mistakes but you will also minimize the chances of harming clients.

We hope you won't be frozen with anxiety over needing to be all-knowing at all times—or afraid to intervene for fear of becoming embroiled in a lawsuit. Perhaps the best way to prevent a malpractice action is by having a sincere interest in doing what is going to benefit your client. We encourage you to ask yourself these questions throughout your professional career: "*What* am I doing, and *why* am I doing it?" "Would I be doing the same thing if my colleagues were observing me?"

By Way of Review

- One of the trends in the helping professions is an increased interest in ethical and professional practice. This trend stems, at least in part, from a rise in malpractice actions against mental health practitioners.

- Ethical decision making is a continuing process. Issues that you look at as a student can be examined from another perspective as you gain experience in your professional specialty.

- Ethical issues rarely have clear-cut answers. Ethical dilemmas, by their very nature, involve the application of professional judgment on your part. It is essential that you be familiar with the professional codes of ethics. However, knowledge of ethical standards is not sufficient in solving ethical problems.

- Ultimately, you will have to make many difficult decisions as a practitioner. Responsible practice entails basing your actions on informed, sound, and responsible judgment. Be open to consulting with colleagues and supervisors throughout your professional career.

- Ethics codes explicitly state that it is unethical to practice outside the boundaries of your competence. It is important to learn what clients you can best work with and to understand when referral is appropriate.

- Either as an intern or on your job, you may be asked to take on clients or to provide therapeutic strategies that are beyond the scope of your training and experience. Learn to be assertive in staying within your limits.

- One way to increase your competence is by seeking supervision whenever it is called for and by remaining open throughout your professional career to learning new skills and techniques. Remember that continuing education is necessary to keep abreast of current developments in your field.

- Many clients have not even thought about their rights or responsibilities. As a helper, you can do much to safeguard your clients by developing informed consent procedures to help them make wise choices.

- Confidentiality is the cornerstone of the helping relationship. Although clients have a right to expect that what they talk about with you in the professional relationship will remain private, there are times when you will have to breach confidentiality. Clients have a right to know from the outset of the relationship the specific grounds for divulging confidences. It is essential that you know and follow the laws pertaining to confidentiality.

• Confidentiality takes on special meaning if you work with couples, families, groups, and minors.

• At times you will have a professional and legal obligation to warn or to protect clients. It is essential that you know your duties in this area.

• Your job is to teach clients how to help themselves and thus decrease their need to continue seeing you. Encouraging dependency in your clients is unethical, and it does not lead to client empowerment.

• Managed behavioral health care programs have had a major impact on the kinds of psychological and social services that can be delivered and the quality of those services. Ethically, it is important that helpers do what they can to inform their clients about the services available and about potential limitations on the helping relationships due to the focus on cost-effective methods. The helping process itself—therapeutic goals, length of treatment, and intervention options—is influenced by the limitations imposed by managed care programs.

• Although it is important to know how to deal with unethical behavior on the part of your colleagues, it is even more important to recognize your own potential unethical behaviors. These unethical acts are often subtle. Maintain a stance of honest self-exploration to ensure ethical behavior.

• Malpractice actions are on the increase. Understand what can lead to being sued, and learn practical ways to lessen the chances of this happening.

What Will You Do Now?

1. Find at least one person in the helping professions to interview about ethical issues in practice. Focus on the major ethical problem that this person has faced. How does this helper deal with this ethical concern? What are their concerns, if any, about malpractice suits?

2. Visit a community agency (such as a Child Protective Service agency) and ask about ethical and legal situations that are being reported. What are some key ethical concerns with which this agency has to cope? Are the staff members concerned about malpractice issues? How does the current malpractice crisis influence what they do in their agency?

3. Think about a particular ethical dilemma that you have experienced in one of your field placements. How did you deal with the situation? If you could replay the situation, would you do anything differently?

4. Identify what you consider to be the most pressing ethical issue you expect to face, and write about your concerns and ideas in your journal. If you are involved in fieldwork, keep journal entries about any potential ethical dilemmas, and bring your concerns to your supervision sessions or class meetings. You might write down specific ways you can increase your likelihood of becoming an ethical practitioner. What can you do now to move in this direction?

5. Structure a class debate around the arguments for and against suicide prevention. Failure to prevent suicide is one of the main grounds for successful malpractice suits against mental health professionals and institutions (Szasz, 1986). Consider debating a specific case of a client who is terminally ill with AIDS and decides that he wants to end his life because of his suffering and because there is no hope of getting better. Divide the class into teams for an exchange on the therapist's responsibility to prevent this suicide.

6. In small groups discuss specific circumstances in which you would break confidentiality, and see whether you can agree on some general guidelines. In your groups, explore ways you might teach clients about the purposes of confidentiality and the legal restrictions on it. Discuss how you would do this in various situations, such as school counseling, group work, couples and family counseling, and counseling with minors.

7. For the full bibliographic entry for each of the sources listed here, consult the References and Reading List at the back of the book. A useful handbook on the grounds for malpractice suits in the mental health professions is Austin, Moline, and Williams (1990). For an ethical decision-making manual, see Steinman, Richardson, and McEnroe (1998). For a casebook geared to the ACA's code of ethics, see Herlihy and Corey (1996a). For a casebook geared to the APA's ethics code, see Canter, Bennett, Jones, and Nagy (1994). For a comprehensive handbook that deals with a wide range of topics in ethics, see Bersoff (1999). For a concise guide for helpers in managed care, see Davis and Meier (2001). For a book on ethics and the law in counseling practice, see Remley and Herlihy (2001). Consult Corey, Corey, and Callanan (2003) for a textbook dealing with ethical issues in the helping professions.

8. We recommend that you familiarize yourself with the basic standards for ethical practice of the various mental health professions. You can obtain the codes and guidelines listed here as a packaged supplement to this textbook, entitled *Codes of Ethics for the Helping Professions*. Compare two or more of these documents and identify concerns that are common to mental health professionals despite differences in specialization.

- *Codes of Ethics and Standards of Practice*, American Counseling Association (1995)
- *Ethical Principles of Psychologists and Code of Conduct*, American Psychological Association (1992)
- *Code of Ethics*, National Association of Social Workers (1999)
- *AAMFT Code of Ethics*, American Association for Marriage and Family Therapy (2001)
- *Ethical Standards of Human Service Professionals*, National Organization for Human Service Education (2000)
- *Ethical Standards for School Counselors*, American School Counselor Association (1998)
- *Ethical Code for the International Association of Marriage and Family Counselors*, International Association of Marriage and Family Counselors (2000)
- *Code of Ethics*, American Mental Health Counselors Association (2000)
- *Code of Ethics*, American Rehabilitation Counseling Association (1999)
- *Ethical Guidelines for Counseling Supervisors*, Association for Counselor Education and Supervision (1993)
- *Best Practice Guidelines for Group Workers*, Association for Specialists in Group Work (1998)
- *Principles for Diversity-Competent Group Workers*, Association for Specialists in Group Work (1999)
- *Professional Standards for the Training of Group Workers*, Association for Specialists in Group Work (2000)
- *Code of Ethics for National Board of Certified Counselors*, National Board for Certified Counselors (1997a)
- *Standards for the Ethical Practice of Web Counseling Guidelines*, National Board for Certified Counselors (1997b)
- *Ethical Standards for Internet On-Line Counseling*, American Counseling Association (1999)

Ethics in Action CD-ROM Exercises

9. In role-play segment 1, Teen Pregnancy, in Part One [Ethical Decision Making] on the CD-ROM, the client is a 13-year-old who just found out she is pregnant. She begs the counselor not to tell her parents. In this situation, what are the rights of the minor client? What rights do the parents have for access to certain information? What ethical and legal issues are involved in this case? What kind of informed consent process would you implement if you were counseling minors?

10. In role-play segment 4 on the CD-ROM, on divorce, the client says that she has decided to leave her husband and get a divorce, and the counselor's line of inquiry is about who will look after the welfare of her children. This case raises some interesting points about the rights of clients to know about your values as a counselor if these values influence your approach to counseling them. If you were counseling couples or families, what would you want to tell clients about your values pertaining to matters such as faithfulness in relationships and divorce? In

class, role-play a situation in which you are meeting a client (or a couple) for the first session. What would you want to tell them about your role as a counselor? Would you discuss core values you hold that could either enhance or interfere with therapeutic progress?

InfoTrac College Edition Resources

For additional readings, explore InfoTrac College Edition, our online library. Go to http://www.infotrac.college.com/wadsworth and select these key word searches:

ethical decision making model*
community W1 standard*
community W1 standard* ethical
standard* practice psych*
aspirational W1 ethic*
mandatory W1 ethic*
informed consent AND psych*
record AND couns*
record AND therap*
ethical managed care of mental health
managed W1 care psych*
malpractice AND psych*
confidentiality AND psych*
confidentiality AND couns*
privileged W1 communication
privacy AND couns*
privacy AND psych*
duty to warn
duty to protect
suicid* client*
suicid* AND therap*
suicid* AND threat* AND therap*
suicide W1 prevention
confidentiality AND HIV
confidentiality AND AIDS
referrals couns*
referrals psych*
education mental W1 health

Key words are listed in a form that enables the search engine to locate a wider range of articles in the online university library. Key words should be entered exactly as shown, including asterisks, "W1," "W2," "AND," and other search engine tools.

Managing Boundary Issues

Focus Questions

1. What problems, if any, might you expect to encounter in establishing boundaries with your clients?

2. If a client lost her job and could no longer afford to pay you for counseling services, would you be willing to enter into a bartering arrangement if she suggested bartering as an alternative to terminating her sessions? What other alternatives can you think of in her case?

3. If a client offered you a gift at the termination session and explained how important it was to him that you accept this gift as a token of his appreciation for your help, what would you be inclined to do?

4. Dual relationships exist when professionals assume two roles simultaneously or sequentially with a person seeking help. Do you believe dual relationships fundamentally unethical, or are such relationships inevitable and not always problematic?

5. What kinds of dual or multiple relationships do you see as being problematic and why? Can you think of any kinds of dual or multiple relationships that you might be willing to engage in with a counseling client?

6. How might you deal with an unavoidable dual relationship with one of your clients?

7. If a client was interested in forming a social relationship with you, what would you say? If this person was a former client, would that make a difference?

8. If a client expressed sexual attraction to you, what would you be likely to do or say? What would you do if *you* experienced sexual attraction to a client?

9. What ethical, legal, and clinical issues would you consider before entering a dual relationship (social, sexual, business, professional) with a *former* client or student?

Aim of the Chapter

Regardless of which helping profession you enter, you will be faced with learning to define and maintain appropriate boundaries with your clients. As will become clear in this chapter, part of becoming a helper involves being able to establish both personal and professional boundaries in a variety of situations. In this chapter we introduce you to an array of ethical concerns that helpers encounter in keeping relationships professional with their clients. In many ways, the topics covered in this chapter are a continuation of the discussion of ethical decision making in Chapter 9. Learning to deal with a range of boundary concerns is a key ethical issue that practitioners in all settings have to address.

It is sometimes difficult to understand the rationale behind prohibitions and boundary limitations that may seem arbitrary. Many of the ethics codes are based on reactions to ethical violations rather than on factors such as the client's issues and the nature of the so-called dual relationship. Codes alone will not keep helpers from behaving in unethical ways. Good judgment, the willingness to reflect on one's practices, and being aware of one's motivations are critical dimensions of being an ethical practitioner. Mental health professionals oftentimes get into trouble by not heeding warning signs in their relationships with clients. They may not have paid sufficient attention to potential problems involved in boundary crossings. Practitioners may innocently cross boundaries that lead to problems for both the client and themselves.

The underlying theme of this chapter is the need for helpers to be honest and self-searching in determining the impact of their behavior on clients. Some of the issues and cases we present may seem clear-cut, but others are not. Resolving the ethical dilemmas we pose requires personal and professional maturity and a willingness to continue to question your own motivations.

Self-Inventory on Managing Boundaries

What are some of your major concerns about establishing appropriate boundaries with clients? Perhaps at this point you have not even raised this question. We hope you will broaden your awareness of the importance of creating and maintaining appropriate, flexible, and realistic boundaries in the helping relationship. For each of the following statements, indicate the response that most closely identifies your beliefs and attitudes. Use this code:

5 = I *strongly agree* with this statement.
4 = I *agree* with this statement.
3 = I am *undecided* about this statement.
2 = I *disagree* with this statement.
1 = I *strongly disagree* with this statement.

_____ 1. It will be relatively easy for me to establish clear and firm boundaries with my clients.

_____ 2. At times I am concerned about my ability to keep relationships with my clients professional.

_____ 3. I am not sure how I would respond to a *current* client who asked me for a date or wanted some other social involvement with me.

_____ 4. I might be willing to consider a social relationship with a *former* client if both of us were interested in meeting on a social basis.

_____ 5. I don't think my training has prepared me to deal with sexual attractions in the helping relationship.

_____ 6. Because dual relationships are so widespread, they should not be considered as either inappropriate or unethical in all circumstances but should be decided on a case-by-case basis.

_____ 7. Dual or multiple relationships are almost always problematic and therefore should be considered unethical.

_____ 8. If I were a truly ethical professional, I would never be sexually attracted to a client.

_____ 9. If I were counseling a client who was sexually attracted to me, I might refer this client to another counselor.

_____ 10. I might be inclined to barter my therapeutic services for goods if a client could not afford my fees.

_____ 11. If a client initiated the possibility of exchanging services in lieu of payment, I would consider bartering as an option.

_____ 12. Sexual involvement with a client is never ethical, even after therapy has ended.

_____ 13. I would never accept a gift from a client, for doing so constitutes crossing appropriate boundaries.

_____ 14. It is essential to consider the cultural context in deciding on the appropriateness of bartering, accepting gifts, and the helper assuming multiple roles with a client.

_____ 15. I would have no trouble accepting a close friend as a client if we had a clear understanding of how our personal relationship could be separated from our professional one.

Once you have finished this inventory, spend a few minutes reflecting on any ethical concerns you have at this time. This reflection can help you read the chapter more actively and formulate ethical questions. Identify a few of the areas where you are uncertain about your position, and bring this ambiguity up in class discussions.

Establishing Personal and Professional Boundaries

Codes of ethics caution against forming dual or multiple relationships with clients. Such relationships occur when professionals assume two or more roles simultaneously or sequentially with a person seeking their help. Helpers establish a dual relationship in cases where they have another, significantly different relationship with one of their clients, students, or supervisees. In these situations, the potential for a conflict of interest and for exploiting those seeking help cannot be ignored. Consider these examples of ethics codes on dual relationships. The American

Counseling Association's (1995) code stresses the risk of impaired professional judgment:

> Counselors are aware of their influential positions with respect to clients, and they avoid exploiting the trust and dependency of clients. Counselors make every effort to avoid dual relationships with clients that could impair professional judgment or increase the risk of harm to clients. (Examples of such relationships include, but are not limited to, familial, social, financial, business, or close personal relationships with clients.) When a dual relationship cannot be avoided, counselors take appropriate professional precautions such as informed consent, consultation, supervision, and documentation to ensure that judgment is not impaired and no exploitation occurs. (A.6.a.)

NASW's *Code of Ethics* (1999) focuses on the risk of exploitation or potential harm to clients:

> Social workers should not engage in dual or multiple relationships with clients or former clients in which there is a risk of exploitation or potential harm to the client. In instances when dual or multiple relationships are unavoidable, social workers should take steps to protect clients and are responsible for setting clear, appropriate, and culturally sensitive boundaries. (1.06.c.)

NOHSE's ethical standards (2000) highlight the power and status differential between helper and client:

> Human service professionals are aware that in their relationships with clients power and status are unequal. Therefore they recognize that dual or multiple relationships may increase the risk of harm to, or exploitation of, clients, and may impair their professional judgment. However, in some communities and situations it may not be feasible to avoid social or other nonprofessional contact with clients. Human service professionals support the trust implicit in the helping relationship by avoiding dual relationships that may impair professional judgment, increase the risk of harm to clients or lead to exploitation.

Recent revisions of codes of ethics deal more specifically and extensively with setting appropriate boundaries, recognizing potential conflicts of interest, and taking ethical approaches in managing dual or multiple relationships. Codes of ethics that address these issues include those of the American Counseling Association (1995), the American Psychological Association (1992), the National Association of Social Workers (1999), the American Association for Marriage and Family Therapy (2001), and the National Organization for Human Service Education (2000). Although codes may function as guidelines, dual relationships are frequently not a clear-cut matter. Ethical reasoning and judgment come into play when ethics codes are applied to specific situations.

The Dual Relationship Controversy

The helping professions have become increasingly concerned about the ethics of dual relationships. During the 1980s, the issue of sexual dual relationships was given considerable attention in the professional literature. It is now clear that sexual dual relationships are unethical, and the all of the professional organizations now prohibit sexual relationships between client and therapist.

Nonsexual dual and multiple relationships came under increased scrutiny in the 1990s, but little consensus has been reached with regard to a determination of ethical practice. Nonsexual dual relationships are discouraged, however, and helpers are cautioned about the dangers of exploitation of clients. Nonsexual dual or multiple relationships tend to be complex, and few of the questions surrounding them have simple and absolute answers. Helpers cannot always perform a singular role when working with clients or in the community, nor is it always desirable that they limit themselves to one role. Many times, helpers will be challenged to balance multiple roles in their professional relationships. Examples of nonsexual dual relationships include accepting clients who are family members or friends, bartering for services, accepting gifts from clients, combining the roles of supervisor and therapist, forming business arrangements with therapy clients, or combining personal counseling with consultation or supervision.

Herlihy and Corey (1997a) point out that some behaviors helpers may engage in have a potential for creating a dual relationship, but they are not, by themselves, dual relationships. Examples of these behaviors include accepting a small gift from a client, accepting a client's invitation to a graduation ceremony, accepting goods rather than money as payment, or engaging in nonerotic touching when this is appropriate. Some writers (Gabbard, 1995; Smith & Fitzpatrick, 1995) suggest that these incidents might be considered boundary *crossings* rather than boundary *violations*. A boundary crossing is a departure from standard practice that could potentially benefit clients, whereas a boundary violation is a serious breach that causes harm to the client. Even though boundary crossings may not be harmful to clients, these crossings can lead to blurring of professional boundaries and can result in dual relationships that do have a potential to be harmful.

There is considerable disagreement about the appropriateness of dual relationships. Some in the helping professions want to see stricter laws and ethics codes prohibiting dual relationships, whereas others see this trend as an erosion of confidence in individual practitioners. Not all dual relationships can be avoided, and some believe these relationships are not necessarily harmful, unethical, or unprofessional (Herlihy & Corey, 1997a). This is particularly true in small, isolated communities. In many rural communities there is a high likelihood that helpers will be involved in multiple relationships.

Schank and Skovholt (1997) conducted interviews with psychologists who lived and practiced in rural areas and small communities. They found that all of the psychologists in their study acknowledged concerns involving professional boundaries. Some of the major themes were the reality of overlapping social or business relationships, the effects of overlapping social relationships on members of the psychologist's own family, and the dilemma of working with more than one family member as clients or with clients who have friendships with other clients. Although the psychologists knew the content of the ethics codes, they admitted that they often struggled in choosing how to apply those codes to the ethical dilemmas they faced in rural practices.

Sleek (1994) describes ethical dilemmas that plague rural practice. The local pharmacist, physician, mechanic, banker, carpenter, or beautician might be a client of a particular helper. Furthermore, rural professionals see clients in the local store and ponder whether to acknowledge the person in the presence of others. If they are in local organizations such as the Chamber of Commerce or if they attend the same church, they may worry about conflicts with some fellow members who are also clients. There is also the problem of mixing business with the therapeutic endeavor in rural communities. For example, if a therapist shops for a new tractor, he or she risks violating the letter of the ethics code if the only person in town who sells tractors happens to be a client. However, if the therapist were to buy a tractor elsewhere, this could strain relationships with the client because of the value rural communities place on loyalty to local merchants. Or consider clients who wish to barter goods or services for counseling services. Some communities operate substantially on swaps rather than on a cash economy. This does not necessarily have to become problematic, yet the potential for conflict exists in the therapeutic relationship if the bartering agreements do not work well. In rural settings, helpers typically play multiple roles and are likely to experience more difficulties maintaining clear boundaries than do their colleagues who practice in urban areas. Practicing in an urban versus a rural setting must be taken into account in assessing ethical practices pertaining to multiple relationships.

We find it useful to frame the discussion of dual or multiple relationships within the context of boundaries. If you have developed clear boundaries in your personal life, you are less likely to have trouble with dual relationships professionally. If your boundaries are ill defined or if you attempt to blend roles that do not mix well, such as therapy and friendships or therapy and business, you are likely to stumble into an ethical dilemma.

We do not think that prohibiting all forms of multiple relating is a realistic answer to the problem of exploitation of clients. Zur (1999) writes that during his graduate school training he was warned over and over never to engage in any kind of dual relationship. Some of the "nevers" that he heard were never indulge in boundary crossing, never touch a client, never go to coffee or have lunch with a client, never treat a spouse or a friend of a client, never meet clients in social situations, and never join the same synagogue or church as a client. We agree with Zur's (2000a) contention that the professions have gone too far in the direction of discouraging practitioners from engaging in any form of dual relating.

Zur (1999) makes some excellent points about nonsexual dual relationships:

- Nonsexual dual relationships do not necessarily pave the way to exploitation or harm.
- Rather than mandating a blanket avoidance of dual relationships, most codes of ethics only prohibit exploitation and harm to clients.
- Exploitative helpers will exploit with or without prohibitions against dual relationships.
- Avoiding all dual relationships keeps practitioners in unrealistic and inappropriate power positions, which increases the likelihood of exploitation.
- The prohibition of dual relationships leads to increased isolation.
- Many therapeutic approaches view dual relationships as an important and integral part of therapy.
- Graduate education tends to escalate students' fear of licensing agencies and lawsuits.

- Some dual relationships can alter the power differential between helpers and clients in a way that results in healing.

Zur (2000b) believes the ban and demonization of dual relationships has led to a simplistic solution to a complex problem and has increased the chance of exploitation and decreased the effectiveness of treatment. Zur concludes: "We have been frightened into accepting the ban, but now it is time to think critically, be courageous and dare to be known by our clients. If we dare to cultivate multiple, non-sexual and non-exploitive relationships with our clients when appropriate, we can be better, more effective therapists" (p. 100).

We appreciate Lazarus's (1994, 1998, 2001) reasonable perspective on therapeutic boundaries. Lazarus contends that a general prohibition against dual relationships has led to unfair and inconsistent decisions by state licensing boards, brought sanctions against practitioners who have done no harm, and often tended to impede a practitioner's ability to perform optimum work with a client. Lazarus takes the position that certain boundaries and ethical rules actually diminish therapeutic effectiveness. He contends that some well-intentioned ethical standards can be transformed into artificial boundaries that result in destructive prohibitions and undermine clinical effectiveness. Moreover, he believes some dual relationships can enhance treatment outcomes. Lazarus argues for a case-by-case, nondogmatic evaluation of boundary questions that involves a selective process of deciding when it may be appropriate to enter into a secondary relationship. He contends that it is essential to consider individual client differences rather than to be subjugated to rigid standards.

Lazarus (2001) admits that some well-intentioned guidelines can backfire. He has socialized with some clients, played tennis with others, taken walks with some, respectfully accepted small gifts, and given gifts (usually books) to some of his clients. Lazarus makes it clear that he is opposed to any form of disparagement, exploitation, abuse, harassment, or sexual contact with clients. He is not advocating elimination of all boundaries, for he sees certain boundaries as being essential. Rather than being driven by rules, however, Lazarus calls for a process of negotiation in many areas of nonsexual multiple relationships that some would contend are in the forbidden zone. Lazarus emphasizes that boundary crossings should not be undertaken without serious consideration. "A clear rationale is necessary, a risk-benefit analysis may need to be factored in, roles and expectations should be quite clear, and possible power differentials must be kept in mind" (p. 16).

Guidelines for Setting Boundaries

Although there are divergent viewpoints on dual relationships, most professionals will agree that blending the roles of counselor and employee or counselor and lover is not appropriate. Whenever helpers play multiple roles, there is a potential for conflict of interest, loss of objectivity, and exploitation of persons who have sought help. Ethical practitioners must take appropriate precautions to ensure that the best interests of their clients are maintained. Herlihy and Corey (1997a) provide these guidelines in cases where professionals are operating in more than one role:

- Set healthy boundaries from the outset. In your informed consent document, it is wise to state your policy pertaining to professional versus social or business relationships.
- Involve the client in setting the boundaries of the professional relationship. Discuss with clients what you expect of them and what they can expect of you.
- Informed consent is essential when you are playing more than one role with a client. Clients have a right to know about any potential risks associated with dual relationships. Informed consent and discussion of unforeseen problems and conflicts needs to be an ongoing process.
- Consultation with colleagues is most useful in obtaining an objective perspective and identifying unanticipated difficulties. If you are functioning in more than one role or engaging in dual relationships, it is a good policy to consult on a regular basis.
- When dual relationships are particularly problematic, or when there is a high degree of risk for harm, it is wise to work under supervision.
- It is essential that counselor educators and supervisors discuss with students and supervisees topics dealing with balance of power issues, boundary concerns, appropriate limits, purposes of the relationship, potential for abusing power, and subtle ways in which harm can result from engaging in multiple and sometimes conflicting roles.
- From a legal perspective, it is good practice to document any discussions about dual relationships with your clients. Include in your notes any actions you have taken to minimize the risk of harm.
- If necessary, refer the client to another professional.

The controversy surrounding nonsexual dual relationships is likely to continue to be discussed and debated. As with any complex ethical issue, complete agreement may not be reached. Helping professionals need to clarify their stance to a host of boundaries issues they will face in practice and develop a strategy to address these issues.

Herlihy and Corey (1997a) present a decision-making model that can be applied when helpers are confronted with dual relationship issues. If the potential dual relationship is *unavoidable,* helpers would do well to (1) secure informed consent of clients, (2) seek consultation, (3) document and monitor their practices, and (4) obtain supervision. If the potential dual relationship is *avoidable,* helpers should first assess the potential benefits and risks in the case. If the benefits outweigh the risks, the relationship may be justified. However, if the risks outweigh the benefits, helpers might decline to enter the relationship, explain the rationale to the client, and offer a referral to another professional.

In your struggle to determine what constitutes appropriate boundaries, you are likely to find that certain role blendings are inevitable. Therefore, it is crucial to learn how to manage boundaries, how to keep boundary crossings from turning into boundary violations, and how to develop safeguards that will prevent exploitation of clients. Think about these general themes and the guidelines we have discussed, and apply them to each situation presented in this chapter. Ask yourself how you would proceed in resolving any ethical dilemmas over conflicting roles with your clients.

Combining Professional and Personal Relationships

You may be tempted to form social relationships with clients who admire you excessively and who invite you to develop a friendship. This lure can be especially strong if you like your client and if you have a limited circle of friends. You may also be afraid to deal with your clients' potential feelings of rejection if you tell them that a personal or social relationship is not possible. Balancing a professional and a personal relationship with a client is a tricky business.

As a helper you may not be inclined to challenge clients lest you endanger your personal relationship with them. Or you may experience difficulty in separating yourself from your clients. Even if you are able to maintain your objectivity, provide an optimal balance between confrontation and support, and still be a therapeutic agent, your clients may have difficulty keeping the two relationships separate. One factor to consider is that no matter how you look at this issue, the relationship is bound to be unequal. The client/friend pays you for your time and attention. Even if you don't charge a fee, the relationship is still unequal because you are likely to be doing more of the listening, giving, and challenging. In an equal friendship, both partners are giving and receiving.

At times, social relationships between helpers and their clients may occur. When you find yourself in this position, here are some questions to ponder: "Does the social relationship get in the way of working effectively with my client?" "Does the friendship get in the client's way of working with me?" "Am I retaining enough objectivity to determine any possible negative effects?" We do have concerns about helpers who rely on their clients to make social and personal contacts. If most of your social acquaintances are people whom you serve professionally, we wonder if you are relying on your role as a helper to meet your personal needs.

Case example.   A client whom you have been seeing for some time asks whether you would be willing to meet for lunch. When you ask about the reason for the out-of-office meeting, your client tells you that he (she) would like to get to know you better in an informal setting and would like to treat you to lunch as an expression of appreciation for the help you have provided. To make matters a bit more difficult, one of your client's personal issues is the fear of being rejected. The client tells you that he (she) is taking a chance and a risk by asking you for lunch.

How would you handle this situation? Would it make a difference whether the client was of the same or the opposite sex? Would your own feelings toward your client influence your decision?

Socializing With Former Clients

Although combining personal and professional relationships with current clients is problematic at best, at least one study suggests that friendships between counselors and clients may be acceptable after termination of counseling (Salisbury & Kinnier, 1996). Seventy percent of counselors in this study believed friendships with former clients were acceptable 2 years after termination, and 33% reported that they had engaged in such friendships. The most important concern expressed by counselors in determining the circumstances under which posttermination friendships would be appropriate related to avoiding potential harm to the client. Salisbury and Kinnier state that the present ethics codes offer little guidance about friendships with former clients. They recommend that further research be conducted to delineate what constitutes friendship and to investigate how such friendships affect former clients.

In their study of nonromantic, nonsexual posttherapy relationships between psychologists and former clients, Anderson and Kitchener (1996) found little consensus regarding how ethical these contacts are. Some therapists believe the client-therapist relationship continues in perpetuity. However, many of the participants in Anderson and Kitchener's study did not hold to the concept of "once a client, always a client" when it comes to nonsexual posttherapy relationships. The majority of therapists in this study described nonsexual relationships with former clients as being ethical, especially if some time had elapsed after termination. Others proposed that such relationships were ethical if the former client decided not to return to therapy with the former therapist and the posttherapy relationship did not seem to hinder later therapy with different therapists.

Although making friends with former clients may not be unethical, the practice may be unwise. The safest policy would be to avoid developing social relationships with former clients. In the long run, former clients may need you more as a therapist at some future time than as a friend. If you develop a friendship with a former client, he or she is no longer eligible to use your professional services. Additionally, it is possible that in many situations the imbalance of power never changes. Even in the social relationship, you may be seen as the provider of help, or you may behave as the person in the helping role. You need to be aware of your own motivations, as well as the motivations of your clients before allowing a professional relationship to evolve into a personal one. If you are in the habit of developing relationships with former clients, you may find yourself overextended and come to resent the relationships you sought out or consented to. What is central in this situation is your ability to establish clear boundaries regarding what you are willing to do and not do.

What are your thoughts about developing friendships with present or former clients? Would you be willing to form such personal or social relationships with clients? Why or why not? What issues would you want to discuss with a former client before entering a personal relationship?

Bartering

The practice of bartering psychotherapy for goods or other services has the potential for conflicts. Glosoff, Corey, and Herlihy (1996) identify several potential pitfalls in bartering, even though the helper may have good intentions when forming this dual relationship. When clients are unable to afford the professional services of a counselor, they may suggest a barter arrangement—for example, cleaning house for the helper, performing secretarial services, or doing other personal work. Clients can easily be put in a bind when they are in a position to learn personal information about their helper. This can interfere with the helper-client relationship.

Bartering is an accepted practice in many cultures, but bartering for counseling services is especially problematic. Clients may believe their counseling is not progressing well and accuse the helper of not following through on his or her agreement. Likewise, helpers may be dissatisfied with the lack of timeliness or the quality of goods and services delivered by clients, which can lead to resentment and ultimately interfere with the therapeutic relationship.

Ethical dimensions of bartering.   At the present time, most professional ethics codes have a specific standard pertaining to bartering. Although bartering is not prohibited outright, there are stipulations to the practice.

The APA code of ethics (1992) discourages bartering as a general rule but also delineates circumstances when psychologists might become involved in such an arrangement:

> Psychologists ordinarily refrain from accepting goods, services, or other nonmonetary remuneration from patients or clients in return for psychological services because such arrangements create inherent potential for conflicts, exploitation, and distortion of the relationship. A psychologist may participate in bartering *only* if (1) it is not clinically contraindicated, and (2) the relationship is not exploitative. (1.18.)

ACA's (1995) code also discourages bartering:

> Counselors ordinarily refrain from accepting goods or services from clients in return for counseling services because such arrangements create inherent potential for conflicts, exploitation, and distortion of the professional relationship. Counselors may participate in bartering only if the relationship is not exploitive, if the client requests it, if a clear written contract is established, and if such arrangements are an accepted practice among professionals in the community. (A.10.c.)

NASW (1999) has the following guideline on bartering:

> Social workers should avoid accepting goods or services from clients as payment for professional services. Bartering arrangements, particularly involving services, create the potential for conflicts of interest, exploitation, and inappropriate boundaries in social workers' relationships with clients. Social workers should explore and may participate in bartering only in very limited circumstances where it can be demonstrated that such arrangements are an accepted practice among professionals in the local community, considered to be essential for the provision of service, negotiated without coercion and entered into at the client's initiative and with the client's informed consent. Social workers who accept goods or services from clients as payment for professional services assume the full burden of demonstrating that this arrangement will not be detrimental to the client or the professional relationship. (1.13.b.)

We agree with the general tone of these standards, although we would add that bartering should be evaluated within a cultural context. In some cultures and in certain communities, bartering is an accepted practice. Bartering is an example of a dual relationship that we think allows some room for helpers to use their professional judgment and to consider the cultural context in which they practice.

If you are considering some form of bartering in lieu of payment for your professional services, consult with experienced colleagues or a supervisor. This type of consultation is likely to offer alternatives that you and your client have not considered. Schank and Skovholt (1997) remind us that we all have our blind spots, and trusted colleagues can help us become aware of them and constructively examine them. After reflecting on the relevant issues involved in a situation and consulting others, we highly recommend a straightforward discussion with your client about the pros and cons of bartering in your particular situation. This collaborative discussion with your client, as well as the opinions of others, might assist you in identifying potential problems associated with certain kinds of proposed bartering arrangements. Ongoing consultation and discussion of cases, especially in matters pertaining to boundaries and dual roles, provide a context for understanding the implications of certain practices.

Before bartering is entered into, both parties should talk about the arrangement, gain a clear understanding of the exchange, and come to an agreement. It is also important that potential problems that might develop be discussed and that alternatives be examined. Using a sliding scale to determine fees or making a referral are two possible alternatives to bartering that might have merit. Perhaps the safest course to follow as a general rule is to refrain from accepting goods or services in exchange for professional services because of the potential for conflicts, exploitation, and strain on the helping relationship. However, you will have to assess the real-life situations that confront you in your professional practice.

Legal aspects of bartering.   Bartering is not prohibited by ethics or law. As a helper, you may face situations where you will need to decide whether you will use bartering as an alternative, especially when clients can no longer afford to pay for services. If you were to consult with Robert Woody, who is a counselor educator and an attorney, he would likely advise you to stay clear of any bartering arrangements. Woody (1998) argues against the use of bartering for psychological services, saying that a case could be made that bartering is below the minimum standard of practice. If you enter into a bartering agreement with your client, you will have the burden of proof to demonstrate (a) that the bartering arrangement is in the best interests of your client; (b) that it is reasonable, equitable, and undertaken without undue influence; and (c) that it does not get in the way of providing quality psychological services to your client. Because bartering is so fraught with risks for both client and therapist, Woody believes prudence dictates that it should be an option of last resort. He concludes that bartering is a bad idea and should be avoided.

Case example.   For several months you have been seeing Wayne, who has consistently paid for your services and who is currently making excellent progress in counseling. Wayne comes to a session very depressed because he lost his job as an auto mechanic at a large dealership. He can see no way of continuing to see you because of his other pressing financial commitments. Knowing that you have had some car problems, he proposes that he do a complete engine overhaul as a way of making payment for some counseling sessions. He asks if you would be willing to go along with this arrangement because he really does not want to interrupt counseling at this point. On top of his other problems, he is now unemployed. Assuming that your car was in desperate need of major work, consider what you would do.

- Would you be inclined to enter into some form of a bartering arrangement with Wayne? Why or why not?
- Would your decision be dependent on whether you were practicing in a large urban area or a rural area?
- How might you take the cultural context into consideration when making your decision?
- Assume that you engaged in this exchange of services and that your car died on you on a busy freeway. How might this affect your work with Wayne, especially if the car problem was due to inferior work on his part?
- Assume that you told Wayne that you did not feel comfortable bartering and that he told you that he felt you were abandoning him in a time of dire need. How might you respond?
- Besides bartering, what other options might you present to Wayne?
- Would you consider seeing him without payment due to his circumstances?

Accepting Gifts From Clients

Few professional codes of ethics specifically address the topic of giving or receiving gifts in the therapeutic relationship. However, the AAMFT (2001) ethics code does address this issue: "Marriage and family therapists do not give or receive from clients (a) gifts of substantial value or (b) gifts that impair the integrity or efficacy of the therapeutic relationship" (3.10).

Lavish gifts certainly present an ethical problem, but you might have mixed feelings about accepting a small gift from a client or giving a client such a gift. Some practitioners include a policy statement that they do not accept gifts from clients in their informed consent document. We believe this approach is too rigid. Our preference is to evaluate the circumstances of each case because a number of factors need to be considered in making a decision of whether or not to accept a gift from a client. Here are some questions you might explore.

What is the monetary value of the gift? Most mental health professionals would probably agree that accepting a very expensive gift would be inappropriate and unethical. It would also be problematic if a client offered tickets to the theater and wanted you to accompany him or her to this event.

What are the clinical implications of accepting or rejecting the gift? It is important to know when accepting a gift from a client is clinically contraindicated and be willing to explore this with your client. You would also want to explore with the client his or her motivation for presenting you with a gift. A client might be seeking your approval and the main motivation for giving you a gift is to please you. Accepting the gift without adequate discussion would not be helping your client in the long run.

At what phase in the helping process is the offering of a gift occurring? It makes a difference if a client wants to give you a gift during the early stage of the relationship or whether this occurs at the termination of the professional relationship. It is more problematic to accept a gift at the early stage of a counseling relationship because doing so may be a forerunner to relaxing needed boundaries.

What are your own motivations for accepting or rejecting a client's gift? Would you be inclined to accept a gift simply because you do not want to hurt a client's feelings, even though you are not personally comfortable doing so? It could be that you would accept a gift because you are unable to establish firm and clear boundaries. You might also accept a gift because you actually want what a client is offering.

What are the cultural implications of offering a gift? The cultural context does play a role in evaluating the appropriateness of accepting a gift from a client. Giving gifts has different meanings in various cultures. In some cultures, if you were not to accept a gift, it is likely that your client would feel insulted. For example, in Asian culture giving a gift is a common practice to show gratitude and respect and to seal a relationship. Although such actions are culturally appropriate, some helpers believe accepting the gift would distort boundaries, change the relationship, and create a conflict of interest.

If you find a pattern of clients wanting to give you gifts, reflect on the possibility that you might be promoting a sense of indebtedness on your clients' part. If, however, it is rare that clients offer you a gift, you still need to determine a therapeutic way to address the situation. Consider what you feel comfortable doing and what is in the best interests of your client. If you decide not to accept the gift, we recommend that you discuss your reasons with your client. An open discussion is more fruitful and sensitive than simply giving your client a rule or a policy.

Case example.   A Chinese client, Lin, presents you with a piece of jewelry. You have been seeing her for five sessions, and it is likely that you will continue to see her for another five sessions. She says she is grateful for all that you are doing for her and that it would mean a lot to her if you accepted this jewelry, which has been in her family for many years. This is her way of expressing her appreciation.

- What aspects would you want to explore with Lin before accepting or not accepting her gift?
- Do you see a difference between accepting a gift during the therapy or at the end of therapy?
- To what extent would you consider Lin's cultural background and the meaning giving a gift holds for her in making your decision?
- What might you say to Lin if she told you that in her culture it is expected that you will reciprocate in some way if you accept her gift?
- Under what circumstances, if any, might you be inclined to give a client a gift?

Dealing With Sexual Attractions

Some helpers feel guilty over an attraction toward a client, and they feel uncomfortable if they sense that a client is attracted to them. There is a tendency to treat sexual feelings as if they are something that shouldn't exist, which makes attractions difficult for helpers to recognize and accept. Pope, Sonne, and Holroyd (1993) maintain that the lack of research, theory, training, and opportunity to discuss sexual attractions has created a context that does not encourage helpers to explore such feelings when they occur. They add that the topic of sexual feelings in psychotherapy is surrounded by a taboo, which has created a sinister context for the helper's experience of sexual attraction. Typical reactions to sexual feelings in the helping relationship include surprise, startle, and shock; guilt; anxiety about unresolved personal issues; fear of losing control; fear of being criticized; frustration at not being able to speak openly; frustration at not being able to make sexual contact; confusion about tasks; confusion about boundaries and roles; confusion about actions; anger at the client's sexuality; and fear over frustrating the client's demands.

In *Sexual Feelings in Psychotherapy*, Pope, Sonne, and Holroyd (1993) break the silence surrounding the taboo of acknowledging and dealing with sexual feelings in therapy and offer these guidelines:

- Exploring helpers' sexual feelings and reactions should be a key aspect of training programs and continuing professional development.
- Sexual feelings must be clearly distinguished from sexual intimacies with clients.
- It is never permissible for helpers to exploit clients.
- Most helpers have experienced sexual attraction to a client, which often results in their feeling anxious, guilty, or confused.
- It is essential that helpers do not avoid recognizing and dealing with sexual attraction in the helping relationship.
- Helpers are best able to explore their feelings in a context with others that is safe, nonjudgmental, and supportive.
- Understanding sexual feelings is not a simple matter, which means that helpers need to be willing to engage in a personal, complex, and often unpredictable process of exploration.

We do not think that you should be distressed over experiencing sexual or emotional attractions to clients. Being emotionally or sexually attracted does not mean that you are guilty of therapeutic errors or that you are perverse. It is important, however, that you acknowledge your feelings and avoid developing inappropriate sexual intimacies with a client. Although transient sexual feelings are normal, intense preoccupation with clients is problematic. Gill-Wigal and Heaton (1996) identify some warning signs that may indicate you are exceeding appropriate boundaries and should take preventive actions:

- Wanting increased time with a particular client
- Feeling powerful when this particular client is present
- Experiencing increased pleasure with the client
- Enjoying discussion of sexual content
- Persistently engaging in sexual fantasies about the client
- Feeling sexually aroused when the client is present
- Wanting the client's approval
- Desiring physical contact with the client
- Feeling that you are the only one who can help this client

- Experiencing anxiety and guilt when thinking about the client
- Denying harm from turning a professional relationship into a sexual one

Part of learning how to deal effectively with emotional reactions or attractions to clients involves recognizing your own feelings and taking steps to minimize the chances of an attraction interfering with the client's welfare. Gill-Wigal and Heaton (1996) suggest that responsible management of attractions requires acknowledging that attractions must never be acted out, encouraged, or nurtured, and they recommend these strategies for managing an attraction to a client:

- Do not deny feelings of attraction, for responsible management is not possible if these feelings are disowned.
- Seek out a supervisor, a trusted colleague, or a therapist to discuss and come to a clearer understanding of your sexual attractions.
- Accept the responsibility of attending to your own therapeutic needs before your sexual feelings interfere with the progress of a client.
- Recognize that you have the responsibility for maintaining appropriate boundaries by setting clear limits.

Case Examples to Consider

As you read the case examples that follow, consider what you would do in each situation.

A therapist's attraction to a client.   A single male colleague of yours tells you that he is having trouble with one of his female clients, whom he is very much attracted to. He finds himself willing to run overtime in the sessions, and if she were not a client, he would like to ask her out for a date. He is wondering if he should terminate the professional relationship and begin a personal one. He has shared with his client that he is sexually attracted to her, and she admits finding him attractive. Your colleague comes to you for your suggestions on how he should proceed. What do you think you would say to him? What do you think you would do if you found yourself in a similar situation?

A client's attraction to a therapist.   In a counseling session, one of your clients discloses "finding you sexually attractive." The client is uncomfortable making this admission and now wonders what you are thinking and feeling. If you heard this, how do you imagine it would affect you? What might you say in response to your client's concern?

Discussing sexual fantasies therapeutically.   One of your clients describes in detail sexual feelings and fantasies. As you listen, you notice that you are getting uncomfortable and you begin to blush. The client notices that you are blushing and asks: "Did I say something that I shouldn't have?" How would you respond? Would you inquire why your client is telling you this?

A personal request by a client. A client whom you find attractive tells you how accepting, kind, gentle, understanding, and strong you are. This client expresses a desire to hear more about your life. Might you take the focus off the client and engage in self-disclosure for your own needs? Could you see yourself getting carried away with personal conversations that are really not relevant to the therapeutic purpose of your relationship? If this happened, what actions might you take?

Are Counselors Receiving Adequate Training?

Housman and Stake (1999) found that 50% of the doctoral students in their study reported having experienced a sexual attraction to a client; only half of these students had chosen to discuss the attraction with a supervisor. Seeking help from a colleague, supervision, or personal therapy can give students and trainees access to guidance, education, and support in handling their feelings. Pope, Sonne, and Holroyd (1993) maintain that practice, internships, and peer supervision groups are ideal places to discuss sexual feelings about clients, which are often treated as though they were nonexistent. Deliberate attention to sexuality issues during training is essential for the development of competent mental health professionals. This training should involve accurate information and opportunities for experiential practice, such as role-playing difficult situations (Wiederman & Sansone, 1999).

Housman and Stake (1999) surveyed sexual ethics training and student understanding of sexual ethics in clinical psychology doctoral programs and found that 94% of the students had received an average of 6 hours of sexual ethics training. They emphasized the importance of addressing sexual issues in therapy early in students' training as sexual feelings for clients are common among students as well as professional practitioners. It was concluded that most students in training do not understand that sexual attractions for clients are normal. Housman and Stake note that even if students refrain from acting on their sexual feelings for clients, they may withdraw emotionally from clients to avoid feelings they believe are unacceptable. It is crucial that students acknowledge their feelings to themselves and to their supervisors and take steps to deal effectively with them.

In addition to supervisory consultations, Housman and Stake (1999) state that clinical programs should provide all students with some form of planned experiential training for developing skills in clarifying boundaries and setting limits with clients. As a part of this experiential training, Housman and Stake recommend discussion of videotaped scenarios portraying client and therapist sexual feelings, role-playing common scenarios that could result in sexual misconduct, and opportunities to discuss personal cases. They emphasize the importance of broadening sexual ethics training to address both the emotional and cognitive aspects of attractions in the therapeutic relationship.

Hamilton and Spruill (1999) believe it is crucial to increase student awareness of sexual attraction before students begin seeing clients. They recommend the inclusion of how to deal with sexual attractions as a basic component of a preparatory clinical skills course. This training needs to create the expectation that sexual attractions will arise in therapy and to create an atmosphere of trust in which students feel as free as possible to disclose these feelings and experiences in their supervision. If students are not presented with normalizing information, they are likely to continue to regard sexual feelings as rare and as proof of a troubled therapy relationship.

In light of the challenges of dealing with sexual attractions in the helping process, Herlihy and Corey (1997a) recommend that training programs in the counseling and human development fields place increased emphasis on the issue of sexual attraction. Helpers need to be assured that their feelings are natural and that with awareness they can learn to provide professional assistance to clients, even if they might experience sexual attraction at times. Herlihy and Corey stress the value of learning to monitor one's own countertransference, consulting with colleagues, and being alert to the subtle ways that sexual attractions can cross the boundary into inappropriate dual relationships.

Sexual Relationships With Current Clients

Sexual misconduct is one of the major causes for malpractice actions against mental health providers. Those who have studied the sexual relationships between helpers and clients generally report that such misconduct is more widespread than is commonly believed. Studies continue to demonstrate that clients who are the victims of sexual misconduct suffer dire consequences. Sonne and Pope (1991) report that clients who had been sexually involved with their therapists tended to exhibit reactions similar to those of survivors of incest and rape, including intense feelings of betrayal, confusion, and guilt.

In the last few years the greatest single category of complaints to the ethics committee of the APA involved sexual relationships. Judgments against therapists, dismissal of professors, revocation of licenses, and large damage awards are no longer unusual. The literature shows that sexual relationships with clients carry serious consequences in both ethical and legal terms. Among these consequences are being the target of a lawsuit, being convicted of a felony, having their license revoked, being expelled from professional organizations, losing their insurance coverage, and losing their jobs. Therapists may also be placed on probation, be required to undergo their own psychotherapy, be closely monitored if they are allowed to resume their practice, and be required to obtain supervised practice. Sexual misconduct is one of the more serious allegations in malpractice suits. Therapist-client sexual contact is highly disruptive and is the most potentially damaging boundary violation (Smith & Fitzpatrick, 1995).

Pope and Vasquez (1998) have noted a fairly consistent decrease in the self-reported rate of sexual involvement with clients but caution that this trend may reflect either a genuine decrease or increasingly less candid reporting. Most mental health professionals take the position that erotic contact with clients is totally inappropriate and is an exploitation of the relationship by the therapist. They view sexual contact with clients as unprofessional, unethical, and clinically harmful.

As you read this, you may think that you would never become involved in sexual misconduct with any of your clients. The chances are that those practitioners who have engaged in sexual intimacies with clients made the same assumption. Realize that you are not immune to becoming sexually involved with those you help. Knowledge of the possibility of this involvement will at least enable you to be on the alert to your own needs and motivations and how they could get in the way of your work.

As a helper you are likely to receive respect and adulation and to be perceived as someone who can do no wrong. Clients may compare you with their significant others, and many times you will rank higher. As a beginning helper you are especially vulnerable. If clients tell you how attractive, how understanding, and how different you are from anyone else they have met, it may be difficult to resist believing what they say. Without self-awareness and honesty, you may direct the sessions toward meeting your needs and may eventually become sexually indiscreet.

Your clients are usually with you for a short time, and they are probably getting the best side of you. This unconditional admiration can become very seductive. You may learn to like their reactions to you too much. You can get in trouble as a helper if you cease to keep the feelings that your clients express to you in proper perspective.

All of the professional organizations have some specific statement that condemns sexual intimacies in the client-helper relationship. In addition to specifically prohibiting sexual contact, most codes of ethics warn against any activities on the helper's part that could lead to the risk of exploitation. If a therapist has had a prior sexual relationship with a person, many ethics codes specify that this person should not be accepted as a client at a later time. If a client-helper relationship develops into a sexual one, most professional codes require termination of the relationship and a referral to another professional.

The reasons erotic contact is unethical center on the power that helpers have by virtue of their professional role. Because clients are talking about very personal aspects of their lives and making themselves highly vulnerable, it is easy to betray this trust by exploiting clients for helpers' own personal motives. Sexual contact is also unethical because it fosters dependency and makes objectivity on the part of the helper impossible. But perhaps the most important argument against sexual involvement with clients is that most clients report harm as a result. They typically become resentful and angry at having been sexually exploited and abandoned. Clients generally feel stuck with both unresolved problems and unresolved feelings relating to the traumatic experience.

Sexual Relationships With Former Clients

Most of the codes of ethics of the various professions do not currently have an absolute ban on sexual relationships after the end of a professional relationship, but helpers are cautioned against forming romantic relationships with former clients for at least 2 years after termination. However, this does not imply that such relationships with clients are ethical or professional after 2 years have elapsed. The codes of the ACA (1995), NASW (1999), AAMFT (2001), and APA (1992) are quite specific about conditions pertaining to relationships with former clients. For example, it is not considered ethical to terminate with a client because of an attraction, wait the time period, and then begin a romantic relationship. Even after 2 years, it is incumbent upon helpers to examine their motivations, to continually consider what is best for the former client, and to be extremely careful to avoid any form of exploitation. In Salisbury and Kinnier's (1996) study, only 33% of counselors believed a sexual relationship with a former client was acceptable even 5 years after termination of the counseling relationship.

In the exceptional circumstance of a sexual relationship with a former client, the burden of demonstrating that there has been no exploitation clearly rests with the practitioner. The factors that must be considered include the amount of time that has passed since termination of therapy; the nature and duration of therapy; the circumstances surrounding termination of the helper-client relationship; the client's personal history; the client's competence and mental status; the foreseeable likelihood of harm to the client or others; and any statements or actions of the helper suggesting a romantic relationship after terminating the professional relationship. The professional codes pertaining to sexual contact with former clients are explicit:

> Psychologists do not engage in sexual intimacies with a former therapy patient or client for at least two years after cessation or termination of professional service. (APA, 1992)

> Counselors do not engage in sexual intimacies with former clients within a minimum of 2 years after terminating the counseling relationship. Counselors who engage in such relationships after 2 years following termination have the responsibility to examine and document thoroughly that such relations did not have an exploitative nature, based on factors such as duration of counseling, amount of time since counseling, circumstances of termination, client's personal history and mental status, adverse impact on the client, and actions by the counselor suggesting a plan to initiate a sexual relationship with the client after termination. (ACA, 1995, A.7.b.)

> Social workers should not engage in sexual activities or sexual contact with former clients because of the potential for harm to the client. If social workers engage in conduct contrary to this prohibition or claim that an exception to this prohibition is warranted due to extraordinary circumstances, it is social workers—not their clients—who assume the full burden of demonstrating that the former client has not been exploited, coerced, or manipulated, intentionally or unintentionally. (NASW, 1999, 1.09.c.)

> Sexual intimacy with former clients is likely to be harmful and is therefore prohibited for two years following the termination of therapy or last professional contact. In an effort to avoid exploiting the trust and dependency of clients, marriage and family therapists should not engage in sexual intimacy with former clients after the two years following termination or last professional contact. Should therapists engage in sexual intimacy with former clients following two years after termination or last professional contact, the burden shifts to the therapist to demonstrate that there has been no exploitation or injury to the former client or to the client's immediate family. (AAMFT, 2001, 1.5)

In discussing the ethics of sexual contact with former clients, Glosoff, Corey, and Herlihy (1996) point out that the topic is being extensively debated within the helping professions. Most agree that simply because a helping relationship is terminated, in and of itself, does not justify changing the professional relationship into a sexual one. Under the present ethics codes, if a helper considers getting romantically involved with a former client after 2 years have passed, a wise course to follow would be to consult with a colleague or seek a therapy session conjointly with the former client to explore mutual transferences and expectations. It is essential to remain aware of the potential harm that can result from sexual intimacies that occur after termination, of the aspects of the therapeutic process that continue after termination including residual transference, and of the continuing power differential (Herlihy & Corey, 1997a).

Sexual relationships with former clients are strongly discouraged, and an ethics code task force of the American Psychological Association is debating the merits of the current standard that prohibits sexual intimacy for 2 years once a therapeutic relationship ends. The task force is proposing a "perpetuity rule" that would prohibit sexual relationships no matter how much time has elapsed since the last client visit. According to the APA's task force, an absolute ban on post-termination sexual relationships more clearly addresses the inherent power imbalance, which is not erased with termination. Furthermore, the task force believes the public image of the profession would be strengthened by an ethical standard that imposes a lifetime ban on sexual intimacy with former clients (Martin, 1999). In developing guidelines for your own practice, where would you begin in defining appropriate relationships with former clients?

Dual Relationships With Supervisors or Teachers

Those who teach or supervise students in the helping professions owe students and trainees the same kind of explanations they owe clients about the potential problems involved in dual relationships. The ethics codes of both the ACA (1995) and the NCFR (1997) deal directly and clearly with dual relationships in teaching and supervisory relationships. It is the responsibility of educators and clinical supervisors to create and maintain appropriate relationship boundaries with students and trainees. Specifically, professionals in charge of educating and supervising students avoid engaging in sexual relationships with students or supervisees and avoid subjecting them to any form of sexual harassment. In addition, supervisors or counselor educators do not serve as counselors to students or supervisees over whom they have administrative, teaching, or evaluative roles—*unless* this is a brief role associated with a training experience. Although supervisors do have the responsibility to help trainees understand how their personal issues may interfere with working effectively with clients, it is not appropriate for supervisors to change the supervisory function to a therapy function.

Sex in the supervisory relationship or in the professor-student relationship typically results in an abuse of power because of the role differences. If a sexual relationship enters into a supervisory relationship, the entire process is confounded. The chances are that supervisees will not get the supervision they need if they are romantically involved with their supervisors (Herlihy & Corey, 1997a).

The student is extremely vulnerable because of this difference in status. Faced with a faculty member who makes a sexual proposition, the student is likely to feel intimidated by the person with power. Students and interns recognize that their decision to reject a sexual proposition might well have a negative effect on their performance evaluation. There is also the reality of poor modeling for students for their future relationships with their clients.

You have a right to expect a learning environment free from sexual harassment, both in the classroom and at your field placement. Ideally, you should not be expected to deal with situations involving unwanted sexual advances from those who function in teaching, supervisory, or consulting roles. Realistically, however, you need to know what to do in the event that you are faced with sexual harassment. Most agencies and institutions of higher education have specific policies regarding sexual harassment, as well as procedures to follow to report such abuse. Find out what the procedures are at your institution and be prepared to use them should the need arise.

By Way of Review

- A dual relationship may occur whenever you interact with a client in more than one capacity. Be aware of your position of power and avoid even the appearance of conflict of interest.

- It helps to keep your relationships with your clients on a professional, rather than a personal, basis. Mixing social relationships with professional relationships often works against the best interests of both the client and the helper.

- It is probably a good idea to avoid bartering, except in cases where this is the cultural norm. Exchanging services can often lead to resentment on both your part and your client's.

- In deciding whether to accept gifts from clients, consider the cultural context, the client's motivations for offering a gift, and the stage of the helping process.

- Sexual attractions are a normal part of helping relationships. It is important to learn how to recognize these attractions and how to deal with them effectively.

- Sexual misconduct is the leading cause of malpractice actions against mental health providers. Sexual intimacies between helpers and clients are unethical for a number of reasons. One of the main ones is that they entail an abuse of power and trust.

- Sexual relationships between supervisors and supervisees or professors and students are unethical because of the harm that they typically do to the students or supervisees. Such relationships represent a clear misuse of power and also confound the supervisory or learning process.

What Will You Do Now?

1. Some say that dual relationships are inevitable, pervasive, and unavoidable and have the potential to be either beneficial or harmful. In small groups, explore both the potential benefits and risks of dual relationships. Come up with guidelines as a group for how you might assess the balance between the benefits and risks of dual and multiple relationships.

2. Review the discussion on sexual relationships with former clients. Form two teams and debate the issue of whether sexual and romantic relationships with former clients should be allowed a specific length of time after termination of the counseling relationship.

3. Assume that you are a member of a committee with the task of revising ethics codes. What input would you have regarding the appropriateness of social, sexual, business, and professional relationships with former clients? Do you think that each of these relationships should be considered unethical under some or most circumstances? Can you think of exceptions? Can you think of situations where you might accept a social invitation from a former client? Would you see it as appropriate to engage in a business relationship with a former client? Can you think of any times when you might form professional relationships with former clients?

4. In small groups spend some time sharing what you learned about the importance of creating personal and professional boundaries. What difficulties might you expect to encounter in establishing and maintaining certain boundaries with some clients?

5. For the full bibliographic entry for each of the sources listed here, consult the References and Reading List at the back of the book. For a treatment of many facets of the dual relationship controversy, see Herlihy and Corey (1997a) and Corey and Herlihy (1997).

Ethics in Action CD-ROM Exercises

6. Complete the self-inventory [Boundary Issues and Multiple Relationships] before viewing role-play segments 8 through 12. Bring your completed responses to class for discussion.

7. In video role-play segment 8, The Picnic, the client (Lucia) would like to meet with the counselor (John) at the park down the street for their counseling sessions so she can get to know him better and feel closer to him. She suggests that she could bring a lunch for a picnic. John is concerned about creating an environment that would help Lucia the most, and she says "That [meeting in the park] would really help me." Through role playing, demonstrate how you would establish and maintain boundaries with this client.

8. In role-play segment 9, The Friendship, at their last therapy session the client (Charlae) says she would like to continue their relationship because they have so much in common and she has shared things with the counselor (Natalie) that she has not discussed with anyone else. Natalie informs Charlae that this puts her in a difficult situation and she feels awkward. Charlae says, "What if we just go jogging together a couple of mornings a week?" Via role playing, demonstrate how you would handle such a request from a former client who is interested in developing a social relationship with you.

9. In role-play segment 10, The Disclosure, the counselor (Conrad) shares with the client (Suzanne) that he has been thinking about her a lot and that he is attracted to her. Suzanne responds with, "You're kidding, right?" She says she came to him because of having problems with men taking advantage of her and not respecting her. She has bared her soul to him and now she feels devalued. Suzanne suggests possibly seeing another counselor, but Conrad thinks they can work it out. Role-play the way you would deal with a client who disclosed to you that he or she found you "quite attractive." Assume that you also found this client "quite attractive."

10. In role-play segment 11, The Architect, the client (Janice) lost her job and can no longer pay for counseling sessions. She suggests providing architectural services for the counselor (Jerry). Jerry suggests they discuss the pros and cons and that he wants to be sure that this is in her best interests. He mentions the code of ethics that discourages bartering. Jerry talks about issues of value and timeliness of services. In a role play, demonstrate how you would deal with this client. What issues would you want to explore?

11. In role-play segment 12, Tickets for Therapy, the client (John) shows his appreciation for his counselor (Marianne) by getting tickets to the theater for her. John says, "I got tickets for you so you can go and enjoy it and have a good time." Marianne talks about why she cannot accept the tickets, in spite of the fact that she is very appreciative of his gesture. What issues would you explore with John? Might you accept the tickets under any circumstances? Why or why not? Demonstrate, through role playing, what you would say to the client.

InfoTrac College Edition Resources

For additional readings, explore InfoTrac College Edition, our online library. Go to http://www.infotrac.college.com/wadsworth and select these key word searches:

dual W1 relationship* couns*
multiple W1 relationships
barter* couns*
barter* psych*

gift psych*
gift therap*
social W1 relationship* client*
social W1 relationship* therap*
sexual W1 attraction* client*
sexual W1 relationship client*
superv* personal couns*

Key words are listed in a form that enables the search engine to locate a wider range of articles in the online university library. Key words should be entered exactly as shown, including asterisks, "W1," "W2," "AND," and other search engine tools.

Working in the Community

Focus Questions

1. What role would you like to play in your community? To what degree do you think you should focus on the needs of the community as well as on those of individuals?

2. Some helpers direct their efforts to helping clients understand factors within themselves that contribute to their problems. Other helpers focus on the environmental forces that need to be changed that are resulting in an individual's problems. What are the advantages or disadvantages of an integrated approach that combines both individual and environmental factors?

3. Community workers devote some of their attention to educating the community about pressing social problems and about making use of the human services within the community. In what area might you be interested in developing an educational program?

4. Outreach work is a basic community intervention. If you were working in a community agency at this time, what target group would you particularly want to reach? Would you go into the community to provide services for a client population that might not seek out your services?

5. What challenges do you expect to face as a community worker with respect to delivering your services to diverse client groups in the community? What kinds of helping roles might you assume as a worker in a community agency?

6. Crisis intervention is a short-term helping strategy that has particular relevance for dealing with many of the problems individuals in a community face. Are you interested in learning more about crisis intervention? How could crisis intervention methods result in community change or strengthen a community?

Aim of the Chapter

Many people argue that professional helpers can foster real and lasting changes only if they have an impact on the total milieu of people's lives. Working with people who come for individual counseling is one way professionals can use their helping skills, but helpers can foster real and lasting community changes if they use a systems approach. The aspirations and difficulties of individual clients intertwine with those of many other people in a community system. Practitioners can make ripples within factions of the community even in small ways if they are committed to becoming change agents. It is essential that community workers focus on the capabilities and strengths within a community, for doing so empowers people in the community. When we use the term *community agency*, we include any institution—public or private, nonprofit or for-profit—designed to provide a wide range of social and psychological services to the community. Likewise, when we speak of *community workers*, we refer to a diverse pool of human services workers whose primary duties revolve around serving individuals within their community.

In this chapter we focus on the special responsibilities of a community worker. Do you view the community as your client or the individual as your client? Do you believe you have a broader responsibility to address the conditions that create problems for individuals who come to see you? If you adopt the perspective of the community as a "client," you will have many roles to play in helping to improve it. Although some of the issues we present pertain mainly to practitioners employed by a community agency, it is essential that you take steps to avoid working in isolation, regardless of the setting in which you are employed. You can benefit by knowing how to work with community resources.

Examine your own commitment to community intervention by thinking about questions such as these: How are the human services needs in your community met? What are the special needs of low-income people? Where can people go for the social and psychological services they need? If people ask you what resources are available to assist them, can you direct them? What are some of the forces within your community that contribute to the problems individuals and groups are experiencing? What are some of the prevailing attitudes of people in your community about the range of human services? How might you build on these attitudes if they are positive? What can you do to change these attitudes if they are negative? What role would you like to play as a helper in improving your community?

We begin by looking at the community approach, which emphasizes understanding clients by examining their social setting. Traditional psychotherapy focuses on resolution of internal conflicts as a pathway to individual change; the community approach focuses on social change rather than merely helping people adapt to their circumstances. A community orientation requires helpers to design interventions that go beyond the office. Helpers trained in individual helping models who work in the community need to develop a more expansive notion of who the client is. The community approach includes meeting unmet community needs, helping the community identify and develop its resources, and employing other measures that ultimately strengthen the community itself.

The Scope of the Community Approach

The helping process does not take place in a vacuum isolated from the larger sociopolitical influences of society. Many human services specialists see a need for new approaches to augment individual counseling. Some call for developing intervention strategies that deal with the societal factors that adversely affect the lives of many members of minority groups (Sue, Arredondo, & McDavis, 1992). Herr (1991) clearly presents a case for developing broader strategies that do not ignore these environmental factors. The changing nature of client populations, pressing social problems, and the impact of advanced technology present a challenge to human services practitioners to develop problem-solving strategies and techniques with a multidisciplinary perspective. Herr's comments echo the traditional social work perspective of working with the "person in the environment." Rather than focusing on individual dynamics or environmental factors, a process that considers both aspects is often most beneficial to clients.

Many of the problems people face are the result of being disenfranchised as individuals or as members of a community or group from systems that hold valued resources for them. The challenge for community workers is to work toward greater degrees of enfranchisement. Culturally skilled community workers particularly understand how the sociopolitical influences impinge on the experiences of racial and ethnic minority groups. For example, immigration issues, racism, stereotyping, poverty, and powerlessness can all severely damage individuals (Arredondo et al., 1996; Sue et al., 1992).

The traditional approach tends to treat dysfunctions as belonging to the individual, and the helper teaches the individual to adjust to the "realities" of living in a society. In contrast, the community approach assesses these dysfunctions in the context of a larger system; individuals are taught ways of empowering themselves so that they can begin to change some of the inequities in society (Lewis, Lewis, Daniels, & D'Andrea, 1998).

Multiple Roles of Community Workers

Increasingly it has become clear that helpers need to move beyond a problem or deficits approach and begin building on the strengths and resources in the community. By creating opportunities for community members to develop skills and abilities that contribute to the vitality of their community, community workers help to develop the community, not merely attend to some of its problems. This elevates the quality of life in the community and expands the members' capacity to confront current and future challenges.

Working with the community usually means working with a specific group or in a situation in which competing or collaborating groups are dealing with an issue or set of issues in a community. These groups usually have a strong identity or a potential for one and can be readily organized for action. In fact, the work of community change is really the work of small groups. That is, within the community group with whom you are working there will be a smaller group of people who take an active part in change efforts. Most of the work of this group will be done in a small group context. In Chapter 13 on working with groups and families, we will describe how important it is for human services workers to capitalize on the value of using group approaches. In functioning as a change agent within the community, small group skills are essential.

Alternative Helper Roles

Atkinson, Thompson, and Grant (1993) believe the conventional role of psychotherapist is appropriate "only for a client who is highly acculturated and now wants relief from an existing problem that has an internal etiology" (p. 269). Other writers have criticized conventional approaches to therapy because they place undue responsibility on the client for his or her plight. At the extreme, some interventions blame client problems entirely on the individual without regard for environmental factors that may be contributing to the client's problem.

The helping professions must recognize that many problems—such as prejudice and discrimination—reside outside, not within, the person. Community-oriented work emphasizes the necessity of recognizing and dealing with environmental conditions that often create problems for ethnically diverse client groups. Helpers are required to assume nontraditional roles if they hope to make an impact on social systems. Atkinson, Morten, and Sue (1998) suggest that it is appropriate for community workers to assume some or all of the following alternative roles as needed to benefit their clients: (1) advocate, (2) change agent, (3) consultant, (4) adviser, (5) facilitator of indigenous support systems, and (6) facilitator of indigenous healing methods. In selecting a role and strategies to use with racial or ethnic minority clients, it is useful to take into account the client's level of acculturation, the locus of problem etiology, and the goal of counseling. Although these nontraditional roles are often the most effective interventions from a multicultural perspective, most training programs do not provide education and training in these roles. Let's look briefly at each of these alternative helper roles.

• *Advocate.* Because ethnic minority clients are often oppressed to some degree by the dominant society, helpers can speak on their behalf. Helpers especially need to function as advocates for clients who are low in acculturation and who need remediation of a problem that results from discrimination and oppression.

• *Change agent.* Functioning in this role, community workers do what they can to confront and bring about change within the system that contributes to, if not creates, many of the problems clients face. In this role, helpers assist clients in recognizing oppressive forces in the community as a source of their problem and also teach clients strategies for dealing with these problems. As change agents, community workers assist clients in developing power, particularly political power, to bring about change in the clients' social and physical environment. A change agent recognizes that healthy communities produce healthy people. The main purpose of community change is fostering healthy communities (Homan, 1999).

- *Consultant.* Operating as consultants, helpers can encourage individuals to learn skills they can use to interact successfully with various forces within their community. In this role, the client and the helper cooperate in addressing unhealthy forces within the system. As consultants, helpers can work with racial and ethnic minority clients to design preventive programs to reduce the negative impact of racism and oppression.

- *Adviser.* This role is similar to that of consultant, except the community worker as adviser initiates the discussion with clients about ways to deal with environmental problems that contribute to their personal problems. For example, recent immigrants may need advice on immigration paperwork, coping with problems they will face in the job market, or problems that their children may encounter at school.

- *Facilitator of indigenous support systems.* Many ethnically diverse clients, people in rural environments, and older people would not consider seeking professional help in the traditional sense. However, they are willing to turn to social support systems within their own communities. Community workers can play an important role by encouraging clients to make full use of resources within their own communities, including community centers, churches, extended families, neighborhood social networks, and ethnic advocacy groups. Community workers can work with church leaders in influencing social policy and community change.

- *Facilitator of indigenous healing systems.* In many cultures human service professionals have little hope of reaching individuals with problems, for these people are likely to put their trust in folk healers. If helpers are aware of what kinds of healing resources exist within a client's culture (indigenous resources), they can refer a client to a folk or spiritual healer from his or her culture. At times it may be difficult for helpers to adopt the worldview of their clients. In such instances it could be helpful to work with an indigenous healer.

Mobilizing Community Resources

In *Promoting Community Change: Making It Happen in the Real World,* Homan (1999) suggests that if you want to assume an active role in mobilizing the resources within a community it is useful to have certain knowledge and skills. To maximize your efforts in a community, hone your skills in these areas:

- Achieve credibility and standing within the community.
- Promote meaningful involvement of members of the community being served in community change efforts.
- Develop and build on the strengths or capabilities of members of the community.
- Know your target, your issue, your troops, and your resources.
- Identify the stakeholders, those who are potential allies and opponents.
- Establish and maintain a personal network, especially involving people who may be in a position to assist client groups.

- Understand the transferability of skills used in working with individual clients to working with the community.
- Understand planning and its relationship to action.
- Acknowledge that power is used to maintain or change conditions within the community.
- Learn that power *with* is at least as important as power *over.*
- Assist the community to declare its needs in a way that enables people to act on them.
- Keep people who are involved in the change effort connected to one another.
- Make sure that your strategies and tactics fit the situation.
- Understand that people must *feel* something before they will *do* something.
- Use the "cycle of empowerment": involvement, communication, decisions, action.
- Listen as assertively as you speak.
- Assume responsibility for instigating change.
- Avoid setting arbitrary limits on yourself. Believe in your own capabilities.
- Commit yourself to learning—about yourself, your community, your issue, your strategies and tactics.
- Focus on the commonalties among community members rather than on their differences.
- Remember that it's not only "they" who need to change but "we" who must change what we are doing.
- Accept the reality of certain problems or conditions without letting these barriers stop productive efforts.
- Address ethical issues in the delivery of services.
- Believe in the rights of members of the community to lead full and satisfying lives.

The most successful programs involve community members in determining the direction their communities need to take. As a community worker you will assume an active role, but remember that it is the community members themselves who are the "experts" on their own needs. Viewing community members as the experts is a way of fostering a sense of empowerment. Rather than deciding for a community what is needed, your role might be more to facilitate connections within a community and to help individuals learn to use available resources to effect changes in their community.

Some uncertainty is natural when you are trying to decide how you can make a difference in your community. Remember, you already have many of the skills you will need to analyze situations and build relationships. It is also important to recognize that idealism can be a valuable asset. Like any other asset, it is strengthened when put into practice.

Take a moment to reflect on what you have already read about the community approach. Think about your educational background, level of professional training, and work experiences. If you plan to go into the human services field, you are likely to spend some time working in a community agency setting, and you will be working with many different groups within the community. If you were working in such a setting at this time, how prepared are you, both personally and academically, to assume a broader view of helping that encompasses being an agent for change within the community? How can you learn what you will need to know to assume the role of a helper in the community? What specific skills do you need to acquire? What fears would you need to challenge to work effectively in the community? How might you translate your idealism into a practical set of strategies to bring about constructive change within the community?

The Community Approach to Helping

Community counseling is "a comprehensive helping framework of intervention strategies and services that promotes the personal development of all individuals and communities" (Lewis et al., 1998, p. 5). The activities that make up a comprehensive community perspective have four components: (1) direct client services, (2) indirect client services, (3) direct community services, and (4) indirect community services.

Direct client services focus on *outreach activities* to a population that might be at risk for developing mental health problems. Community workers provide help to clients either facing crises or dealing with ongoing stressors that impair their coping ability. There is a growing need to provide programs for populations such as school dropouts, alcohol and drug abusers of all ages, the homeless, victims and perpetrators of child and elderly abuse, suicidal individuals, victims of violent crimes, elderly people, persons with AIDS, and adolescent mothers. By reaching out to those schools and communities that would be receptive to help, community workers can offer a variety of personal, career, family, and counseling services to at-risk groups (Lewis et al., 1998).

Indirect client services consist of *client advocacy,* which involves active intervention for and with an individual or a group. The community agency works to empower disenfranchised groups that have become split off from the mainstream community. These include, but are not limited to, the unemployed, the homeless, the elderly, the handicapped, and persons living with AIDS. Helpers need to become advocates, speaking up on their clients' behalf and actively intervening in their clients' situation (Lewis et al., 1998). Advocacy consists of those focused efforts to change existing policy or to influence proposed policy on behalf of specific underrepresented groups (Ezell, 2001). The advocacy process is best conceived of as a way to assist groups who typically do not have power to move in the direction of acquiring tools to find and use resources, both within the community and within themselves.

Direct community services in the form of *preventive education* are geared to the population at large. Examples of these programs include life planning workshops, AIDS prevention workshops, the creative use of leisure, and training in interpersonal skills. Because the emphasis is on prevention, these programs help people develop a wider range of competencies.

Indirect community services are attempts to *change the social environment* to meet the needs of the population as a whole and are carried out by influencing public policy. Community intervention deals with the victims of poverty, sexism, and racism, which typically leave people feeling powerless. The focus is on promoting systemic change by working closely with those in the community who develop public policy. The overall goal is the reduction of health problems, both mental and physical.

Community intervention calls for helpers who (a) are familiar with resources within the community that they can refer clients to, when necessary, (b) have a basic knowledge of the cultural background of their clients, (c) possess skills that can be used as needed by clients, (d) have the ability to balance various roles as professionals, and (e) have the willingness to be advocates for policy changes in the community.

Outreach

As mental health professionals have become more aware of the need to provide services to a wider population, effective outreach strategies have received increased attention. These strategies are particularly useful for reaching ethnic minorities because of the traditional mistrust of primarily white mental health professionals who have often mislabeled minorities and excluded them from services. Many people of color perceive counseling as a process that the dominant society employs to forcibly control their lives and well-being (Lee, 1997c). As you saw in Chapter 8, if practitioners hope to reach and effectively deal with a cultural group different from their own, they must acquire a broad understanding of culturally diverse client populations. It is essential that helpers use intervention techniques that are consistent with the life experiences and cultural values of culturally diverse groups in the community if they hope to succeed in their outreach efforts (Sue et al., 1992).

The community psychology model, with its emphasis on creating responsive social systems, is perhaps best suited for people of color. White and Parham (1990) write that this kind of outreach model differs from the traditional model used in the helping professions in the sense that the community worker does not wait for people to come in for help. Instead, the worker reaches out to the community with a coordinated package of preventive mental health services aimed at improving the psychological health of people throughout the life cycle.

White and Parham (1990) view the community as the client and the community worker as a social engineer who orchestrates a variety of functions involving various levels of the social system that impinge on the psychological well-being of minority groups. It is essential that the community perspective be reflected in the design and delivery of psychological services.

The Right of Passage program (cited in Marino, 1996) is an excellent example of an outreach effort that is exposing a community to counseling and developing a community program for preventing potential problems with young people. Ron Coley and Thomas Parham are both very active in developing the Right of Passage, which is part of the Passport to the Future program organized by the 100 Black Men of Orange County. The Right of Passage program includes counseling for a group of African American young men, ages 14 and up, on a variety of issues. The students in this program meet every other week until they are 18, and the program includes discussion of these pertinent issues:

- Self-awareness
- History of African American culture
- Relationships with family, women, and other men
- Skill development, including conflict resolution and career development
- Leadership skills such as economic empowerment
- Community service

Parham (cited in Marino, 1996) hopes that the program demonstrates how counseling can become more relevant to the reality of these young men. Parham sees this program as an example of how helpers can design interventions that address specific needs within a community.

The outreach approach includes developmental and educational efforts, such as skills training, stress management training, education of the community about mental health and the benefits of counseling, and consultation in a variety of settings. These efforts must be made in a way that makes sense to the community, not just the practitioner. If people in the community do not utilize services, it is appropriate to question the value of the services or the appropriateness of the way these services are delivered. Community workers need to be willing to learn *from* and *with* the community when organizing services.

You do not have to be all things to potential clients in the community. If you work in a community agency, you will most likely be part of a team working with individual clients. The case management approach involves a number of helping professionals, each with a different specialty. Managed care systems also utilize a team approach, so you need to learn how to build collaborative relationships with the members of a professional team at your agency. Once a need is identified within a community, a group of workers has more power to reach client groups than does a single worker functioning in isolation.

Ask yourself what kind of outreach work you might be inclined to do in your own community. If you have a field placement or a job in a community agency, what ideas do you have for outreach projects? Can you seek out mental health professionals in your community, or faculty members at your college, who have the expertise to provide you with direction in meeting critical needs of certain client groups? How might you and some fellow students combine your talents and efforts to develop a program for reaching a neglected segment of your community? What agencies and resources within your community could you use in developing an outreach project? Your program does not have to involve a grand design; even a small change can help individuals who are not likely to ask for the assistance they need.

Educating the Community

Educating the community includes educating the professionals regarding the existence and dimensions of problems as well as some steps for dealing with them; educating the broad community about the same things and, in addition, about the costs to the community of maintaining the problem; and educating the potential consumers about the availability of services as well as their right to demand that they be delivered with quality.

There are many reasons people do not make use of available resources: they may not be aware of them, they may not be able to afford these services, they may have misconceptions about the nature and purpose of counseling, they may be reluctant to recognize their problems, they may harbor the attitude that they should be able to take charge of their lives on their own, they may believe professional helpers are attempting to control their lives, they may perceive that these services are not intended for them because they view such services as culturally insensitive, or they may believe they are not worthy to receive services. There are also practical limiting factors that make it difficult to use community services. For example, if clients are required to travel to the agency to receive services, community members without access to transportation may be unable to make use of the programs.

One goal of the community approach is to educate the public and attempt to change the attitudes of the community toward mental health programs. Perhaps the most important task in this area is to demystify the notion of mental illness. Many people still cling to misconceptions and archaic notions of mental illness. Professionals face a real challenge in combating these faulty notions. Helpers also need to be able to present the array of services they offer to the community in terms that the target groups can understand. Many people still consider seeking any form of professional psychological treatment as something only for those who are seriously mentally ill. Others see professional helpers as having answers for every problem a client brings to the agency. And others hold the belief that professional help is only for the weak or for those who simply cannot solve their own problems. Unless professionals actively work on presenting helping services in a way that is understandable to the community at large, many people who could benefit from professional help may not seek it out. Educating the community can awaken people to what is available to empower various groups.

One small, grass roots nonprofit agency in Orange County, California, has applied outreach strategies to educate the community and meet critical needs in the community (Hogan-Garcia & Scheinberg, 2000). The Coalition for Children, Adolescents and Parents (CCAP) is a community agency aimed at the prevention of adolescent pregnancy. For the past 20 years, CCAP has provided after-school recreational services, tutoring, academic enrichment programs, physical examinations, parenting education, conflict resolution, cultural diversity training, school-based group counseling, a homeless shelter, drug abuse prevention, and child care training—to mention a few services. All members of the agency staff have demonstrated a commitment to clarifying and understanding personal values, beliefs, and behaviors. Because the individuals on the staff believe in the value of understanding cultural diversity, they have been able to serve as a bridge between mainstream and non-mainstream segments of their community.

One of the early projects designed by CCAP involved outreach and education in the Latino community to prevent the spread of HIV. A Latina staff member conducted interviews with 30 mothers in the community regarding their understanding of HIV, human sexuality, and teen pregnancy. From this contact with these mothers, a group of leaders (comadres) was formed, and they took steps to educate the community. The women who served as leaders met for monthly meetings, which were held at a neighborhood center. Eventually, the women invited their husbands into the classes.

This is an example of an effective collaborative effort by an agency that is committed to ensuring that the members of the community have a full voice in determining the nature of the services. The projects that are a part of CCAP are based on a set of culturally competent practice principles in a culturally diverse community. These principles have been identified by Hogan-Garcia and Scheinberg (2000) and can be applied to a variety of community agencies:

- Be willing to examine your assumptions and personal values.
- In an agency, bring together an ethnically diverse staff and board.
- Develop and maintain positive relationships with key people in the community.
- Ask community members about their perceptions of what is needed in the community.
- Bring community members and agency staff together in genuine dialogue.
- Design a program based on the community's definition of their needs.
- In implementing a program, be sensitive to the pace of the community.
- Advocate for the needs of the community and serve as a bridge between cultural groups.
- Translate the progress of the community in terms that the funders of the project will understand.

Client Advocacy

It is our view that an increasing number of people are unable to cope with the demands of their environment and are receptive to the idea of professional assistance. As more people overcome the stigma attached to seeking help, the demand for community services increases. Helpers need to assume an advocacy role for disenfranchised clients whose backgrounds make it difficult for them to utilize professional assistance. They need to challenge long-standing traditions and preconceived notions that stand in the way of optimal mental health and development.

This challenge might take the form of social and political activism to help client groups learn how to overcome barriers and empower themselves (Lee, 1997c). For example, today's older people were raised in a time when helping services were available only to people with severe impairments, and thus they often attach a negative stigma to receiving such services (Myers, 1990). The elderly are more difficult to reach, for they may not be so likely to seek help when they are facing problems. They may be more skeptical about the effectiveness of counseling than are other populations, and it may take special efforts and more time to establish trust. A coordinated effort is needed to remove the stigma that older people have often associated with helping relationships and to stimulate community practitioners in designing appropriate programs for the elderly (Weikel, 1990).

Another example of an advocacy role that helpers might assume involves the civil rights of gay and lesbian clients. Dworkin and Gutierrez (1992) challenge mental health professionals to inform lawmakers and government administrators who determine public policy about the reality of the lesbian, gay, and bisexual population so that decisions will not be based on fears, misconceptions, and stereotypes. Dworkin and Gutierrez present some steps that helpers can take as agents of social change within the community and as advocates for the rights of lesbian, gay, and bisexual people:

- Helpers can demonstrate a spirit of activism by becoming involved with special interest groups of professional organizations that are designed to examine lesbian, gay, and bisexual issues.
- Practitioners can become activists on the local, state, and national levels. For example, school counselors can work with school boards to bring about in-service education and training pertaining to the needs of gay and lesbian youths.
- Mental health professionals can assist in the struggle for recognition of gay and lesbian couples and families by supporting bills that provide equality for them.
- Helpers can play a crucial role in advocating fairness in housing and employment, regardless of sexual orientation. An example might be assisting in the national movement to change the discriminatory policies of the military against gay and lesbian people.

Other groups also face discrimination, and helpers can exert their influence in changing discriminatory policies toward these special populations as well. Some of the special client populations who could benefit from activism on the part of the mental health professions are discussed in more detail in Chapter 12.

It is essential for helpers to demonstrate a willingness to deal with clients' economic survival needs from the outset. Too often practitioners ignore the fact that before people can be motivated toward growth and actualization their basic needs must be met. Mental health services can no longer be tailor-made for the upper middle class. People who are unable to afford the services of professionals in private practice are equally entitled to high-quality treatment programs. Consequently, the community approach is needed to serve people of all ages and backgrounds and with all types and degrees of problems. To be able to effectively serve various client populations, practitioners will need to develop culturally diverse competencies (Hogan-Garcia, 1999). Community workers may find themselves performing some or all of these duties:

- Helping to support the needs of minority groups in the community
- Assisting client groups to become true partners with professionals in the development and delivery of services
- Promoting community organization and development activities as fundamental agency responsibilities and seeing that this is reflected in agency budgets
- Actively reaching out to people with special needs and initiating prevention programs for drug and alcohol abuse, child sexual and physical abuse, and domestic violence
- Drawing on and improving the skills of community workers and laypeople to help meet the diverse needs of clients

- Developing strategies that will empower the disenfranchised in the community
- Consulting with a variety of social agencies about programs in gerontology, welfare, child care, and rehabilitation
- Evaluating human services programs for effectiveness
- Advocating and assisting with public and private initiatives that promote the total well-being of clients
- Working with members of a particular community to develop and build on community assets to promote communities and instill self-reliance

Homan (1999) admits that community workers may not be able to exert a major role in changing conditions for clients, but they can take specific actions that will help their clients. For example, helpers can assist clients in understanding the forces in the environment that are causing or contributing to their distress and help clients develop skills to confront these forces.

Influencing Policymakers

The need for community-based programs is compounded by such problems of our contemporary society as poverty, homelessness, crime, drive-by shootings, gang activities, AIDS, absent parents, divorce, domestic violence, child abuse, unemployment, tension and stress, alienation, addictions to drugs and alcohol, delinquency, and neglect of the elderly. These are just a few of the major challenges that communities need to address in preventing and treating human problems. One role that community helpers can assume is shaping social policy. Helpers need to work within the sociopolitical arena to instigate change. For instance, research into the prevention of AIDS has come about largely through lobbying efforts and political pressure.

It is critical that professional training programs prepare helpers to become competent advocates for at-risk individuals and groups and that they teach students the skills they will need to influence policymaking. If helpers are to be competent in these areas, they will need planning and consultation skills, and they will need to study organizational systems and community resources. They will also need to know (1) what affects policy at the state, local, or national level, (2) what laws or regulations can be applied to gain services for at-risk individuals, and (3) what processes are involved in bringing programs and services to at-risk clients (Hanson, Skager, & Mitchell, 1991).

Community workers can easily feel overwhelmed, and community agencies are often underfunded and understaffed. Without adequate funding, creative programs can only remain on the drawing board, and agencies often resort to crisis work and treat rather than prevent problems. Because helpers are frequently overworked and have many conflicting demands on their time, it may be difficult for them to do much work in the areas of education, influencing policymakers, outreach, and advocacy. However, helpers must find a way to legitimize the use of time for these activities.

Mobilizing Nonlicensed Helpers

How best to deliver services to the people who are most in need of them is a controversial question. Many in the mental health field have concluded that entry-level human services workers could be given the training and supervision they need to provide some psychological services. Formerly labeled paraprofessionals, these nonlicensed helpers have demonstrated a positive influence in the human service field, effectively carrying out roles and assuming responsibilities that were not anticipated (Woodside & McClam, 2002).

Nonlicensed workers have a variety of job titles, a few of which include community support worker, human services worker, social work assistant, alcohol or drug abuse counselor, mental health technician, child care worker, community outreach worker, and case manager (Woodside & McClam, 2002). Another example of nonlicensed workers include volunteers from the community who receive training and supervision in therapeutic intervention with a wide range of clients. These volunteers work on hot lines, co-lead groups, and engage in other supportive activities.

Former patients, who are in their own recovery from chemical dependency, now assume a helper's role in substance abuse programs mentoring others who are chemically dependent. Besides helping to alleviate the shortage of personnel, these nonlicensed practitioners may actually be more effective in reaching certain people because they have experienced similar problems and learned to deal with them successfully.

Service agencies have discovered that nonlicensed helpers can indeed provide some services as effectively as trained professionals—for much less cost. Tan (1997) asserts that nonlicensed helpers are able to provide support through fostering a sense of community and decreasing the isolation that many clients experience. He writes: "Paraprofessional helpers can make unique and significant contributions in treatment planning and implementation, and paraprofessionals and psychologists can work collaboratively to benefit their communities" (p. 371). Trull and Phares (2001) believe there is a vital role for nonlicensed helpers in the mental health field today and that they may be as effective as licensed professionals when performing some tasks.

Not all mental health professionals are enthusiastic about the increased use of nonlicensed workers. Some point to the danger that inadequately trained people might do more harm than good. Others contend that the poor will receive inferior service. Still others fear that more and more helpers will be allowed to practice without supervision and necessary training. Some fear that their own jobs or income may be jeopardized if nonlicensed helpers are allowed to provide services similar to those rendered by professionals.

The trend toward the increased use of nonlicensed workers means that licensed mental health professionals will have to assume new and expanding roles. Tan (1997) observes that mental health professionals can be expected to spend less time providing direct services to clients and more time teaching, supervising, and consulting with community workers. In-service workshops for entry-level human service workers and volunteer workers, educating the public about the nature of mental health, consulting, working as agents for change in the community, designing new programs, conducting research, and evaluating existing programs may all become part of the job for traditional mental health professionals.

Crisis Intervention in the Community

Crisis intervention work is one of the main models utilized in community agency work. You will learn methods of dealing with a variety of crisis situations in your supervised field placements, and chances are that you will have many opportunities to practice these skills. In writing about the development of the crisis intervention model, Kanel (1999) shows how this model is linked to community-based mental health programs. The community mental health movement emphasized prevention programs, and much of crisis intervention theory is based on interventions aimed at minimizing psychological impairment and promoting psychological health.

Although the Community Mental Health Centers Act of 1963 was originally intended to serve chronically mentally ill patients, community workers soon began seeing clients who were experiencing psychological problems that were typically dealt with in the private practices of therapists. Later, the Lanterman Petris Short bill of 1968 established more specific requirements for providing mental health services in the community, emphasizing short-term crisis intervention for people who were not chronically mentally ill. The short-term crisis intervention model is considered more cost effective than traditional forms of psychotherapy, which made crisis intervention a preferred approach by most health maintenance organizations (Kanel, 1999).

Think about some of the recent crisis situations you have read about in the daily newspaper or seen on television. Reflect on the direct impact that crises on the international, national, and state levels have had on the functioning of your community. Newspaper headlines reveal tragedies that generate multiple victims and affect entire communities. As disasters have escalated, helping professionals have had to develop quick and effective intervention strategies to deal with the disruption in the community (Modrak, 1992). When entire communities experience major disequilibrium, members of those communities need immediate and effective intervention to help them rally their resources. Modrak cites lessons that have been learned about the importance of being prepared to deal with tragedies. In some communities, crisis teams meet regularly to update information and work out procedures for responding. It is clear that those in the helping professions need to have the knowledge, skills, and training to provide immediate assessment, intervention, referral, and follow-up.

The Context of Crisis

Crisis intervention has been defined as "a helping process aimed at assisting a person or a family to survive an unsettling event so that the probability of debilitating effects (e.g., emotional scars, physical harm) is minimized, and the possibility of growth (e.g., new skills, new outlook on life, more options in living) is maximized" (Slaikeu, 1990, p. 6). The crisis model can be applied to working with the community as the "client" as well as working with individuals who are in crisis.

Crisis intervention is a short-term approach to helping that is the treatment of choice in cases where clients are experiencing a state of acute psychological disequilibrium. Individuals in crisis, or a community that is faced with a crisis, are temporarily disrupted cognitively, emotionally, and behaviorally, and they are in need of immediate and skilled help. This helping process should last as long as it typically takes people to bounce back to their pre-crisis level of functioning, which is generally up to 6 weeks.

Most clients who come to a community agency will be experiencing either a developmental or a situational crisis. A *developmental* crisis pertains to some expected difficulty at a particular stage of life. As you saw in Chapter 4, Erikson's developmental stages present opportunities for transformation and also represent a potential crisis. Some examples of developmental crises include the trauma of early childhood, getting married or divorced, the stresses of parenthood, coping with children's leaving home, finding meaning in life after retirement, and adjusting to the death of friends and family members. Events such as these do not necessarily lead to crises, for the person's interpretations and responses to these life transitions are the determining factors.

In crisis theory, the term *crisis* is not considered negative; rather, it is an essential ingredient in human growth and development. Crisis is a time in one's life for making choices. Situations do not merely happen to us. The stance we take toward life situations is what determines the quality of life. The word *crisis* is derived from the Greek word *krinein,* which means "to decide." The Chinese symbol for *crisis* represents both danger and opportunity. For example, being confronted by a serious illness can result in a reevaluation of one's priorities and a major change in the way one is living. How people respond to these critical turning points is what makes the difference. A utopian existence is not one without any crises, for crisis is an essential element in human development. The crises that we face at various phases of life are frequently catalysts that awaken us to the richer possibilities awaiting us if we have the courage to go through a transformation.

In addition to the expected developmental crises associated with the various stages of life, we also must endure unexpected events that can have the impact of paralyzing our will to act or can result in new directions for living once the crisis situation is over. Such *situational* crises can include sexual assault, discovery of a serious illness in oneself or a loved one, the breakup of an intimate relationship, a serious financial setback, or a natural disaster. As a helper employed in a community agency, you may be called on to counsel suicidal clients, deal with clients with posttraumatic stress disorders, help those with severe physical limitations, or offer strategies for those who abuse drugs and alcohol.

The Process of Crisis Intervention

There are two levels of crisis intervention. First-order intervention can be thought of as psychological first aid. This level of intervention is carried out by mental health professionals and a network of others such as ministers, judges, police and fire personnel, nurses, paramedics, physicians, school counselors, parole officers, teachers, and a wide range of human services workers. Second-order intervention, or crisis therapy, requires considerably more specialized training and expertise.

First-order intervention involves immediate assistance and often takes only one session. The major goal of this level of intervention is to reestablish an individual's immediate coping capacity. To accomplish this goal, helpers offer support, do what they can to reduce the chances of death, and link people in crisis to other helping resources. There are many settings where the staff must be equipped to handle a wide range of crises, such as the hospital emergency room or the crisis intervention hot line. Staff members and nonlicensed workers can be given training to respond quickly and effectively when they initially encounter people in crisis.

Helpers understand that the outcomes of a crisis can be for better or worse. As a result of a crisis, a person can return to an old level of coping, assume a new way of dealing with life, or ultimately decide on suicide. The task of helpers who offer psychological first aid is to help individuals tap any resources available to them to restore a sense of equilibrium, which will eventually enable them to work through their reactions so that they can meet future challenges.

Helpers create support through their attitudes and behaviors. Perhaps what helpers most have to offer is their gift of presence. This is the capacity "to be fully there" for individuals in crisis as they tell their story and seek human connection to guide them to some sense of stability amid the temporary chaos they are experiencing. In your initial encounter with a client in crisis, you can give the gift of presence partially by what you say but even more by a manner that reflects genuine caring and a deep sense of compassion. You may often feel helpless to change a tragic situation, and you could burden yourself with thoughts that what you are *doing* is not enough. Yet presence is powerful and often transcends what you can actually do to change the situation. Your willingness to be fully in contact with others as they strive to put their lives back together can be most healing and necessary.

It is important that your clients feel invited to tell their stories and also that you avoid assuming that you know exactly what they need or what is best for them. As they tell their stories, listen with as much understanding as possible. The real task is for you to encourage them to talk and for you to understand what they are going through from their perspective. Try to get a sense of where your clients want to go and what options for action they are open to. As clients express themselves, it is important that you also make an assessment of the immediate situation, especially of their coping resources.

Your primary task in crisis intervention is to ensure your clients' safety. Some clients may feel so distraught and so unable to cope with the crisis that they see suicide as their only way out. Suicidal urges may last for only a short time in the face of despair, and it is your job to intervene to prevent any deadly actions. People in crisis frequently provide clues to the depth of their despair. In making an assessment of the client's potential for taking lethal action, you must know the appropriate questions to ask as well as be aware of danger signs. Develop contracts with clients who pose a danger to themselves, and plan specific methods of follow-up after a session. Arranging for referrals is a very important part of this work. Ask yourself if you have enough knowledge and skill to assist your crisis clients. Know your limits and the resources within the community that can serve as a lifeline for those working through a crisis.

The first-order level of crisis intervention often entails a short-range plan of what to do next. People in crisis may overwhelm themselves with feeling that everything has to be attended to at once. You can help clients focus on what must be done now and what can wait until later. Clients often feel immobilized to the degree that they cannot see any options or have difficulty knowing which are the best options. You can calm them and help them identify a network of resources available to them, such as family, friends, and community.

Through the process of receiving psychological first aid, people often get the understanding, support, and guidance they need to avoid harm to themselves or others. At this level, one of your tasks is to help clients identify and examine possible routes they can later use to work through the crisis. This initial level of intervention does not resolve their crisis, for the effects of the crisis linger, and vestiges must be worked through. This is where second-order intervention, also known as *crisis therapy,* becomes necessary. This is a short-term therapeutic process that goes beyond immediate coping and aims at crisis resolution and change. The main goals of this level of intervention are to help people in crisis better face their future and to minimize the chances of their being a psychological casualty. It is critical that clients learn from the crisis and that they be given opportunities to work through unfinished business. Ideally, they will be given the assistance that will result in their remaining open to life and to new choices rather than closing themselves off to the vast range of future possibilities.

In crisis counseling, clients are encouraged to express and deal with feelings, some of which may have been locked up. It can be very freeing for clients to let go of trapped feelings, which can be converted into positive emotional energy that can be used constructively. Typically, the feelings that are denied expression (such as guilt or anger) are the ones that cause people grave difficulties. Venting pent-up feelings in itself often facilitates psychological healing.

Another task of second-order crisis intervention consists of helping clients attain a realistic perspective on the crisis event. There is a need to develop an understanding of how the event has affected them, including the meaning of the crisis in their lives. Clients typically must rebuild cognitions that have been damaged by the crisis. Part of the process of crisis therapy involves clients' learning how their thought patterns have resulted in certain behaviors. Clients are helped to cognitively reframe events, which allows for a new range of behavioral possibilities. As can be seen, this advanced phase of crisis work demands a great deal of expertise. Crisis therapy is provided by helping professionals who have specialized knowledge and skills.

How Crisis Work Can Affect the Helper

One young social worker we know did crisis intervention primarily with the family members of murder victims. Although she Ãÿowed concern and empathy for her clients, the nature of her work was "getting to her" to the extent that she was planning to change jobs. Like other crisis workers, she learned that burnout is an occupational hazard. According to Brown and O'Brien (1998), crisis intervention and other frontline mental health workers experience sources of stress that often lead to burnout. Some of these include lacking full involvement in the decision-making process related to work; feeling that their abilities are not being fully utilized on the job; being taxed by regulations, procedures, and paperwork; and being exposed to discomfort and dangers in their work setting. Sapienza and Bugental (2000) believe one of the main causes of burnout is the pressure of solving the problems that clients bring to therapy. Crisis workers often try to assume the responsibility of curing the client. This is a fundamental error in all approaches to helping, but it is particularly burdensome for crisis intervention workers.

Joining a group of peers who are also doing crisis intervention is one of the best ways of dealing with the emotions that surface as a result of crisis intervention. If you are carrying around excess psychological baggage, the crises of your clients can soon become your crises. It is absolutely essential that you retain your sensitivity to the ways in which this work is affecting you personally and that you pay attention to what is emerging within you. If you forget to take care of yourself or if you delude yourself into thinking that you don't have time for yourself, you can be certain that you will not be able to function very long in the demanding work of helping others through their crises. You will have become stuck in the quagmire of your own crisis.

By Way of Review

- The community perspective emphasizes social change rather than merely helping people adapt to their circumstances.

- It is not useful to focus on individual client treatment and neglect the institutional or social conditions that contribute to an individual's problems. A process that considers both the internal conflicts of the individual and the social factors within the community will provide a balanced perspective for helpers.

- It is essential that training programs prepare students to assume a proactive stance toward community intervention, especially with reference to early prevention approaches for at-risk groups in the community.

- A comprehensive community counseling program has four aspects. Direct client services that focus on outreach activities for at-risk groups in the community. Direct community services in the form of preventive education geared to the population at large. Indirect client services that consist of intervening actively for an individual or a group. And indirect community services that focus on influencing policymakers and bringing about positive changes within the community.

- Helpers need to assume an advocacy role for disenfranchised clients whose background makes it difficult for them to utilize professional assistance.

- Because helpers are frequently overworked and have many conflicting demands on their time, it may be difficult to do much work in the areas of education, influencing policymakers, outreach, and advocacy.

• You do not have to be all things to potential clients in the community. If you work in a community agency, you will most likely be part of a team working with individual clients.

• One way to meet the mental health needs in the community is to move toward a cooperative effort on the part of licensed mental health professionals and a variety of entry-level human service workers.

• Crisis intervention is one of the main modalities in community agencies. Many at-risk groups are in need of immediate and short-term help in working through both situational and developmental crises.

What Will You Do Now?

1. Select an at-risk population in your community. As a class project, you and several classmates can explore strategies for dealing with a particular client population by using a community approach. What can be done to awaken people in your community to the needs of the at-risk group that you have identified?

2. Spend some time thinking about how you might get involved in your community by doing some kind of volunteer work or selecting a field placement that will get you directly involved in community projects. Brainstorm possible ways of making even small changes in some facet of your community. How can you involve yourself in projects that are already under way or with fellow students who are doing some form of work in the community? Write ideas in your journal of how you can use your interests and talents in the service of others in your community.

3. Investigate the services available in your community for people in crisis. Look into what is offered in your own college or university. Ask about the crisis services provided by one of your community agencies. Inquire about what is being done by way of training volunteers for crisis intervention, such as working on a telephone hot line. You might consider doing volunteer work in your community as part of a crisis team. Ask about training programs and the possibility of serving as an "on-call" worker in times of special need.

4. For the full bibliographic entry for each of the sources listed here, consult the References and Reading List at the back of the book. Homan (1999) views the community as the client and offers the basic knowledge and skills needed to face the challenge of community change. For a treatment of multicultural social work practice with culturally diverse clients in family service centers, hospitals, and mental health centers, see Lum (1999, 2000). See Lewis, Lewis, Daniel, and D'Andrea (1998) for a comprehensive description of the community counseling perspective. For a variety of topics pertaining to community agency counseling, see MacCluskie and Ingersoll (2001). For a good overview of community psychology, with discussion of

community and social change, see Dalton, Elias, and Wandersman (2001). For an excellent resource outlining the theory and practice of crisis intervention, see James and Gilliland (2001); for a practical guide to crisis intervention techniques, see Kanel (1999); and for assessment in crisis intervention, see Myer (2001).

InfoTrac College Edition Resources

For additional readings, explore InfoTrac College Edition, our online library. Go to http://www.infotrac.college.com/wadsworth and select these key word searches:

community W1 outreach
prevention W2 education
client W1 advocacy
client W1 empowerment
community W1 counsel*
mental health paraprofessional
community mental health movement
crisis W1 intervention

Key words are listed in a form that enables the search engine to locate a wider range of articles in the online university library. Key words should be entered exactly as shown, including asterisks, "W1," "W2," "AND," and other search engine tools.

CHAPTER *12*

Understanding Special Populations

Focus Questions

1. AIDS continues to be an increasing problem in all our communities. What kind of education or action program is needed for a community? What role would you want to play in this endeavor?

2. What are some common themes with clients who seek counseling after receiving an antibody positive test result, and how can mental health professionals best work with HIV-positive clients?

3. What ethical, legal, and clinical dilemmas might you face in working with HIV-positive clients who question whether to tell others about their status?

4. Helpers who work with people with HIV/AIDS face a demanding set of challenges. If you choose to work with this population, what are some countertransference issues you might encounter? How might this work affect you personally? What might you do to prevent burnout?

5. How have you been involved with people with disabilities? How do you generally feel in their presence? What personal characteristics or experience do you have that might facilitate your work with this special population?

6. What are some societal stereotypes pertaining to people with disabilities? How might you work to change these beliefs in your community?

7. Have you been involved with older people? How do you generally feel in their presence? How do they generally respond to you? What personal characteristics could enable you to work effectively with the elderly?

8. What are some myths and stereotypes pertaining to the elderly? Can you think of some ways to go about correcting the negative perceptions of the elderly in your work setting?

Aim of the Chapter

In this chapter we focus on several special populations—people with HIV/AIDS, people with disabilities, and the elderly—as examples of target populations for which programs may be designed in your work setting. Regardless of the setting in which you work, you need to educate yourself about the characteristics of the client population and find ways to combine forces with other helpers and organizations so that you won't be a single voice in the wind as you attempt to bring about change within your agency. In the previous chapter on the community you saw how essential it is to work with individuals and groups in a manner that will increase their chances of becoming empowered rather than depending on you for answers to their concerns. This chapter is a continuation of the principles of the community chapter in that we focus on developing prevention programs in the community to address the needs of special populations. A key message of this chapter is the importance of seeking guidance from experts within your community who can provide special knowledge and make suggestions for how you can best serve various client groups.

AIDS: A Contemporary Crisis

Because the AIDS crisis shows no signs of easing, education to stop the spread of the disease is becoming a priority in many of the helping professions. We encourage you to think about your role and responsibility in dealing with the issues surrounding this crisis.

If you have not already done so, you will inevitably come in contact with people who have tested positive for HIV, people who have AIDS, people who have had sexual contact with someone who has tested HIV-positive, and people who are close to individuals with HIV or AIDS. You simply cannot afford to be unaware of the many issues that have emerged from the AIDS epidemic. You might be expected to offer direct services to clients with the disease or to provide indirect services in the community geared to education and prevention. You will not be able to educate those with whom you come in contact unless you are educated about the problem yourself. Keep yourself up to date on recent findings as they affect clinical practice. Although it is not realistic to expect that you will have in-depth knowledge of the range of problems confronting a community, you can have a general knowledge of these problems and familiarize yourself with resources valuable to people with specific needs. In working in a community you will probably be part of a team of human services professionals. Each member of the team will have different areas of expertise, and through interprofessional collaboration the combined strengths of practitioners can bring a diverse range of resources to a problem such as preventing HIV/AIDS.

We have decided to give prominence to this disease because of the ignorance and fear surrounding the AIDS crisis, both within the community and among members of the helping professions. Remember that there are conflicting reports and evidence about this disease. The changing nature of information about AIDS and misinformation about the ways in which the disease is spread result in apprehension and frustration among helping professionals. We encourage you to explore your own attitudes, values, and fears about working with people with AIDS-related concerns and how working with this client population might affect you personally.

Acquired immunodeficiency syndrome (AIDS) is the last stage of a disease caused by the *human immunodeficiency virus* (HIV), which attacks and weakens the body's natural immune system. Without a working immune system, the body gets infections and cancers that it would normally be able to fight off. By the time an individual develops AIDS, the virus has damaged the body's defenses (immune system). People who have AIDS are vulnerable to serious illnesses that would not be a threat to anyone whose immune system was functioning normally. These illnesses are referred to as "opportunistic" infections or diseases. AIDS weakens the body's immune system against invasive agents so that other diseases can prey on the body. Research suggests that the course of HIV infection is unpredictable. Some individuals progress to full-blown AIDS and die within several months. Others have no symptoms for as long as 10 years or more after being infected with HIV (Edlin, Golanty, & Brown, 2000).

At this point, those who carry the virus are likely to have it for the rest of their lives. Currently no drugs are available that will completely destroy HIV, although some drugs and vaccines are being developed with that goal in mind. Certain drugs are available that appear to retard the progress of the disease in some patients. Although optimism for treating HIV infections has increased, a cure for AIDS is still a remote hope (Edlin, Golanty, & Brown, 2000). Several experimental drugs have also shown potential efficacy in delaying the onset of AIDS. According to Edlin, Golanty, and Brown (2000), the majority of HIV-infected patients require powerful drugs to keep HIV in check and prevent progression to AIDS. The cost of these drugs is high, however, and may be beyond the reach of low-income clients. In this case, community resources need to be mobilized to bridge this gap.

Upon learning that they are HIV-positive, it is not uncommon for people to experience a range of painful emotional reactions from shock, to anger, to fear and anxiety, to grieving for the loss of sexual freedom, to alarm over the uncertain future. Some feel that they have been given a death sentence. Clients who seek counseling after they receive an HIV-positive test result often experience anxiety, depression, distress, hopelessness, numbness, and feeling like they are out of control. Typically these clients report feeling both overwhelmed and emotionally numbed. Seropositive clients (those with a positive HIV-test) must make many critical decisions in the context of uncertainty about medical prognosis, health care options, planning for the future, and disclosing their condition to others (Silven & Caldarola, 1993). These individuals will need to find a support system to help them cope with the troubled times that lie ahead.

It needs to be emphasized that HIV-positive individuals can live long and relatively symptom-free lives for many years. Many new medications are now available to treat the opportunistic infections that often kill people with AIDS. Today, much more is known about the disease than was the case when AIDS was first discovered.

HIV/AIDS already affects a wide population and will continue to be a major health problem. You simply cannot afford to be unaware of the personal and societal implications of this epidemic. Accurate information is vital if you are to deal with the personal and societal implications of the AIDS epidemic. You need to be able to differentiate between fact and fiction about the virus and about this disease.

The Helper's Role and Responsibility in the AIDS Crisis

The AIDS crisis has created anxiety among many medical personnel and helping professionals. Never before have helping professionals had concern that they would be infected with a fatal disease that their clients were carrying. This fear brings such helpers into a real conflict. Although they have dedicated their lives to helping those in need, helpers may find a variety of reasons to justify their unwillingness to help people afflicted with the HIV virus or AIDS-related problems.

Helpers will likely have to deal with their own countertransference issues in working with seropositive clients related to the high level of ambiguity surrounding HIV disease itself. If you have difficulty dealing with ambiguity, you might inhibit your client's freedom to recognize and cope with the uncertainty of the situation. These clients are likely to resist the painful awareness of the uncertainty of their situation and search for clear-cut and immediate answers. In turn, you need to monitor the pressure you might feel to produce quick solutions to very complex problems (Silven & Caldarola, 1993).

Much ignorance and fear of AIDS is fueled by conflicting reports. Misinformation about the ways in which the disease is spread results in apprehension among many people. Helping professionals may say "I don't know anything about this disease, and I'm not competent to deal with people who are affected by the problem." If you find yourself identifying with this statement and feeling somewhat overwhelmed, it is not necessary to remain this way. Today there is no reason to remain ignorant because you can get the basic information you need about this disease from current literature. You can also attend a workshop on AIDS or contact clinics all over the country for resources. You do not have to burden yourself with the demand that you are the only resource for your client. One very important aspect of being informed about HIV consists of knowing which people or organizations to refer clients to for further assistance.

In addition to this basic information about AIDS, it is imperative that you have skills in crisis intervention. Hoffman (1991a) maintains that offering services to individuals who are infected with the human immunodeficiency virus will challenge helpers to rethink typical therapy goals and instead develop a framework for utilizing strategies such as reducing stress, helping victims cope, promoting healthful behaviors, and promoting active change. She points out that helpers need to address a range of common issues with these clients, such as sexuality and sexual practices, drug practices, anticipatory grief, declining abilities in daily functioning, spirituality, death, and loss. Perhaps the major challenge is helping persons with AIDS come to terms with loss: "At its simplest, AIDS is about loss. It is about loss of one's health, vitality, sensuality, and career—and most profoundly, the letting go of the future as one had envisioned it" (Hoffman, 1991a, p. 468).

Both those who have tested positive and those who have contracted AIDS are typically in need of short-term help. They will surely need to find a system to support them through the troubled times that lie ahead. Not only can you be of support by listening to them and helping them deal with their immediate feelings, but you can assist them in finding a broader network. This may take the form of a support group at the agency where you work or a support system among friends and family members.

Some topics frequently shared and explored in an AIDS support group are the grief and loss process, assertiveness training, family issues, spirituality, medication and other health care concerns, nutrition and exercise, learning ways of being sexually safer, coping with homophobia and discrimination, and coping with depression. A group experience teaches people that they are not alone in their plight. For a description of how an AIDS support group can be initiated and maintained in the community, see Steven Lanzet's "One Counselor's Story: Starting an HIV/ AIDS Support Group," in M. Corey and G. Corey (2002).

Lanzet began AIDS support groups in his community by consulting with other health care professionals in the community. He worked with a nurse epidemiologist at the local health department who was administering HIV tests. To find out what help was available in his community, he called the National HIV and AIDS Hotline at 800-342-AIDS. He then looked for a suitable location to hold the group meetings and eventually decided to use the YMCA. He found the Gay Community Center to be a helpful resource in spreading the word about the group he was forming. Lanzet suggests that in a large community it is possible to create different groups to meet the specific needs of people at various stages such as those who are HIV-positive with symptoms, those with terminal-stage AIDS, those who have been newly diagnosed, and family and friends. Perhaps the key to success in a project like Lanzet's is to realize that relevant people and organizations within a community need to be contacted for their support. An individual practitioner who works in isolation will not have the rich range of resources that is available in many communities. It is the mobilization of these resources that can provide the team effort needed to launch and successfully implement any program in the community.

Special Needs of Clients with the AIDS Virus

The stigma of AIDS. Both those who have AIDS and those who discover that they have the virus within them struggle with the stigma attached to this disease. People who are HIV-positive live with the anxiety of wondering whether they will come down with this incurable disease. Most of them also struggle with the stigma attached to AIDS. They live in fear not only of developing a life-threatening disease but also of being discovered and thus being rejected by society in general and by significant persons in their life. Of course, those who develop AIDS must also deal with this stigma.

The stigma is attached to the fact that most of those in the United States who have contracted AIDS are either sexually active gay or bisexual men or present or past abusers of intravenous drugs. For some, the stigma may be worse than the diagnosis itself. Yet it is a mistake to identify the problem of AIDS with any particular group. AIDS has been called an "equal-opportunity disease," for it affects a wide segment of society. It is a myth that AIDS is a disease that is restricted to the gay male population. Indeed, in many parts of the world AIDS is spreading rapidly through the heterosexual population as well.

Many of the social fears felt by people with HIV or AIDS are realistic. Among the mainstream population, there is still a general negative reaction toward lesbians, gay men, and bisexuals. Educational programs must be directed at challenging and changing stereotypes, misconceptions, and negative attitudes toward these groups. Typically, people who develop AIDS are afflicted with a double-edged stigma, one due to their lifestyle and the other due to the disease, which is often seen as the result of their homosexual activities or drug behavior. People who learn that they are HIV-positive often stigmatize themselves and perpetuate beliefs such as "I feel guilty and ashamed," "I feel that God is punishing me," "I am a horrible person, and therefore I deserve to suffer," and "I am to blame for getting this disease."

AIDS patients' anger.   In addition to feeling different and stigmatized, those with AIDS typically have a great deal of anger. They often feel left alone and without support. This feeling is frequently grounded in reality. In some cases family members actually "disown the outcast." Patients often feel a sense of disillusionment, for after getting better for a time, they become sicker. They also feel isolated. For some, this isolation is expressed through their feeling of utter rejection by others: "I'm gay, and now I've got AIDS. No one wants anything to do with me." "I'm a drug user, and I engage in criminal and deviant behavior." It is hard for them to see any meaning in their plight, and thus they often slip into depression. Consequently, they develop anger at having a life-threatening condition. They express this anger by asking over and over: "What did I do to deserve this? Why me?" This anger is sometimes directed at God for letting it happen, and then they may feel guilty for having reacted this way. Anger is also directed toward others, especially those who are likely to have given them the virus. Anger is aimed at health professionals as well. Patients are angry because their lives have been unalterably changed.

If you expect to provide help to HIV-positive individuals, people with AIDS, and their loved ones, it is critical that you confront any biases and misconceptions you may have. If you have negative views toward people with the virus, the chances are slim that you will be able to work effectively with this population. It is essential for you to carefully examine your own attitudes and assumptions about homosexuality, IV drug use, and death and dying, so that you will not form an unconscious collusion with clients about any self-ridicule they may have about any of these issues. You are called upon to monitor your own attitudes and anxieties about HIV/AIDS so that both you and your client might have an opportunity to develop an enhanced sense of purpose and meaning within a crisis situation. Even though the crisis brings about emotional turmoil, it can be the catalyst for making significant positive life changes. Some clients will make the decision to get involved in therapy, which can transform the crisis into a profoundly life-enhancing experience (Silven & Caldarola, 1993).

How You Are Affected as a Helper

In our earlier discussion on AIDS, we mentioned that one helper, Steven Lanzet, organized and led AIDS support groups in his community. In writing about how his work affected him personally, he indicated that dealing with the crises of others had led to a sense of burnout tapping on his shoulder. He learned how to take care of himself by reducing the frequency of the groups he led and by taking periodic breaks from facilitating groups. He dealt with his personal reactions to his work by joining a support group with fellow counselors (see M. Corey & Corey, 2002). If you are involved in providing help and support for people who have developed AIDS, many of these clients will be dying, which will certainly have an impact on you. Reflect on the following questions:

- Your clients may well displace some of their anger onto you. How do you think you will handle such anger?
- Your clients will probably be affected by relationship issues and shifts in roles. How will they adapt to these changes? How might you be affected by their struggles to adapt?
- How do you prepare yourself as a helper to respond to questions such as "Why did this happen to me?"
- How might the hopelessness that your clients feel affect you? Could their despair lead you to feel that your work with them was futile?
- As your clients bring up unfinished business with key people in their lives, how might it affect you?
- What specific values and biases might you hold that could make it difficult for you to be objective in working with people who have AIDS? Are you open to examining and changing these attitudes?
- Your clients are likely to bring up the issue of meaning in their lives now that they are unable to do many of the things that gave their life meaning. How might their crisis in discovering meaning have an impact on you?
- Many times these clients will say: "I simply can't see any point in living anymore. I can't do anything. All I have to look forward to is suffering." What would you have to offer them?
- If clients bring up their fears of dying or what lies beyond death, do you see yourself as able to assist them in giving expression to their fears? Will their fears trigger your own fears?
- How do you think losing relatively young AIDS patients is likely to affect you?
- In working with clients who are at risk for contracting AIDS, you cannot avoid talking about sexually explicit topics. Do you feel able to discuss such topics?
- If you do a good deal of work with AIDS patients and their family members, what concerns do you have about burnout? How will you work to prevent it? Are you willing to ask for support from others as you work with this difficult population? Do you have a support group?

- Assume that you are working with people who had tested HIV-positive or who have AIDS and were confronted with the question "How can you possibly understand what I am going through; you haven't walked in my shoes?" How would you respond?

The Helper's Role in Educating the Community

Regardless of what type of helper you happen to be, one of your most important functions is to dispel myths and misconceptions about HIV/AIDS and to help the community acquire realistic knowledge and attitudes. As we have mentioned, to be able to carry out this function effectively, you need to differentiate between fact and fiction about this disease.

Education of various target groups is the key in preventing sharp rises in the number of people with HIV/AIDS. To educate various segments of the community, you will need to know your community and be aware of the values, mores, and cultural backgrounds of the various groups you serve. In attempting to change the habits of racial, cultural, and religious groups, you are likely to run up against considerable resistance unless you are able to "speak their language." Furthermore, in educating members of the community, it is important to realize that HIV/AIDS patients can easily become the scapegoats of people's projections of their unconscious fears and hatred. People who are highly intolerant of those who are different from them often engage in denial and seek a target for their resentments. Any educational program must be directed toward minimizing denial and homophobia. This also involves education of HIV-positive clients themselves. For the gay man, learning of his antibody status may trigger internalized homophobia whereby he blames his being infected on his homosexuality (Silven & Caldarola, 1993).

Because information is changing rapidly, it is difficult for people who are at risk to trust what they hear from the medical profession. They may be defensive about further education because they don't believe what is presented to them. They may also remain in a state of denial because they do not want to change their sexual behavior. Education is only one step in the change process, and information alone is not sufficient to bring about change. Behavior change is not easy, especially when dealing with highly personal behaviors such as sexuality. These difficulties will challenge you to find a meaningful way to provide education. A few key elements of the educational effort are listed here:

- As a helper, explore your own attitudes, and work assiduously at challenging and eliminating those beliefs that make it difficult for you to make contact with those who need your help.
- Take steps to understand HIV/AIDS yourself. Learn updated information on both the medical and the psychological aspects of the disease.
- Emphasize prevention. A comprehensive sex education program, for all age groups, is essential if HIV/AIDS is to be prevented.
- Although HIV/AIDS has created a tremendous amount of fear for most people, it can be reassuring to know that it is unprotected sex that can lead to HIV infection, not any and all sexual experiences.

- Rather than thinking in terms of "safe sex," consider practices that are "unsafe," "relatively save," and "safer." If people are going to be sexually active, they will not be safe, and they need to recognize the risks of infection. "Safer" behavior includes choosing not to be sexually active; restricting sex to one mutually faithful, uninfected partner; and not injecting drugs. Whether or not they are infected with the virus, clients should be informed and encouraged to adopt safer sex practices to reduce risks.
- Effective and consistent use of latex condoms and spermicidal barriers will reduce the possibility of transmitting the virus, but they are not one hundred percent effective in preventing HIV. It is essential that latex condoms be used correctly from start to finish with each act of intercourse. When condoms are used reliably, they provide a high degree of protection against a variety of sexually transmitted diseases, including HIV infection.
- Seek training in crisis intervention in the issues facing HIV-positive individuals and people with AIDS.
- Community efforts need to be made to care for people with AIDS. Part of your job as a helper could be to mobilize people in the community to become active and to serve in various capacities as volunteers.

In developing educational programs, keep in mind the special needs of minority groups. Many minorities are not responsive to education as it is typically presented. Alternatives to the usual means of education might include training ministers to work with their congregations, using a spokesperson or a role model to whom young people can relate, creating videos with educational goals, and using HIV-positive individuals and persons with AIDS as resources to teach others about the disease.

Advances in medical technology, birth control, and artificial reproduction methods allow for an increased range of sexual choices. At the same time, AIDS and other sexually transmitted diseases make the consequences of sexual choices more serious than at any time before. Human services professionals have an ethical responsibility to help their clients identify and explore any sexual issues that are relevant to their lifestyle or to refer clients to helpers who are prepared to address sexual concerns. Helpers will not be able to carry out this responsibility if they are lacking in knowledge about human sexuality. If helpers are uncomfortable dealing with sexual matters with their clients, the helping relationship may be sabotaged.

Case Example of AIDS Education

You are working in a community mental health agency, and the director asks you and several of your colleagues to design a comprehensive education program to promote awareness of AIDS in the community. The director tells you that her goal is to do everything possible to prevent people from contracting AIDS and that she would like members of the community to develop a realistic understanding of the issues involved in this major health problem. She wants people to have detailed information about AIDS and would like to see them discuss the issue at community meetings in the center. Once you and your colleagues have written up a proposal, she wants your group to make a presentation to the board members of the agency, who represent a range from very conservative to very liberal.

Your group works diligently and comes up with a comprehensive program. Your proposal calls for focusing on the schools from elementary to community college. Your group is suggesting workshops and short courses to be conducted by community workers and health care providers. Although your program involves a frank and comprehensive discussion of all major issues pertaining to AIDS, it also calls for dealing with the topic in a manner that is sensitive to the community and that is appropriate for the target groups. The key features of your proposed workshops include the following: information on the state of the disease, identification of who is at risk, psychosocial dimensions of the disease, attitudes toward those who have contracted AIDS, ethical and legal issues, medical facts and concerns, prevention of AIDS, and implications for the future. You intend to have AIDS patients talk to classes at the schools, along with physicians and other professionals with knowledge about this disease. Your program will also focus on teaching specific methods of "safer sex" and encouraging these practices.

After your group finishes presenting its findings to the board of directors, several members loudly and passionately protest on the grounds that your group is promoting immorality and interfering with their rights as parents. They don't want schools to encourage their children to practice "safer sex" when in their home they are teaching them how to live morally decent lives. They attempt to convince you that AIDS is a natural consequence of rampant immorality that has been spreading throughout the country.

On the basis of your values, what arguments might you give these board members? How would you answer their opposition? Would you be willing to omit the more controversial aspects of your program? Would you be willing to make room in your program for advocates of abstaining from sexual relationships outside of marriage? Would you be willing to give equal time to representatives who opposed your point of view? Your values will certainly enter into the picture as you develop your views toward your responsibilities in dealing with the AIDS crisis.

Understanding People With Disabilities

People with disabilities have to face prejudice, hostility, lack of understanding, and discrimination on the basis of their physical, emotional, or mental handicap. Nondisabled individuals frequently view this group through the same distorted spectacles with which they see others who differ from them. The clarity of a helper's vision can be impaired by myths, misconceptions, prejudices, and stereotypes about people with disabilities.

Our discussion focuses on recognizing the potential of people with disabilities. Helpers' attitudes are a key factor in successfully intervening in the lives of people with disabilities, and some guidelines are given for better serving this diverse group. Dispelling myths and misconceptions and helping people with disabilities achieve their goals can be highly rewarding.

Challenging Stereotypes

People with physical disabilities do not want to be labeled in a general way as "handicapped." Individuals with disabilities may be physically challenged in some way, but these disabilities can often be overcome. Some paraplegics are concerned that others may view them as being paralyzed from the neck up as well as from the waist down. Nonhandicapped individuals often try to hide their feelings of awkwardness in the presence of a person with a disability through exaggerated attention and kindness. It is essential for helpers to demonstrate a willingness to examine their own attitudes when they are working with people who have any kind of disability. Helpers need to avoid categorizing individuals as all being the same, even though they have some common concerns due to their disability (Vacc & Clifford, 1988).

As with any special population with which you work, it is important that you identify your assumptions pertaining to people with disabilities. For example, you could assume that certain careers might be out of reach for a client with a disability. But to make this assumption without checking it out with your client is tantamount to limiting his or her options. This would be a good time for you to reflect on any stereotypes that you may have toward this group and to challenge your assumptions. A few examples of myths and misconceptions associated with this special population are:

- If you are physically disabled, you are also mentally and emotionally disabled.
- People with disabilities do not have the same feelings as the nondisabled.
- Individuals with a disability have a limited capacity to be normal.
- People with disabilities are totally dependent on others.
- They are disabled as people, and their goals should be modest.

In addition to these misconceptions, common societal stereotypes that human service practitioners may bring to their work with persons with disabilities include perceiving persons with disabilities as objects of pity, as menaces to society, as sick, as incompetent, as curses from God, as tests from God, and as freaks (Mackelprang & Salsgiver, 1999):

> Stereotypical attitudes are pervasive in society, and human service professionals are as susceptible to them as anyone. Close monitoring of personal reactions to people with disabilities can help professionals identify and deal with their personal attitudes based on stereotypical beliefs. (p. 9)

As a helper, you need to be aware of these societal stereotypes so you are better able to challenge these misconceptions and come to view people with disabilities as unique individuals.

A major role of practitioners who work with people with disabilities is to help these clients to understand the prejudice and discrimination that surrounds disability. If helpers lack insight into their own preconceived notions and stereotypes regarding disability, they will not be able to assist their clients who have a disability to understand the impact that societal stereotypes have on their view of themselves (Mackelprang & Slasgiver, 1999).

Pushing Through Perceived Limitations

If you work with people with disabilities, it is essential that you develop attitudes and intervention skills that will enable your clients to recognize the strengths and resources they possess. As a helper, you may encounter clients who have been disabled from birth, adolescents recently disabled due to traumatic injury (perhaps a sports injury or an automobile accident), adults who have had a stroke or heart disease and have suffered rapid onset disabilities that may or may not be permanent, or adults who have been diagnosed with a chronic degenerative condition such as Parkinson's disease or diabetes.

The kinds of help these individuals need may encompass a broad range of services. Some clients may need help finding community resources to enable them to participate fully in the workforce. Others may need counseling to overcome the shock and depression often present when it looks like all of life has been turned on its head in a moment. Some clients can be encouraged to pursue their former fitness levels through rehabilitation and counseling. And finally, some clients will need your help to accept and plan for a life with gradual but increasing challenges in the performance of daily living tasks. Persons with disabilities come in all guises; do not be too quick to judge these clients or their needs based on your first meetings with them.

Some guidelines for practice with persons with disabilities are provided by Mackelprang and Salsgiver (1999):

- Operate on the assumption that people are capable or potentially capable.
- Critically evaluate the assumption that the problem with disability lies with the person and that individuals with disabilities must be changed before they can function adequately in society.
- Recognize that people with disabilities often face discrimination and oppression, as do other minority groups. Realize that your interventions might well involve political advocacy and actions on your part to eliminate policy barriers that prevent individuals from accessing society's benefits.
- Develop interventions that are based on the assumption that persons with disabilities have the right to control their own lives.

Reflect on these basic assumptions and principles as you strive to formulate your own guidelines for effective practice with people with disabilities.

Real Examples That Challenge Our Perceptions

I (Marianne) gave a talk to people with disabilities at a residential facility. The kinds of questions they raised were not any different from those of other groups that I have addressed, and many of the residents emphasized that they were no different from people without disabilities. Later, I asked a staff member at this institution to ask a few residents this question: "What would you like to tell helpers in training about yourself to assist them in better dealing with special populations?" Some of the residents gave these responses:

- "I would like them to know that I want to be treated as a normal person even though I am in a wheelchair. Look at the person, not at the wheelchair. Don't be afraid of us."
- "I'm a very good person. I'm a very smart person. I have a disability, but I also have intelligence."
- "I can think and feel just like a normal person."

The staff member said a great deal in very few words in a letter to me about her perceptions of the people she helps:

> They have lived in institutions for most of their adult lives. They say they are no different from people without disabilities, but I think that they have enormous hearts. The people I have known have no prejudice and are very loving and giving. They also have a greater appreciation for the very simple things in life that most of us take for granted each day. They are unique individuals and I feel fortunate to have worked with them.

Societal attitudes are slowly changing as well-known individuals demonstrate a basic truth—having a disability does not mean that the person is disabled. One example is Christopher Reeves, a silver screen hero who has become a real-life hero, showing us that determination can go a long way in pushing one's limits. Although Reeves suffered a major neck and spinal cord injury, he continues his slow process of recovery and teaches us that hope can lead to a meaningful life.

In *Touch the Top of the World* (2001), Erik Weihenmayer—born with a degenerative eye disorder that resulted in losing his sight by age 13—chronicles a life of determination that led to accomplishing incredible physical feats. Weihenmayer is a world-class athlete, acrobatic skydiver, long-distance biker, marathon runner, skier, mountaineer, ice climber, and rock climber. He was the first blind man to gain the summit of Mt. McKinley and to scale the 3,300 foot rock wall of El Capitan. In the spring of 2001 he earned the distinction of being the first blind person to climb above 29,000 feet to reach the summit of Mount Everest. So far he has climbed five of the seven highest mountains in the world, and his goal is to reach all seven summits on each of the seven continents. Weihenmayer is living proof that physical disabilities do not necessarily limit a person's ability to reach his dreams. His story and the stories of others, though less dramatic, demonstrate that misconceptions regarding disabilities can be challenged. Weihenmayer's accomplishments give new meaning to the term "physically challenged."

Most of us are familiar with the Special Olympics, in which people with physical disabilities compete at the highest levels. Indeed, many people who are not so well known are challenging themselves to reach phenomenal goals in their daily lives. Such individuals continue to teach us about ourselves and the capacity of the human spirit to overcome any obstacle.

What about clients who have a disability but who lack hope and want to give up? If helpers accept their hopelessness and despair, they will be of little therapeutic value to these individuals. Human service professionals need to discover their clients' strengths and work toward empowerment. Consider these words from Judy Heumann, Assistant Secretary for the Office of Special Education and Rehabilitation Services, Washington, D.C. (cited in Mackelprang & Salsgiver, 1999):

If you [professionals] don't believe that disabled people can achieve, get out of the way. They [the professionals] need to learn as much as they can to help assure that disabled people are given the tools we need in order to move ahead in our lives. Professionals who work with kids need to give their parents positive images of their children's abilities and possibilities. They should not limit people's thinking; they should help expand people's horizons. They need to understand the implications of discrimination and bias in order to allow people to remedy those problems. They need to be part of the solution, not part of the problem. (p. 241)

Helpers who hope to make a difference with clients with disabilities need to acquire the attitudes and beliefs illustrated by Judy Heumann. Operate from a diversity-affirming approach and be willing to adopt a variety of professional roles, some of which include counselor, teacher, broker, and political activist or advocate (Mackelprang & Salsgiver, 1999).

Understanding the Special Needs of the Elderly

The way you approach aging has a great deal to do with how you will treat older people. Rather than focusing on old age as being exclusively a time of loss, you can see it as a time of both positive and negative transformations. Be open to what older people can teach you, even if you are in the role of helping them. Elderly people have a vast wealth of life experiences and coping skills, which they are likely to share with you if they sense that you have a genuine interest in them. They can draw on their experiences as they are deciding on ways to respond to the circumstances of later life.

The elderly have special needs and problems that cannot be ignored by helping professionals who have the role of assisting elderly people in finding meaning in their lives after retirement. As helpers become involved with the elderly, their challenge is to do more than add years to an individual's life—they are called to assist individuals in leading richer and more productive lives.

Key Themes in the Lives of the Elderly

Working with the elderly demands an awareness of the particular life issues they face. Prevalent themes for people during late adulthood include loss; adjusting to decreased physical and sensory capacities; loneliness and social isolation; feelings of rejection; the struggle to find meaning in life; dependency; feelings of uselessness, hopelessness, and despair; fears of death and dying; grief over others' deaths; and regrets over past events. Today, many of these themes characterize people in their mid-80s more than people in their 60s and even 70s.

In many countries, those age 75 and older are the fastest growing portion of the population. America is aging, yet it is just one of the many countries whose populations are growing older. As is the case for earlier developmental stages, there is a great deal of individual variance at this final stage of life. Many 70-year-old people have the energy of middle-aged people. How people look and feel during late adulthood is more than a matter of physical age; it is largely a matter of attitude. To a great degree, vitality is influenced more by a state of mind than by chronological years lived.

A basic task of late adulthood is to complete a life review in which we put our life into perspective and come to accept who we are and what we have done. This is a time for both consolidation of experiences and resources and a reorientation toward one's later years. This is also a time in life when spirituality may take on a new meaning and provide us with a sense of purpose, even as we face a growing dependence on others (McGoldrick & Carter, 1999).

Old age does not have to be something we look toward with horror or resignation; nor must it be associated with bitterness. However, many elderly people in our society do feel resentment, because we have generally neglected this population, treating them as an undesirable minority that is merely tolerated. Their loss is doubly sad, because the elderly can make definite contributions to society.

Elderly people have a wealth of life experiences and coping skills, and they are likely to share this wisdom if they sense that others have a genuine interest in them. Many elderly persons are still very capable, yet the prejudice of younger adults often keeps us from acknowledging the value of the contributions the elderly offer us. Perhaps because we are afraid of aging and confronting our own mortality, we "put away" the elderly so they won't remind us of our future.

Challenging Myths and Stereotypes

If you are working with the elderly, one of your first tasks is to debunk some of the myths and negative perceptions about the elderly that you may have incorporated, either consciously or unconsciously. If you accept the many misconceptions about older people, there is little chance that your behavior with them will be helpful. Not only do you need to explore your own beliefs about the elderly, but it would be well to think of ways in which you could educate the community about the aging process. It is also important in your work with the elderly to find ways of helping them question any self-limiting beliefs they may have accepted from society. Here are some stereotypes associated with older people that need to be challenged:

- All elderly people eventually become senile.
- Old people are nonproductive and cannot contribute to society.
- Most older people are depressed.
- Growing old always entails having a host of serious physical and emotional problems.
- Older people are set in their ways, are stuck in rigid patterns of thinking and behaving, and are not open to change.
- Retirement is the next step before death.
- Old people are not creative.

- When people grow old, they are no longer capable of learning.
- Old people are no longer beautiful.
- Most elderly people are lonely.
- Old people are no longer interested in sex.
- Most older people live in institutional settings.

These negative perceptions and stereotypes of older people are common in our society. According to Myers (1990), those in the mental health professions are not exempt from such stereotypical thinking about the elderly, which discourages many helpers from working with older clients. Myers describes the interaction of negative societal perceptions and the psychological functioning of older people within the framework of the *social-breakdown syndrome.* This model holds that as people age they become more vulnerable to perceptions and definitions of themselves by society. The social-breakdown syndrome involves a downward spiral in which older people increasingly internalize myths and negative perceptions, resulting in a view of themselves as incapable of experiencing a rich life. This self-perception leads to decreased attempts to control their environment. As they appear to have less control, negative input from society reinforces their shaky perceptions of self, and the downward spiral continues. Although during most of their adult years people may have had an internal locus of control, they may shift to an external locus when they are faced with crises of later life that they feel powerless to control.

Guidelines for Effectively Reaching Older People

We do not think that there is one kind of person, one set of personal characteristics, or one style of helping that makes for effective involvement with older people. But effective helping of the elderly demands a knowledge of their special needs and the ability to form working relationships with them. Let's examine some ways you can increase your capacity for understanding and working with older people.

Young people sometimes put older people in a very different category from themselves. In reality, there are more similarities than differences between older and younger people. Both age groups have a need for support and challenge, respect, understanding, and acceptance. A way to treat elderly people is to consider them as having the same feelings, wishes, and thoughts as many younger people.

Elderly clients can activate the helper's recollections of parents and grandparents. At times, helpers avoid dealing with the elderly because of the stark reminders of their own inevitable aging and death. If helpers are unaware of the reactions that are being stimulated within them as they work with elderly clients, their efforts at helping will be thwarted.

Realize that there is a continuity in life patterns, and help clients discern these themes. Individuals who are chronically unhappy in their youth also stand a good chance of remaining unhappy as they age, unless they make a decision to do something to change certain patterns.

Older people often have youthful feelings and wish they had a youthful body. Treat them as though they were young. Don't treat them as pitiable old people, and don't become overly focused on age. Believe in their capabilities rather than dwelling on their limitations.

Babies have a need to be held; adolescents have a need to be let go of; older people have a need to be seen and heard. Typically, elderly people need to reminisce and reflect, and they need to be listened to and understood. Through talking and being heard, they are able to put facets of their lives into perspective. If you demonstrate a genuine interest in them, they will reveal a great deal of themselves through their stories. You can show respect by being patient and by accepting them through hearing their underlying messages.

Don't get caught up in listening only to the content of what the elderly reveal, but listen for the deeper messages that they often convey nonverbally. Let them know how you are being affected as you listen to them.

As a way of establishing rapport, remember that kindness goes a long way in building bonds. Touch is a meaningful way of contacting elderly people. A touch on the arm or shoulder can signify warmth. Although hugging and touching may be meaningful, this contact should be used only when it is deemed acceptable by the older person. In touching it is absolutely critical to be real. Do not use touching as a technique but only as an extension of concern you are feeling.

Many elderly people suffer from confusion and forgetfulness. Strive to be patient, because their symptoms tend to worsen if you are impatient with them. They are probably frustrated with themselves over their symptoms. They have a need for self-pride, which is difficult to maintain as they face being dependent.

Be open to understanding the ways in which older clients' cultural backgrounds continue to influence their present attitudes and behaviors.

Your personal characteristics will influence the quality of your contact with elderly clients. Some of the qualities that are essential to cultivate are humor, a sense of playfulness, enthusiasm, patience, respect, caring, courage, endurance, hopefulness, tolerance, nondefensiveness, freedom from prejudices, and a willingness to learn. Your gift of presence and the understanding that flows from this presence can be powerful ways to make connections with the elderly. It is essential that you have an ability to be both gentle and challenging. It requires sensitivity to know when it is therapeutic to provide support and when to challenge.

Not everyone can work effectively with the elderly. However, before you conclude "I could never work with old people," test your assumptions and any conclusions that you might have made. Just because you may be uncomfortable in relating to older people does not mean that you cannot change. You do not have to be elderly to appreciate the difficulties of this time of life. Through your active caring, you can build a bridge between yourself and those who are considerably older. If you are open to your own feelings—over painful events, experiences of sadness, times of uncertainty, hopes and fears, and times of loneliness—these feelings can be your best tools in touching people who are older than you. As an adolescent you might well have struggled with finding meaning in your life. You might have felt stifled by your limited control at this time of your life. Many elderly people are also stifled in their attempts to realize their full potential, and they often struggle with finding meaning in the face of many losses. You can use your experiences as an adolescent to get a better sense of the nature of an elderly person's world. It is not necessary to share identical experiences with your clients but, rather, to find a way to tap into similar feelings over different life experiences. What is important is that you do what you can to learn about the worldview of clients who are different from you and at the same time use your universal life themes as a way of building bridges between you and those who differ from you.

How to Work With Other Special Populations

We encourage you to think about other neglected or unpopular client groups within your community and to apply our discussion about people with disabilities, elderly people, and people with AIDS to them. Keep in mind the importance of being willing to pay attention to similar feelings you are experiencing with your clients, even if you have not experienced their same problems. This principle is true not only in working with older people and those with disabilities but also in relating to individuals in other special client groups who are likely to differ from you in a number of significant respects.

Learn to work with the community as well as for the community. Any program that you design must incorporate ways of reaching out to the target population as well as ways for potential clients to gain access to your services. How might you develop educational programs in your community to provide services to these client groups? Realize that education is only a first step and that educational efforts must be directed toward action programs that will bring about community improvement. How might you mobilize the community to take action that will improve the plight of certain at-risk groups? It is essential to identify the principles relevant for community action that we developed in the section on AIDS. Regardless of the client population, these questions illustrate principles that you can apply in understanding and working with any target group:

- What specific populations in your community are most in need of help? What kind of help do they need?
- To what degree do you understand the special needs of these target groups? What resources and capabilities of the community can be brought to bear on resolving the plight of a target group?
- What are your assumptions and attitudes toward this target group? What possible prejudices, biases, and stereotypes might you harbor toward this group?
- Identify some of your fears or concerns in working with a client group. How will you deal with your own fears?
- How might you deal with the strong reactions of those within the community who may be shocked that you are working with such unpopular client populations?
- In what ways might society stigmatize at-risk groups such as the homeless? substance abusers? veterans? children from alcoholic families? the unemployed?
- In what ways might individuals within certain groups continue to stigmatize themselves?
- As a helper, how can you remove stigmas that block effective programs?

By Way of Review

- The AIDS crisis challenges professional helpers to acquire basic information about the disease and also to develop strategies for helping those who are infected. Your attitudes, assumptions, and values will influence your stance toward AIDS education and counseling.

- AIDS has been called an "equal-opportunity disease," for it affects a wide segment of society. To educate various segments of the community, you will need to know your community and be aware of the values, mores, and cultural backgrounds of the various groups you serve.

- There is much ignorance and fear of AIDS, fueled by conflicting reports. Misinformation about the ways in which the disease is spread results in apprehension among many people.

- Regardless of what type of helper you happen to be, one of your most important functions is to dispel myths and misconceptions about special populations, such as people with HIV/AIDS, people with disabilities, and older people. Help the community acquire realistic knowledge and attitudes about these special populations.

- As a helper it is essential that you demonstrate a willingness to examine your own attitudes when you are working with people who have any kind of disability.

- Many individuals with disabilities achieve extraordinary success; keep your focus on clients' potential rather than their perceived limitations.

- As you become involved with the elderly, your challenge is to do more than add years to an individual's life—you are called upon to encourage individuals to lead richer and more productive lives.

- Your personal characteristics will influence the quality of your contact with elderly clients. Confront your own feelings about aging and evaluate your assumptions about the limits of the elderly.

What Will You Do Now?

1. As a way to educate yourself about HIV/AIDS, obtain more information by contacting your state or local health department, your local chapter of the American Red Cross, and the Public Health Service's toll-free HIV and AIDS hot line (1-800-342-AIDS). This national hot line is for anyone with questions about HIV and AIDS, and it functions 24 hours a day in every state. These information specialists are well trained, respect privacy, and can provide referrals to appropriate sources.

The National AIDS Clearinghouse (1-800-458-5231) also provides information on HIV/AIDS. Updated pamphlets can also be requested by contacting either of these hot lines. Additional sources of information on HIV/AIDS and other STDs include these agencies:

- HIV/AIDS Treatment Information Service 1-800-HIV-0440
- National Gay and Lesbian Task Force AIDS Information Line 1-800-221-7044
- AIDS National Interfaith Network 202-546-0807
- Public Health Service AIDS Hotline 1-800-342-AIDS
- National Institute on Drug Abuse Hotline 1-800-662-HELP
- National Sexually Transmitted Diseases Hotline 1-800-227-8922
- Centers for Disease Control and Prevention 404-639-3534
- American Red Cross 1-800-375-2040
- World Health Organization 202-861-4354

As a class project, you and several classmates can make a brief presentation in class about the various facets of AIDS and what can be done to mobilize community action to prevent the spread of the disease.

2. Imagine that you are doing an intake interview with a man who has just found out that he tested HIV-positive. He is seeking counseling to deal with his high anxiety over fears of death and is in a crisis state. What might you feel? What might you say to this individual? How well prepared are you to listen to this man and help him through this crisis? If you do not feel adequately prepared to take this person as a client, consider going to an AIDS center and asking for information. Talk with someone about this disease, especially its social and psychological aspects. Find ways to challenge any of your biases, misconceptions, assumptions, and values that could render you ineffective in helping HIV-positive individuals who are in crisis.

3. Helpers are likely to encounter clients with a variety of disabilities. Some broad types of disabilities include mobility disabilities, visual disabilities, deafness, developmental disabilities, psychiatric disabilities, and cognitive disabilities. In groups of three or four, select a broad category and research the kinds of help available in your community for persons with this disability. What additional services would benefit this special population? Present your findings in class.

4. If you are interested in working with the elderly, it would be valuable to become involved not only with older people but also with their families. Consider taking any of these steps to better prepare yourself to work with the elderly:

- Take courses and special workshops dealing with the problems of the aged.
- Get involved in fieldwork and internship experiences with the elderly.
- Investigate institutes and conferences that provide training for helpers who work with the elderly.
- Explore your feelings toward your own aging and toward the older people in your life.

5. For the full bibliographic entry for each of the sources listed here, consult the References and Reading List at the back of the book. Three of the most useful books about the counseling aspects of HIV/AIDS are Dilley and Marks (1998), Dilley, Pies, and Helquist (1993), and Kain (1996). For information on working with persons with disabilities, see Mackelprang and Salsgiver (1999); and, for an inspirational look at one man's accomplishments in the face of physical limitations, see Weihenmayer (2001). Refer to Tice and Perkins (1996) for prevention of mental health problems of older persons and methods within a community-based practice.

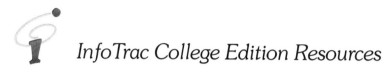

InfoTrac College Edition Resources

For additional readings, explore InfoTrac College Edition, our online library. Go to http://www.infotrac.college.com/wadsworth and select these key word searches:

> late W1 adulthood
> acquired immunodeficiency syndrome AND AIDS
> human immunodeficiency virus AND HIV
> physically W1 challenged
> people with disabilities AND disabled

Key words are listed in a form that enables the search engine to locate a wider range of articles in the online university library. Key words should be entered exactly as shown, including asterisks, "W1," "W2," "AND," and other search engine tools.

CHAPTER *13*

Working With Groups and Families

Focus Questions

1. Have you participated in any kind of group? If so, what was this experience like for you? What did it teach you about groups? about leading groups? about being a member? about yourself?

2. What value do you see in group work for meeting the needs of the various client populations that you hope to serve?

3. If you were to organize a group, what kind of group would you most like to get started? What would you most want to accomplish?

4. In designing a group, where would you begin? What specific actions would you take to start your group? What colleagues or other sources might you consult in getting this group going?

5. How prepared do you think you are to lead or co-lead a group? What personal qualities do you have that might help or hinder you as a group leader? What knowledge and skills do you possess that will enhance your ability to lead groups? What do you still most need to learn?

6. If a supervisor or the director of the agency where you work approached you and encouraged you to start groups in your agency, how would you respond? What are the supervisory and consultation issues you would need to resolve with your supervisor?

7. How would you decide if a co-leader was necessary or appropriate? If you were to select a colleague to co-lead a group or a family counseling session with you, what kind of person would you select? What characteristics would you look for?

8. What characteristics of a group would you look for to differentiate between a productive and a nonproductive group?

9. If you were asked to work with families, how ready would you be to take on this task? How would you assess the progress of family counseling sessions?

10. What are some advantages of working with an entire family rather than restricting your services to one-to-one counseling?

11. When would you consider working with a family? What kinds of problems of an individual do you think would be particularly useful to explore in the context of a family system?

Aim of the Chapter

Group work is becoming an increasingly popular helping modality. For example, group work is recognized as the appropriate modality to be used most frequently by professional school counselors, and groups are often found in agency settings specializing in treatment of substance abuse as well as with other populations. Your supervisor or the director of your agency may ask you to start a group for a particular at-risk population, and you are likely to feel anxiety over not knowing where to begin. If you are like many other helpers, you may feel unprepared to organize and lead a group, or you may be uncertain about the value of groups for special client populations. The purpose of this chapter is to introduce you to the distinct values of working with groups and families, to the advantages of specialized groups and family therapy, and to the merits of your becoming involved as a member in a therapeutic group. Our intention is not to teach you how to lead groups or to conduct family therapy sessions. Instead, we present a perspective on ways of working with people in groups and families.

You will be introduced to the characteristics that make groups productive and powerful. Guidelines are given for deriving the maximum benefit from a group experience. Some key ethical and professional issues are outlined, as are suggestions for acquiring the basic skills required for effective group leadership. We also present a rationale for co-leading groups. You are encouraged to think about how to get the skills you need to organize and facilitate groups for some of the diverse client populations that you will serve.

This chapter provides a brief overview of a systems approach, by identifying the themes that characterize a family-systems perspective and showing how this view differs from an individual counseling perspective. Key concepts of family therapy are also described, providing a clearer picture of how practitioners work from a family-systems perspective.

Group Work as the Treatment of Choice

In the past decade group work has been enjoying a resurgence of interest. In the 1960s and 1970s encounter groups and personal-growth groups were considered one pathway for making human connections and for moving toward greater self-actualization. Today the focus has changed, and the groups that have been springing up in all settings are short-term groups designed for specific client populations and remediation of specific problems.

One American Psychological Association *Monitor* lead article describes an expanding array of group techniques that are affordable and effective in overcoming a range of psychological and medical problems (Sleek, 1995). The crux of the article is that group therapy fits well into the managed care scene because groups can be designed to be brief, cost-effective treatments. Sleek summarizes studies giving evidence that, in general, group counseling is as effective as individual counseling in bringing about change. The focus of these groups is definitely time-limited, and they have fairly narrow goals. Many of the time-limited groups are aimed at symptomatic relief, teaching participants problem-solving strategies and interpersonal skills. The interpersonal learning that occurs in groups can accelerate personal changes.

Some helpers view groups as a second-best treatment modality. They are convinced that interventions for individuals, couples, and families are the most valuable and appropriate strategies. If groups are used in their work setting, these helpers believe cost factors are the primary consideration. When budgets are tight and personnel are overworked, the economics of group treatment could seem paramount.

From our perspective, groups are the treatment of choice, not a second-rate approach to helping people change. We hold this view, not just because the dollars are stretched but because inherent values in the group process result in self-understanding, healing, and change on the part of participants.

Groups are being designed for all kinds of settings today and for many different client groups. Many of the problems that bring people to counseling are interpersonally rooted, and people often seek professional assistance because of difficulties forming or maintaining intimate relationships. Clients feel that their problems are unique and that they have few options to get out of bland ruts. They may be at a loss in knowing how to live well with the ones they love. Groups provide a natural laboratory that demonstrates to people that they are not alone and that there is hope for creating a different life. Groups provide a sense of community, which can be an antidote to the impersonal culture in which many individuals live. Groups are powerful because participants can experience some of their long-term problems being played out in the group sessions. At the same time, the group gives members opportunities to design and try out more effective ways of behaving.

Groups have immense power to move people in creative and more life-giving directions. Most client populations can benefit from a properly designed group with a qualified leader or co-leaders. If a group is hastily thrown together, or if it is led by someone without proper training, however, it may be more damaging than beneficial.

The Value of Group Work

Groups do not represent the "only approach" or the "best way" of helping clients understand and cope with their problems. In some cases, groups may be the most appropriate intervention in a client's life. In other cases, group work may be used as a supplementary form of treatment or as the next step a client takes after completing some individual counseling. In our own practice, we find groups to be powerfully effective and to offer unique advantages for new learning.

Through the unfolding of the group process, members can observe how others interact, and they can learn something about themselves by joining in the interaction. The group experience serves as a living laboratory, for it becomes a mirror in which members see themselves as they are. For instance, Luigi tends to keep himself isolated in the group, and in many ways he makes it difficult for others to get close to him. Through the feedback of other members and the leader, he has a chance to learn about his part in contributing to his own isolation, not only in the group but also in his everyday life. The safety of the group affords him opportunities to experiment with being different. Instead of holding in his feelings, he can begin to let them out. Rather than being quickly defensive, he can open himself to really hearing others. He can experiment with reaching out to others and asking for what he wants. Others in the group profit from Luigi's work, because it enables them to evaluate how they are like him.

People who are beginning to deal with their problems often feel that they are alone in the way they think and feel. Groups offer a forum in which members share their confusion, anger, helplessness, guilt, resentment, depression, and panic. By sharing their feelings, members feel less alone. If some members in the group have difficulty expressing their feelings, they are likely to find comfort in listening to others who are able to express the range of their emotions. For example, Carola has adopted a stoic attitude, thinking that her situation will be more tolerable if she contains her feelings. She may not realize the stress to which she is subjecting herself by denying her emotions. Generally, as she begins to share her concerns, she will probably realize that others also experience some of her pain and that she is not alone in what she feels. Her sharing can help tear down some of the walls that keep her isolated.

Some universal human themes typically become apparent through a group experience. It is true that clients are separated by differences in age, gender, sexual orientation, social and cultural background, and experience. Yet as people risk revealing their deeper concerns and feelings, they typically comment on how they are more alike than different. Although the circumstances leading to pain over disappointment may be different for each person, the emotions associated with certain events have a universal quality. In groups composed of people with a common struggle, such as a support group for women survivors of incest, the sharing of feelings is often even more intense. Before joining the support group, they probably felt alone in their feelings of hurt, sadness, fright, guilt, resentment, and anger. As each woman reveals her story and her feelings about her situation, others are able to identify and come to understand a pattern that unites them. The bonding that builds within the group creates an atmosphere in which women can see more clearly how they have been affected by incest. It also leads to insights into how their earlier experiences have set the stage for the way they now think, feel, and behave.

Another commonality of groups is the hope they offer to members that a new life is possible. For example, groups for people who admit that their lives are out of control when they use alcohol offer steps leading to recovery. When these clients were caught in drinking patterns, they were convinced that they were powerless to change and that they were hopeless. But the modeling of others who are learning to take control of their lives one day at a time is living proof that there is hope for a better life.

The caring and acceptance that develop in a group are powerful healing forces. In a group for children of divorce, compassion and support are given not only by the leader but also by other children. Individuals within this group are able to risk being vulnerable as they sense that what concerns them has importance to others.

A distinct advantage of groups is the opportunity for learning from the feedback of many others. If reactions are given with sensitivity, members come to realize the ways in which their behavior affects others. The process of interpersonal feedback shows people how they contribute to both favorable and unfavorable outcomes, and it also gives them new possibilities for relating to others.

How Groups Can Help You

Take a few moments to reflect on how open you are to being a group member. How willing are you to define goals that will enable you to participate actively and fully in learning about yourself and others? Are you willing to recognize your own vulnerabilities and to share them in the context of the group? As you think about yourself as a group member, let yourself imagine that you are leading a group in which all the members are very much like yourself. What might it be like for you to lead such a group?

If you participate in experiential groups as a part of your training, you can use your experience for personal change and also for working on concerns you have as a helper. Other members can help you take an honest look at yourself, which can also teach you how to confront yourself. Your own honesty about who you are is the most significant factor in your ability to change. We would encourage you to do what you can to make any group you enter as personally meaningful as possible.

In Chapter 6 we went into detail about dealing with the transference reactions your clients may have to you, as well as ways of recognizing any countertransference reactions you may have to them. A group is an ideal place to explore your feelings toward clients and the effects that their behavior has on you. The group can be useful in bringing about an awareness of blind spots that make it difficult for you to be objective. A group experience that is connected with your training program may not be an appropriate place to work through unfinished business from your past, but it can serve you by sensitizing you to how your vulnerabilities could interfere with your work as a helper. For instance, assume that you discover that you act somewhat like a child seeking approval of your parents when you are in the company of certain older persons. You will probably need to work outside the group in your own therapy to understand these early wounds associated with your parents. However, the group can reveal when you tend to revert to less mature ways of responding. In a group you can learn a great deal about your resistance when you feel vulnerable, and this awareness of your own defenses can be extremely useful in teaching you how to work with clients who exhibit resistant behaviors.

In several previous chapters, we alluded to thought and feeling patterns with which many helpers struggle during their training. For instance, you may have a sense of not knowing enough to really help others. You may be overly cautious lest you make mistakes that your clients will see. Or you may find yourself overly sensitive to anything that sounds like criticism. Refer to some of the common concerns of helpers that we examined in Chapter 6 for other examples of places where you might get stuck yourself. Being in a group as a part of your program affords you an avenue for talking about the feelings, fears, and uncertainties that characterize the developing helper you are becoming.

You don't have to be psychologically disturbed to profit from a group experience designed for personal growth. Instead, your willingness to seek input from others and to consider feedback can start a pattern that will encourage you to continue seeking out others when the demands on you in your helping role are great. Your capacity to receive support and challenge from others can better equip you to give quality service to clients. If you are a reluctant client yourself, you will probably have trouble inspiring others, especially clients who seem reluctant.

Getting the Most From a Group Experience

How can you get the most from a group experience? How can you maximize your learning? If you are able to become an active group member yourself, you can use this experience later in teaching members in the groups you lead how to make the most of their group experience. We are convinced that those who participate in groups will get more from the experience if they are given some instructions. After all, the norms that govern group process are somewhat different from the norms of some other social situations. We offer some recommendations here that you can apply both to yourself as a member and to teaching others about groups. For a more detailed discussion, we refer you to *Groups: Process and Practice* (M. Corey & Corey, 2002).

1. Recognize that trust is not something that "just happens" in a group; you have a role in creating this climate of trust. If you are aware of anything getting in the way of a sense of safety, share your hesitations with the group.

2. Commit yourself to getting something from your group by focusing on your personal goals. Before each meeting, think about how you can get involved, what personal concerns you want to explore, and other ways to use the time in group meaningfully.

3. Although it is useful to have a tentative agenda of what you want to discuss, do not cling inflexibly to your agenda if you are affected by what others are exploring and if this suggests moving in a different direction.

4. If the work other members are doing is affecting you, it is useful to let them know in what ways you are being affected. If you are able to identify with the struggles or pains of others, it generally helps both you and them to share your feelings and thoughts.

5. Decide for yourself what, how much, and when you will disclose personal facets of yourself. Others will not have a basis for knowing you unless you tell them about yourself. If you have difficulty sharing yourself personally in your group, begin by letting others know what makes it hard for you to self-disclose.

6. Avoid getting lost and overwhelming others with detailed information about you or your history. Share your struggles that are significant to you at this time in your life, especially as these concerns pertain to what others in the group are exploring.

7. Express persistent feelings that you are having that pertain to what is emerging in the group in the here and now. For example, if you are feeling intimidated by other people in the group, announce that you feel this way. If you feel somewhat isolated, share this. If you are not wanting to be a part of the group, it is essential that you talk about this.

8. Realize that others will not know you if you do not let them know what issues are important to you, nor will they realize you identify with them or feel close to them unless you let them know.

9. Practice your attending and listening skills. If you can give others the gift of your presence and understanding, you are contributing a great deal to the group process.

10. Try to challenge yourself if you sense that you are "taking too much group time for yourself." If you become overly concerned about measuring how much you are taking and receiving, you will inhibit the spontaneity that can make a group exciting and productive.

11. Use your group as a place to experiment with new behaviors. Allow yourself to try out different ways of being to determine ways that you may want to change. Think of ways to carry any new ways of thinking, feeling, and acting into your outside life. Give yourself your own homework assignments and let others in your group know how you are applying in-group learnings to your behavior with family, friends, and associates.

12. Understand that making changes will not be instantaneous. You can also expect some setbacks in the progress you make. Keep track of any progress you are making, and remember to give yourself credit for your efforts and the subtle changes that you are making.

13. Avoid giving others advice, or giving intellectualized interpretations of their behavior, or of using questioning as your main style of interacting with others. If you are inclined to ask a question, let others know why you are interested in hearing their answer. Or if you want to give advice, reveal to others what your investment is in giving this advice. Learn to speak *for* yourself and *about* yourself.

14. Concentrate on making personal and direct statements to others in your group. Direct communication with a member is more effective than "talking about" that person through the leader.

15. In giving feedback to others, strive to avoid categorizing or labeling them. Instead of telling others who or what they are, tell them what you are observing and let them know how they are affecting you.

16. Pay attention to any consistent feedback you might receive. For example, if you hear that others perceive you as being somewhat judgmental and critical, do not be too quick to argue and convince others that you are open and accepting. Instead, take in what you are hearing and consider their input to determine the degree to what they are saying might fit for you.

17. Respect your defenses and understand that they have served a purpose for you. However, when you become aware of feeling or acting defensively in your group, challenge your defenses by seeing what will occur if you strive to be less guarded.

18. Provide support for others by expressing your care for them, but do not quickly intervene by trying to comfort others when they are experiencing feelings, such as expressing pain over an event. Let them know how their pain is affecting you.

19. Take responsibility for what you are accomplishing in your group. Spend some time thinking about what is taking place in these meetings and evaluating the degree to which you are attaining your goals. If you are not satisfied with your group experience, look at what you can do to make the group a more meaningful experience.

20. Be aware of respecting and maintaining the confidentiality of what goes on inside your group. Even though you may not maliciously breach others' confidences, recognize how easy it might be to inappropriately talk to others who are not in the group about what others have revealed. The way that you handle confidentiality says a great deal about your professional character. If you have any concerns that what you are sharing is staying within the group, be willing to bring this matter up in a session.

21. Keep a personal journal in which you record impressions of your own explorations and learning in your group. A journal will be invaluable in keeping track of your progress and noting changes in your ways of thinking, feeling, and acting.

The Ethical and Professional Group Leader

In our view, the best way to ensure that your groups will be productive for your clients is to strive to follow ethical and professional standards in your practice of group work. The Association for Specialists in Group Work (ASGW) has developed and published the "Best Practice Guidelines" (1998), which provide group workers with suggestions aimed at increasing ethical and professional behavior. What follows is an overview of some of the qualities that we think reflect such standards.

You first spend time thinking about what you most want to accomplish through a group format. If you intend to co-lead your group, you arrange to carve out time before you even meet potential members to discuss with your colleague general group goals and an overall plan for getting your group into motion. You will not be getting a group together simply because groups are fashionable but because you believe that your group has real potential for making a difference to those who join.

You then provide information to prospective group candidates. Realizing that some of the people who need your group the most may be reluctant to seek your services, you are willing to make some provisions for outreach work and getting the word out to a particular target population that could most benefit. You make arrangements for some orientation sessions where potential members can find out more about the group and decide whether it is what they need. You also make some provision for screening prospective group members. In the screening sessions, you give consideration to selecting members whose needs and goals are compatible with the goals of the group, those who will not impede the group process, and those whose well-being will not be jeopardized by the group experience. You explore with the members the risks of potential life changes, and you help them explore their readiness to face these possibilities. In short, before your group ever meets, you will have spent time laying a foundation and preparing members for a successful learning experience.

Once the group begins to meet, you assess the degree to which its purposes are being met. If you are co-leading the group, you arrange to meet with your colleague regularly so that your efforts are coordinated. Ideally, these meetings take place both before and after each group session.

Because you are aware that confidentiality is the cornerstone of any group, you make sure that the participants know what it implies, and you encourage them to bring up any concerns they might have about maintaining confidences. You make some effort to teach the members how to become active participants so that they can get the most from the group sessions and also how to apply their newly acquired interpersonal skills in everyday living.

If you have an open group, one characterized by changing membership, you help members who are ready to leave the group integrate their learning, and you allow those who are staying to talk about their feelings about losing a member. As new members join, you attend to them so that they will be able to make use of the group resources. Although members ultimately have the right to leave a group, you discuss with them the possible risks of leaving prematurely, and you encourage them to discuss their reasons for wanting to quit. If your group is made up of involuntary members, you take steps to enlist their cooperation and their continuation on a voluntary basis.

Just as you take care not to impose your values on those clients you see individually, you are also sensitive to the ways in which your own values and needs have an impact on the group process. You exert care not to coerce participants to change in ways they have not chosen. Although you avoid imposing your values on members, you are willing to expose your beliefs and values if doing so is likely to benefit the members. Although you are able to meet your needs through your work, you do not do so at the members' expense. You also protect members' rights against coercion and undue pressure from other participants. You teach the members that the purpose of the group is to help them find their own answers rather than yielding to pressure from others.

For the duration of the group, you monitor your own behavior and become aware of what you are modeling to the members. You recognize the importance of teaching members how to evaluate their progress in meeting their goals, and you also design follow-up procedures.

You recognize and respect diversity within the group. You also encourage members to be sensitive to cultural, racial, religious, lifestyle, age, sexual orientation, disability, and gender differences. Indeed, group workers need to acquire diversity competence if they expect to effectively reach a wide range of client populations. The ASGW has adopted the "Principles for Diversity-Competent Group Workers" (1999), which spells out beliefs and attitudes, knowledge areas, and skills and intervention strategies of diversity-competent group practitioners. You are able to recognize the limits of your multicultural competency and expertise when working with a diverse range of group members. It is not necessary to expect that you will know everything about the cultural background of members in your groups. There is a good deal to be said for inviting members to share what they deem to be significant aspects of their culture with you and other members.

Many individuals live in two cultures. Oftentimes they have allegiance to their own home culture but find certain aspects of their new culture appealing. These members may experience conflicts in their attempt to integrate the values from the two cultures in which they live. These core struggles can be productively explored in an accepting group if you and other members respect this cultural conflict. If you are a diversity-sensitive group practitioner, the techniques that you employ are appropriate to the cultural background and needs of the members in your group. Depending on the type of intervention, you are aware of the limits of your competence. You avoid using potentially powerful techniques unless you are trained in their use under supervision. You are willing to seek out consultation or supervision when encountering ethical concerns that could interfere with the functioning of the group.

Just as you prepare members for entering a group, you also prepare them for termination from the group in the most efficient period of time. You help members pull together what they have learned from their group experience and assist them in developing an action plan for the period after they leave the group. If possible, you arrange for some method of follow-up with individuals or with the entire group to assess the outcomes. You are knowledgeable about the resources within your community that can assist members in their special needs, and you help members seek any professional assistance they need. As the group comes to an end, you encourage members to find resources that will enable them to continue the growth they have begun through the group.

Developing Skills as a Group Leader

Many institutions now use groups as their primary approach in helping clients resolve their problems. If these groups are led by practitioners who are not competent in group work with a given population, more harm than good can result. One of the most important ethical helping principles pertains to obtaining the necessary knowledge and skills to lead groups effectively. Supervised training is an indispensable element in becoming a competent leader of groups. You are faced with an ethical dilemma if a supervisor asks you to design or lead certain kinds of groups when you have not had the proper educational preparation. Not infrequently, we find that professionals who attend our workshops recall negative experiences with their one and only group course. This experience sometimes sours them on wanting to conduct groups themselves or makes them skeptical about the value of groups.

In Chapter 5 we described some of the helping skills that are basic to interviewing, assessing, and counseling individuals. Some of these skills include active listening, providing support, challenging clients when appropriate, responding with empathy, clarifying feelings and thoughts, helping clients formulate goals, reflecting feelings, reframing problems in a new light, and helping clients develop action plans. All of the skills that are needed for individual counseling are also required of group workers. Your knowledge of the major theories and techniques of counseling, as well as your familiarity with what it is like to be a member of a group, will be most useful as a background for developing group facilitation skills.

Effective group leaders are aware of group processes and know how to tap the healing forces within a group. Leading a group is far more complex than merely counseling individuals in a group setting. In addition to the basic skills for individual counseling, group leadership skills include helping members create trust, linking members' work, teaching members how to give and receive feedback, facilitating disclosure and risk taking, intervening to block counterproductive group behavior, identifying common themes, setting up role-playing situations that help members dramatize their struggles, and preparing members for closure. Although it may seem beyond your reach to know enough and be skilled enough to lead a group, you can learn a great deal about how groups function by participating in them, as we discussed earlier. Course work in group process, opportunities to co-lead groups under adequate supervision, and participation in training groups will give you many opportunities to acquire, practice, and hone the essential skills needed to facilitate the various kinds of groups.

The ASGW has developed and published the "Professional Standards for the Training of Group Workers" (2000), which are a specific set of core competencies in general group work. Be sure that your training program includes these core competencies. Both direct participation in supervised small groups and clinical experience in leading various groups under careful supervision are needed to equip leaders with the skills to meet the challenges of group work.

Groups for Various Populations

The various kinds of groups differ with respect to goals, techniques used, the role of the leader, training requirements, and the people involved. The range of groups designed to help people cope with specific problems or those aimed at particular client populations is limited only by a practitioner's imagination. We find that such special groups are mushrooming and that they frequently arise from the needs of a particular group or from the interests of the professional who is designing them.

Many groups have both an educational and a therapeutic dimension. These groups are often short term, have some degree of structure, deal with a particular population, and focus on a specific theme. They can serve a number of purposes, such as giving information, sharing common concerns, teaching coping skills, helping people practice better ways of interpersonal communication, teaching problem-solving techniques, and assisting people once they leave the group.

Eventually, as a part of your job as a professional helper, you may be asked to set up and lead one or more groups. Depending on the age and population with which you work, you are likely to find yourself looking for resources that will help you design a group. Many creative groups are designed to meet the special needs of children, and you may be expected to form a group to help children in your community. These groups are generally structured by focusing on a theme such as surviving divorce, controlling acting out, dealing with abuse or neglect, enhancing self-esteem, or coping with terminal illness.

For adolescents, you may be asked to organize a group program for alcohol and drug rehabilitation, a growth group to meet normal developmental needs, a group for young women with eating disorders, a group for school dropouts, or a group to help young people cope with the aftermath of some crisis. For adults, there are groups for single parents, for middle-aged people contemplating a career change, for couples who hope to improve their relationship, for people who have tested HIV-positive, for people who are diagnosed with cancer, and for the physically challenged. Increasing in popularity are groups for women and groups for men, which allow for the exploration of gender-identity concerns and issues pertaining to gender-role conditioning. There are many different groups designed for specific skills training or learning to manage particular problem areas.

Structured groups, sometimes referred to as psychoeducation groups, generally have an educational focus in that they are designed to teach participants a variety of coping skills. These groups, which tend to focus on a particular theme, are being increasingly used by agencies, schools, and college counseling centers. Generally, the sessions are about 2 hours each week for 4 to 15 weeks. Depending on the population, some group sessions may be as short as 30 to 45 minutes, especially with children or clients with a short attention span.

At the beginning of these structured groups it is common to ask members to complete a questionnaire on how well they are coping with the area of concern. Such groups make use of structured exercises, readings, homework assignments, and contracts. When the group comes to an end, another questionnaire is often used to assess the members' progress.

This list will give you some idea of the scope of topics for structured groups:

- Stress management
- Weight control and body image
- Women in transition
- Dealing with an alcoholic parent
- Dealing with chemical dependency
- Learning coping skills

- Groups for re-entry students
- Managing relationships and ending relationships
- Parenting skills groups
- Groups for the elderly
- Support groups for victims of crime
- Support groups for persons with AIDS

In reality, the kinds of groups you might design are limited only by your ingenuity. For most client populations, a support or structured group can be organized that combines educational and therapeutic aims. Once you determine some areas of need within the community or at the agency where you work, you and your co-workers can launch short-term groups to address these needs.

Working With Co-Leaders

In our practice of group work, in teaching and supervising group practitioners, and in conducting group-process workshops for students and professionals, we favor working as a team. Although our preference is for the co-leadership model, this is not the only acceptable model of leadership. Many people facilitate a group alone quite effectively. Realistically speaking, however, there are many institutional barriers to the practice of co-leadership of groups. For example, in many hospital settings where groups are used, it is common to be understaffed in behavioral health and community counseling. Using co-leaders for some of the groups in a hospital setting would place a strain on staffing requirements in other domains at the hospital. Budgetary concerns are an ever-increasing barrier to co-facilitated groups. A hospital administrator is likely to ask the question: "Why should we pay two staff members to facilitate a group that could be led by one person?"

Although there are restrictions on co-led groups in some settings, this does not imply that such a practice is nonexistent in most agencies. There are a number of advantages to co-leading groups for all concerned: the group members can gain from the perspectives of two leaders; depending on their styles, the co-leaders can each bring a unique focus to the session and can complement each other's facilitation; and the co-leaders are able to consult before and after a group and learn from each other.

Careful selection of a co-leader is essential. A major factor should be mutual respect. Two leaders working together may have differences in leadership style, and they are not likely to always agree or share the same perceptions or interpretations. If there is mutual respect and trust, however, they will be able to work cooperatively instead of competitively, and they will be secure enough to be free of the constant need to prove themselves. If the two leaders are incompatible, their group is bound to be negatively affected. For example, if one is jealous of the other and tries to discount the other's interventions, the group members will sense the tension, and their cohesion will suffer.

We cannot stress enough the importance of co-leaders' making a commitment to meet regularly. We encourage those who co-lead groups to spend some time both before and after each session discussing their reactions to what is going on in the group as well as their working relationship. One of the benefits of co-leading is that your relationship with your co-leader can be nourishing, both personally and professionally. The chances of burnout can be reduced, especially if you are working with a demanding and draining client population.

Not infrequently, a group session is characterized by the expression of intense emotions. If you or your co-leader is strongly affected by what occurred in a session, your own meetings allow for the exploration of any feelings, impressions, or reactions. The two of you can use each other as sounding boards, can check for objectivity, and can offer useful feedback. However, it is often necessary for leaders to express and deal with such feelings in the session itself. For example, if you are aware that you are consistently feeling put off by a particular member, it would be best for you to deal with your reactions to this person in the group itself. In certain cases a group member's concerns may touch your own "unfinished business," and you may explore your personal issues, either within or outside of the group, depending on which would be more appropriate. This is a time when a competent and trusted co-leader is especially important.

You can see that one of the advantages of co-leading is that it can help you identify and work with countertransference that emerges within the group. As you recall from our earlier discussion of countertransference in Chapter 6, this phenomenon can distort your objectivity to the extent that it interferes with effective counseling. For example, your co-leader may typically react with great impatience to men who are reluctant to express their feelings. You may be better able to make contact with such a man. You can also help your co-leader identify his or her reactions and attachments to a certain member.

Even with a co-leader whom you respect and like, there are likely to be occasional disagreements. These differences need not necessarily pose a problem; rather, they can keep both of you professionally alert. Moreover, if you deal with your differences constructively during the session, you are providing excellent modeling on how to work with conflicts. Most of the disadvantages in co-leading groups have to do with poor selection of a co-leader, random assignment to a co-leader, or failure of the two leaders to meet regularly.

Although we like a co-leading model, we think it is important that the two leaders have some say in deciding to work as a team. Otherwise, there is a potential for harm for both members and leaders. In addition to the values we have mentioned, co-leading can keep your work interesting, and it can be fun.

Working With Families

Families are a particular kind of group that is best approached from a systems perspective. That is, psychological problems arise within the present family environment and the intergenerational family system. In a family-systems approach, symptoms are viewed as an expression of a dysfunction within the family system—not the individual—and dysfunctions are often passed across several generations.

Family therapy involves a conceptual shift from individual dynamics to inter-action within the system. A systems perspective views the family as a functioning unit and as an entity unto itself that adds up to more than the sum of its members. The family provides the context for understanding how individuals behave. Ac-tions by any individual family member will influence all the other members, and their reactions will have a reciprocal effect on the individual. For example, a couple devote most of their energy to their acting-out son. They form an alliance to save him. Once he leaves home and they no longer have control over his ac-tions, they begin to fight with each other. A short time later they file for divorce because of their differences. This example illustrates how a change in one part of the family affects the actions of other family members. It may be possible that the problems existed earlier in the relationship and the son's acting out served the purpose of keeping the parents together.

Another systems principle is that each family member is part of a whole pie, even though it is easy for the members to think of themselves as separate pieces of the pie without an integral connection. The system assumes its own personality. You cannot pluck yourself out of your family system, for you are dynamically re-lated to it. If you restrict yourself exclusively to your internal dynamics, without considering your interpersonal dynamics, you are not getting a full picture of your-self. From a systems perspective, being a healthy person involves both a sense of belonging to your family system and a sense of separateness and individuality.

A Family-Systems Perspective

The family-systems perspective holds that individuals are best understood through assessing the interactions of the entire family. This perspective is grounded on the assumptions that a client's problematic behavior may (1) serve a function or pur-pose for the family; (2) be a function of the family's inability to operate produc-tively, especially during developmental transitions; or (3) be a symptom of dysfunc-tional patterns handed down across generations. All these assumptions challenge traditional individual therapy frameworks for conceptualizing human problems and their formation.

All family therapists subscribe to the basic notion that families are systems. Therefore, a treatment approach that comprehensively addresses the other family members as well as the "identified" client is required. Goldenberg and Goldenberg (2000a) point to the need for therapists to view all behavior, including the symp-toms expressed by the individual, within the context of the family and society. The Goldenbergs add that a systems orientation does not preclude dealing with the dy-namics within the individual but that this approach broadens the traditional em-phasis. Because a family is an interacting unit, it has its own set of unique traits. It is not possible to accurately assess an individual's concerns without observing the interaction of the other family members as well as the broader context in the com-munity and in society. Focusing on the internal dynamics of an individual without adequately considering interpersonal dynamics yields an incomplete picture of that individual.

Family therapy is more than an approach to working with a family; it is a perspective that sheds light on the individual's and the family's development over time. It also provides a lens through which to view connections in the world. It takes into consideration the influence of an individual's neighborhood, community, church, work environment, school, and other systems. Indeed, the family-systems perspective holds that significant change within an individual is not likely to be made or maintained unless the client's network of intimate relationships is taken into account. Systems practitioners assume that even if an individual makes changes they are not likely to endure if there is little support for, or if there is opposition to, these changes from the individual's family and other social relationships.

Family therapists view individuals from a relational, developmental, cultural, and gender perspective. Emphasis is on an individual's relationships with others in the system. The best vantage point for understanding an individual's behavior is by paying attention to what is occurring within the many layers of systems that touch the individual.

An individual's level of functioning can be seen as a manifestation of the way the family is functioning. For example, a young girl who develops ulcers may be signaling not only her own pain but the unexpressed pain of the family. If individual change is a goal of therapy with the daughter, it is essential to understand how the family influences her and how any changes she makes are likely to affect other members of her family. It should also be noted, however, that an individual can have a symptom that may exist independent of the family structure. An example of this is clinical depression, which could be caused by a biochemical imbalance; it is not necessarily a result of some family dynamic.

Key Concepts of Family Therapy

Family therapy is a diverse field with respect to concepts, techniques, and approaches. The key concepts presented here detail some of the themes that unite the many schools of family therapy and look at some of the variations that exist among these theoretical orientations.

Focus of family therapy.   Family therapy tends to be brief, because families who seek professional help typically want resolution of some problematic symptom. In addition to being short-term, solution-focused, and action-oriented, family therapy tends to deal with present interactions. One way in which it differs from many individual therapies is its emphasis on how current family relationships contribute to the development and maintenance of symptoms.

Almost all of the family therapies are concerned with here-and-now interactions in the family system. The role of history is handled in different ways. Some approaches assume that family history is crucial in understanding present functioning, whereas other models make no assumption about history at all. However, by dealing with interactions in the here and now, patterns that have existed over time can be changed.

Another focus that characterizes family therapy is the attention paid to communication. All family therapy orientations emphasize verbal and nonverbal communication. Some approaches to family therapy assume that the central aim of communication is attaining power in interpersonal relationships. Symptoms are seen as ways of communicating with the aim of controlling other family members. For instance, a child who fears going to school might be expressing his or her insecurity about making new friends.

Role of the therapist. Family therapists function as models, teachers, and coaches. What most approaches have in common is their commitment to helping family members learn new and more effective ways of interacting. All family therapists have a keen interest in the process of family interaction and in teaching patterns of communication.

Goals of family therapy. Family or relationship therapy is aimed at helping the members change the patterns of relationships that are not working well and helping the family create new ways of interacting. The general goal is to bring about system change, predicated on the assumption that if a system changes so will the individuals within the system. The specific goals are determined by the practitioner's orientation or by a collaborative process between the family and the therapist.

How families change. An integrative approach to the practice of family therapy must include guiding principles that help organize goals, interactions, observations, and ways to promote change. Theories of family therapy can be grouped into two categories: (1) those that focus on change within the therapy sessions, and (2) those that deal with the occurrence of change outside the therapeutic context in the natural world (Hanna & Brown, 1999). Some theories focus on perceptual and cognitive change, others deal mainly with changing feelings, and others emphasize behavioral change.

Techniques of family therapy. Diverse techniques are available to family therapists, but the intervention strategies they employ are best considered in conjunction with their own personal characteristics. It is essential that therapists use skills and techniques that fit their personality and that are appropriate for the goals of therapy. Goldenberg and Goldenberg (2000a) and Nichols and Schwartz (2001) emphasize that techniques are tools for achieving therapeutic goals, yet these intervention strategies do not make a family therapist. Personal characteristics, such as respect for clients, compassion, empathy, and sensitivity, are human qualities that influence the manner in which techniques are delivered. Faced with the demands of clinical practice, practitioners need to be flexible in selecting intervention strategies that will meet specific therapeutic objectives and contribute to specific outcomes. The central consideration is what is in the best interests of the family. Many therapy procedures can be borrowed from various models, depending on what is likely to work best with a given family.

Key to the family-systems approach is that neither the individual nor the family is blamed for a particular dysfunction. The family is empowered through the process of identifying and exploring interaction patterns. If change is to come about in a family or between individual members of a family, the family must be aware of the systems that influence them. Contemporary approaches to family therapy emphasize understanding the individual within the systems that influence him or her. This sheds an entirely different light on assessment and treatment of individuals and families.

Diversity and the Family Therapy Approach

One of the advantages of the systemic perspective in working from a multicultural framework is that many ethnic and cultural groups place great value on the extended family. If practitioners are working with an individual from a cultural background that gives special value to including grandparents, aunts, and uncles in some form of cooperative family unit, it is easy to see that family approaches have a distinct advantage over individual therapy. Working with families offers some excellent possibilities for consensus building and for networking with members of the extended family.

Today, family therapists explore both the individual culture of the family and the larger culture to which the family belongs. They look for ways in which culture can both inform and modify family work. Interventions are no longer applied universally, regardless of the culture involved, but rather are adapted and even designed to complement the family system within the larger community of which it is a part.

By Way of Review

- For many target populations and certain purposes, groups are the treatment of choice, not a second-rate approach to helping people change.

- Inherent values in the group process lead to self-acceptance, deeper understanding of oneself, and change. Some of these values are learning that one is not alone, receiving feedback from many sources, gaining opportunities for experimenting with new behavior, and using the group as an interpersonal laboratory.

- As a student in a training program, you have a great deal to gain from groups in your personal and professional development. If you expect to make group work or family counseling a part of your practice, training and supervision are essential.

- Helpers are expected to follow ethical guidelines in forming and conducting group counseling sessions.

- It is important to know the limits of your competency if you are asked to work with groups or families.

- Skills in working with groups and families can be acquired and refined. These skills can be applied to working with a wide array of special populations in a variety of settings.

- The practice of working with families rests on the foundation of a systems perspective, which views psychological problems as arising from within the individual's present environment and the intergenerational family system.

- An assumption of the systems approach is that change in any one part of the system affects all parts of that system.

- A family-systems perspective provides a lens through which to view connections in the world by taking into consideration the influence of an individual's neighborhood, community, church, school, and work environment.

What Will You Do Now?

1. Investigate the services that are offered in a local community agency or facility. Ask about how the groups are organized, what services are available to special client groups, and what outcomes these groups have had. If you are doing fieldwork in an agency now, inquire about group work and working with families.

2. If a group experience is not part of your training program, join a group in your college or university, in the community, or through private practice. Even if you decide not to join a group, this exercise can be useful in learning about community resources.

3. If you are working in an agency or if you have a fieldwork placement, see whether you can observe a group. Of course, both the group members and the leader would have to agree before you could visit a session. The purpose of this visit is to acquaint you with the potential of groups for meeting the needs of various client populations.

4. If you are currently involved in a group, or have been in a group in the past, in your journal describe the kind of group member that you are (or were). What might this teach you about your ability to lead or co-lead groups? You might also write about your concerns or fears in doing group work. Let yourself brainstorm as you write about the possible advantages to working with people in groups. Think about your interests, and see if you can identify some general ideas for ways to employ small groups as a vehicle for branching out from your interests.

5. Review the section on understanding your family of origin in Chapter 3. In small groups, spend some time exploring how your experiences with your family are likely to influence your work with families. What are some of your attitudes about family life that will show up in your professional work?

6. In small groups, take some time to discuss what you need to know and specific skills you need to have to be able to effectively work with families. If you were asked by your supervisor in your fieldwork placement to join him or her in conducting family sessions in the agency, what would be your response? How well prepared, both personally and academically, are you to work with families?

7. For the full bibliographic entry for each of the sources listed here, consult the References and Reading List at the back of the book. For a practical handbook on the evolution of a group and key group process issues at each stage, see M. Corey and Corey (2002). For a practical book on ways of creating, implementing, and evaluating techniques for therapeutic groups, see Corey, Corey, Callanan, and Russell (1992). Consult Yalom (1995) for an in-depth treatment of theoretical and practical issues dealing with interpersonal therapy groups. For an overview of ten major theories of group counseling, with practical applications to various groups, see Corey (2000). For an overview of the major theories of family therapy, see Becvar and Becvar (2000); Carlson, Sperry, and Lewis (1997); Goldenberg and Goldenberg (2000a); Hanna and Brown (1999); and Nichols and Schwartz (2001). Goldenberg and Goldenberg (2000a) deal with effective interventions for a range of traditional and nontraditional families that helpers will encounter. Thomlison (2002) is a good source as a family assessment workbook.

InfoTrac College Edition Resources

For additional readings, explore InfoTrac College Edition, our online library. Go to http://www.infotrac.college.com/wadsworth and select these key word searches:

    work W1 group* AND psych*
    group* W2 couns*
    diversity AND psych* AND group*
    group W1 process
    training group leader*
    co-leadership AND group
    ethical issues in training group
    values AND group counseling
    systems W1 approach
    values AND marital W1 family therapy
    gender W1 sensitive AND therapy
    confidentiality AND marital W1 family therapy

Key words are listed in a form that enables the search engine to locate a wider range of articles in the online university library. Key words should be entered exactly as shown, including asterisks, "W1," "W2," "AND," and other search engine tools.

CHAPTER *14*

Stress and Burnout

Focus Questions

1. The assumption is often made that helpers are not good at asking for help for themselves. To what degree are you willing to seek help from others when you are experiencing difficulties?

2. What major stresses do you experience, both at home and at work? How well do you cope with them?

3. What major demands do you expect to face in the organization where you will work? How can you keep your individuality and integrity and at the same time keep your job?

4. Are you concerned about burnout for yourself? If you have experienced burnout as a student, what have you done?

5. What key stresses do you expect to encounter in your work as a helper? How well prepared do you feel you are to deal with such stresses?

6. Becoming a helper is bound to open you up to some of your own unresolved conflicts and personal vulnerabilities. What unfinished business in your personal life could present difficulties for you in working with clients with a range of problems?

Aim of the Chapter

If you choose one of the helping professions, it is valuable to consider the joys and rewards of your work. Your involvement in working intimately in the lives of others can yield many benefits and gifts to you personally. In very few other kinds of work do you have as many opportunities to reflect on the quality of your own life. Helping others can provide you with the satisfaction of knowing that you are making a significant difference to others, which in itself enhances the meaning of life. In their research study, Radeke and Mahoney (2000) indicate that mental health practitioners recognize that the impact of their work makes them better and wiser, and increases their self-awareness. The work that helpers do tends to accelerate their psychological development, amplify their emotional life, and results in them feeling both stressed and satisfied. As a result of their professional commitment, helpers report a deeper appreciation for human relationships, an increased tolerance for ambiguity, a greater capacity to enjoy life, a sense of doing spiritual work, and an opportunity to examine and change their personal values. These are but a few of the psychological benefits often reported by helping professionals.

Along with the rewards you may derive from being a helping professional come certain hazards. As you well know, the demands on you as a student often create stress. In addition, a fieldwork placement or a class that involves an emotional focus is likely to bring out your own anxieties. Such stress, of course, is not necessarily negative. This painful awareness, which is a normal process, can be a vehicle for growth and self-understanding.

When you finish your program and begin practicing full time, new stresses will stem from the nature of your work and from professional role expectations. Helpers in a training program are seldom warned about the hazards of the profession, and many helping professionals are not particularly skilled at recognizing when their own life situation might warrant assistance from others. Helpers have been socialized to think of others, and they have difficulty accepting their own needs. Thus, they often give to the point of depletion and in the process neglect taking care of themselves.

Helpers feel great pressure to perform well. Frequently, the lives and welfare of others depend on the decisions and recommendations they make. All of this work-related stress can result in serious psychological, physical, and behavioral disorders. Radeke and Mahoney (2000) suggest that people considering a career as helping professionals should be informed that it will likely result in changes in their personal lives. Norcross (2000) is another voice claiming that "psychotherapy is often a grueling and demanding calling" (p. 710). A growing body of research reveals the negative toll exacted on mental health practitioners. The literature points to symptoms such as moderate depression, mild anxiety, emotional exhaustion, and disturbed relationships. It is essential to recognize the hazards of helping if we hope to develop effective self-care strategies. A significant benefit that is associated with acknowledging the strains of helping is the realization that virtually all mental health professionals experience similar kinds of pressure (Norcross, 2000).

If you are considering a career as a counselor, you may be looking forward to guiding people to resolution of problems they face and to assist them in dealing constructively with pain in their lives. You are likely to be thinking about the expected satisfaction that comes with knowing that you can be an agent of change for your clients. Yet you may not be fully aware that the commitment to being a helping professional for others is fraught with difficulties. As you saw in Chapters 3, 4, and 6, the process of helping others may open you up to some of your own deepest personal struggles and unfinished business. It also seems impossible to us that you can work intensely with clients week after week and not be affected by their pain. When your old pain surfaces and present struggles become overwhelming, it is essential that you seek help for yourself. There is a steep price to pay for numbing yourself to this pain, and you need to recognize that the nature of your work makes it difficult to hide from yourself. In this chapter we explore how stress can affect you as a helper and how prolonged stresses can lead to burnout. In the final chapter we address the topic of self-care and retaining your vitality as a person and as a professional. Self-care is a basis for utilizing your strengths, which can enable you to deal effectively with the stresses of your work and prevent some of the risk factors listed above.

Sources of Stress for Helpers

The sources of work-related stress for helping professionals fall into two categories: individual and environmental. To understand the dynamics of the stress you will experience as a human services professional, you must understand both the external realities that tend to produce stress and the ways you contribute to your stress by your perceptions and interpretations of reality.

Individual stressors can be discovered by examining your attitudes and personal characteristics as a helper. Think about client behaviors that would represent the most stress to you. Look over the following checklist of client behaviors, and rate them according to this scale:

1 = This would be *highly stressful* to me.
2 = This would be *moderately stressful* to me.
3 = This would be *mildly stressful* to me.
4 = This would *not be a source of stress* to me.

_____ 1. I am seeing a client who seems unmotivated and is coming to the sessions only because he was ordered to attend.

_____ 2. One of my clients wants to terminate counseling, but I don't think she is ready for termination.

_____ 3. A client is very depressed, sees very little hope that life will get better, and keeps asking me for help.

_____ 4. One of my clients makes suicidal threats, and I have every reason to take his threats seriously.

_____ 5. One particular client is angry with me for not doing enough to help her situation.

_____ 6. With this client I feel a great sense of identification, almost to the point of overidentifying with him.

_____ 7. A client tells me that he (she) is sexually attracted to me, and I am not sexually attracted to him (her).

_____   8.   A client tells me that she (he) is sexually attracted to me, and I am sexually attracted to her (him).

_____   9.   My client is very demanding and wants to call me at home for advice on how to deal with every new problem that arises.

_____   10.   This client almost never expresses any appreciation to me, but she often lets me know that I am not doing enough for her and don't seem to care enough about her.

Once you have made your ratings, assess the patterns that emerge. What specific behaviors seem to be the most stressful for you? How does stress affect your self-esteem, both on a personal and a professional level?

In addition to these personal, or internal, sources of stress, external factors can also create stress in helpers. *Environmental* sources of stress include the physical aspects of the work setting or the structure of the position itself. A major stressor is the reality of having too much to do in too little time. Other environmental stresses are organizational politics, restrictions imposed by insurance companies, an abundance of paperwork, and cutbacks in programs. Since managed care programs have come into existence, helpers experience the stress of addressing critical needs of individual clients and families within a few sessions. Yet six or fewer sessions may be far from adequate to effectively help certain clients who require more extensive care. Helpers oftentimes feel personally responsible to provide the level of care that is necessary, but they must work within highly restrictive parameters. Attempting to accomplish the impossible in an unrealistically short time can certainly be highly stressful.

Another potential environmental stressor is the quality of your working relationships with colleagues. Dealing with co-workers and supervisors can be a source either of support or of stress. Some events can be extremely stressful, such as legal actions, financial pressures, major life transitions, threats of layoffs, and change of job responsibilities. Certain client behaviors, such as suicidal threats or attempts and severe depression, are highly stressful. Other client-induced stresses include anger toward the helper, aggression and hostility, apathy or lack of motivation, a client's premature termination, and lack of client cooperation.

Stress in an Agency Environment

Because you may well work for some kind of organization, it is useful to reflect on the major sources of frustration, dissatisfaction, and tension that are likely to be part of this work. It is also beneficial to look at ways that you can retain your power and vitality within an organization. A rehabilitation counselor who worked with veterans told us of the stress he experienced as a result of the demands placed on him by his agency to see more clients in a shorter amount of time. He felt pressured to "close a case quickly and efficiently," yet his clients often wanted more from him than he was giving. In fact, he reported that many of his clients saw him as uncaring in that he did not give them enough time. What he did not tell his clients was that he would have liked to spend more time with them. Instead, he took on full responsibility for how his clients were reacting, and he typically felt unappreciated by both his staff and his clients. Had he said more to his clients about what he was thinking and feeling, they would have had a basis to perceive him differently.

During your initial years of employment as a professional helper in an organization, it is common to experience a high level of stress and anxiety. Many helpers report that they were frustrated and disappointed about their job's unexpected stressors and demands.

We asked former students who had entered the helping professions to identify some of the main frustrations and stresses they were facing. Most of them identified the slowness of the system, the resistance of administrators and fellow staff members to new ideas, and unrealistic expectations and demands. One woman in her mid-20s made this comment:

> I get frustrated with the slow process of the system. New ideas are often overlooked. My age is a source of frustration when working with other people who will not take me seriously. Because of my age, I sometimes have difficulty gaining credibility. My biggest source of dissatisfaction, however, is watching a child that I have worked with and have seen improve go back into the system (or family) and regress to where they started.

A young social worker observed: "My greatest frustration is with the administration and its lack of support, common purpose, or teamwork."

A woman who was managing a volunteer staff of student interns had this to report:

> I am most frustrated when the staff is resistant to new ideas. Dealing with governmental bureaucracy is another major source of stress. They make it very difficult to get things done.

A social worker who was a consultant to senior managers of a bank said that she became frustrated with executives who wanted her to "fix" their employees but were not willing to see their part in the employees' problems.

Agencies often make demands that are unrealistic, especially an insistence that problems be solved quickly. For those who work with clients sent by the courts or those on probation, for instance, the helper is under pressure to see that behavioral changes take place in a specified time, so that more people can be seen, which means more funding.

Organizations tend to make too many demands on workers by reducing their autonomy, by providing little positive feedback for their job performance, and by setting policies that they feel compelled to resist. Poor management and inadequate supervision are other factors that increase workers' stress.

The Stress of Avoiding Responsibility

The impact of agency stress can actually be escalated by denying your part in learning to cope effectively with the demands of an organization. Some helpers have a tendency to blame institutions for failing to implement effective programs. At times we hear the "If only it weren't for ___" argument, which absolves the individual worker of responsibility and diminishes his or her personal power at the same time. Take a moment now to reflect on the following list of typical statements of this kind and apply them to yourself. How likely are you to resort to these statements as a way of deflecting responsibility to external sources?

- You have to play politics if you want to get your programs through.
- I can't do what I really want to do because my director or supervisor wouldn't allow it.
- If my supervisor (or co-workers) were more receptive to mental health programs, my projects would be far more successful than they are.
- I am not succeeding because my clients are not motivated.
- I cannot really say what I think because I would lose my job.
- The bureaucratic system makes it almost impossible to develop innovative and meaningful programs.
- I am not free to pursue my own interests in my job because the institution dictates what my interests will be.
- My own individuality and professional identity must be subordinate to the policies of the institution if I expect to survive in the organization.

What other statements might you make about your difficulties and sources of stress resulting from working in an organization?

Helpers who place the blame on the organization when they fail to act in accordance with their beliefs are bound to experience a growing sense of powerlessness. Some mental health workers have found a niche in the system and have learned to survive with a minimum of effort. To remain comfortable, they continue to do the same thing over and over for weeks, months, and years. They rarely question the effectiveness of their efforts or give much thought to ways of reaching a greater number of people. They neither question the system in which they are involved nor develop new projects that would give them a change of pace. Although we appreciate their difficulties and the reality that organizations can be restrictive, this complacency contributes to powerlessness and ultimately results in job stress.

Retain Power and Vitality

Although we cannot prescribe a universal method for getting along in the agency where you work, we can present some strategies we have found helpful and ask you to determine how appropriate these strategies are for you. In addition, we hope you can think of other ways to cope with the stresses associated with being part of an organization and ways to preserve your individuality.

Your first opportunity to assert your individuality is in the job interview. People being interviewed for a position often confine themselves to answering the questions asked of them. However, job interviews can be mutual exchanges in which you explore the requirements and expectations of a position and assess its suitability for yourself. It is important to recognize that accepting a position with an agency entails agreeing to work within a certain philosophical framework. By asking relevant questions, you begin to assume a stance of power, for you are exploring how much you want a particular job and what price you are willing to pay for it.

Our experience has been that most established organizations resist major attempts at change, yet small and subtle changes can be quite significant. If you devote most of your energy to trying to change the people who defend the status quo, your positive programs may become a lesser priority. You will need to decide for yourself how much energy you are willing to expend on dealing with the resistive forces you encounter. If you attempt radical, systemwide changes, you may feel overwhelmed or paralyzed. If you focus instead on making changes within the scope of your position, you will stand a better chance of extending your influence. For instance, a social worker whose goal is to correct fundamental inequities in the social welfare system may soon feel discouraged and helpless. By directing his attention to ways of dealing more humanely with the people he comes in contact with, he may experience a sense of power and accomplishment as he makes less grandiose but still significant changes. To take another example, a school counselor may give up in exasperation if she directs most of her efforts to changing her colleagues' view of their role. If she concentrates instead on defining her own role so that she can do the kind of counseling she believes in, she may succeed in making a smaller but still meaningful change.

Learn the reasons for the policies of the organization for which you work. Perhaps there are good reasons certain rules have been established, even if they seem to restrict your freedom in your job. However, if a policy is not in the best interest of your clients, you can begin to challenge the assumptions on which it is based. You can suggest alternative policies, and you can find out whether others on the staff share your view. Forming alliances with colleagues can put you in a better position to suggest changes than operating in isolation.

Establish Priorities and Cultivate Support

People often remain powerless because they do not establish their priorities and work on them systematically. We have found it helpful to first determine what we *most* want to accomplish in a given position. By ordering our priorities, we can decide which compromises we can make without sacrificing our integrity and which positions cannot be compromised in good faith. Knowing what we consider to be most important puts us in a much better position to ask for what we want. In addition, good communication with directors and supervisors is essential. We try to keep the people to whom we report informed about how we are using our time and why. Proposals often fail to be accepted not because they are unsound but because the person responsible for approving them has not been adequately informed of the rationale or design. Because supervisors or directors are the ones who will be on the receiving end of any complaints, they may thwart a plan if they haven't been convinced of its merit.

One essential element in learning how to work effectively in any organization is to realize that you are a vital part of that system: "The institution" is not something that can be divorced from you. Your relationships with other staff members are a central part of the system, and ignoring this reality and attempting to function in isolation will probably diminish your effectiveness. More positively, colleagues can be nourishing and supportive, and your interactions with them can give you a fresh perspective on some of your activities. Furthermore, genuine relationships with your co-workers can be a way of gaining power to make changes.

Although interactions with others in the institution can be energizing, they can also be debilitating, draining, and a chronic source of stress. Instead of developing support groups within an agency, some people form cliques, harbor unspoken hostility, and generally refuse to confront the conflicts or frictions that keep the staff divided. There are often hidden agendas at staff meetings, and only superficial matters are discussed while real issues are kept secret. We want to underscore the importance of finding ways to establish working relationships that enrich your professional life instead of draining your energy. It is ironic that professional helpers, who are supposed to be experts in teaching others to establish nourishing relationships, often complain that they miss meaningful contacts with their colleagues. If you feel isolated, you can decide to take the initiative and arrange for helpful interactions with others on the staff. There are resources that can nourish you if you reach out for them.

As you answer these questions, think about how you could increase your chances of assuming power in an organization while remaining true to your principles:

- What experiences have you had in encountering resistance to ideas that you wanted to put into practice?
- What would you do if the organization you worked for instituted some policies to which you were strongly opposed?
- What would you do if you believed that some fundamental changes needed to be made in your institution but your colleagues disagreed?
- What would you do if your supervisor continually blocked most of your activities, despite your efforts to keep him or her informed of the reasons for them?
- How would you attempt to make contact with other colleagues if members of your staff seemed to work largely in isolation from one another?
- If the agency staff seemed to be divided by jealousies, hostilities, or unspoken conflicts, what do you think you would do about the situation?
- If you are being asked to do things that are against your basic philosophy, what do you consider to be the ethics involved in remaining in the organization after you have done everything you can to bring about change but to no avail?

In working in an agency or an institution, your key challenge will be to maintain your own centeredness and a sense of your priorities. It is easy to become engulfed in the stresses and demands placed on you by the agency and, in the process, lose your own perspective on how your professional life fits into your total life plan. Make the time for personal reflection and find ways to keep your centeredness.

Case example.   Agencies can easily be run in dehumanizing ways, and the battle to retain your integrity is often fierce. The following interview with a social worker in a community agency in a large city gives some flavor of how endless demands can wear down a helper's stamina and lead to feelings of futility:

> Seeing clients is my primary interest. I must make progress notes after each client. These notes include descriptions of treatment methods, proof of measurable results, and assessment. We are expected to write specifically and behaviorally. There is a press for constant justification for seeing a client. On one hand, if your client improves, there is pressure from the agency to terminate work with the client. On the other hand, if the client regresses, then treatment is typically judged as ineffective. Thus, there is the hassle with the paperwork game. What some of us write may not be what we are actually doing. In the back of my mind there is the constant stress of unfinished paperwork. The expectation of the agency is that of short-term treatment. I have to deal with edicts from above, which I often find frustrating.
>
> There is also the need for professional consultation. The expectation is that an interview can be completed in an hour, yet this often takes one and a half hours. I attend staff meetings, where we talk about policies. I have to deal with staff issues about clients and case conferencing at these meetings. On top of this there are many unexpected tasks that endlessly come up. There are phone calls, checking up on clients, contacts, and networking. I have to contact parents, teachers, and school counselors in cases involving children. Quality work takes time. There is so much indirect time that does not get recognized by the agency. I spend some time in peer review and in supervising case presentations. Supervising interns is part of my job, which takes much time. I am ultimately responsible for all of the clients my interns are seeing. The push is toward direct service and for seeing many clients. The more clients we see, the more money for the agency.
>
> Part of my work involves community outreach. I must make referrals and then check up on these referrals. This involves talking with personnel at the probation department and at schools. Although much of my time is taken up by many of these indirect services, we don't get credit for these activities. For every client seen, there is much extra work. Listening to tapes of client sessions and to interns' tapes takes time. At times, there are unexpected meetings with the auditors.
>
> Because of the pressure of these unanticipated audits, we must keep current with our paperwork, which is not always realistic or possible. At times I feel overwhelmed by petty policies and procedures. Once I made a mistake on a date on a written report, and I was told that this represented a 5% level of inefficiency. This resulted in me being monitored by my supervisor for a month.
>
> There are ethical issues in submitting to the demands of a system or transgressing the demands of the system. Many of us are guilty of creative lying and stretching the truth. This involves writing reports in ways that we know will be accepted. Working in an agency involves knowing when and how to report clients. Yet reporting always means more work. Because of the extra work and time involved in the process of making reports and following up, some workers tend to avoid reporting in certain cases where they should do so.

After reading this account, consider how you can creatively and successfully cope with the demands that agencies will make on you. How can you do what you believe in and at the same time deal with the multiple demands of your job? What are your reactions to this social worker's personal account?

Understanding Stress and Burnout

When stresses are not coped with effectively, the end result can be burnout. This is a critical problem in the helping professions. Burnout is the result of severe, prolonged, and mismanaged stress. People in many different careers experience burnout, but helpers are especially vulnerable because of the nature of their involvement with people in need. Although there is no guarantee that you will remain immune, if you increase your awareness of the early warning signs of burnout and develop practical strategies for staving it off (see Chapter 15), you will be better able to respond effectively to the situation.

The Nature of Burnout

Burnout has been described as a state of physical, emotional, and mental exhaustion that results from constant or repeated emotional pressure associated with an intense, long-term involvement with people. It is characterized by feelings of helplessness and hopelessness and by a negative view of self and negative attitudes toward work, life, and other people. Maslach and Leiter (1997) define burnout as "the index of the dislocation between what people are and what they have to do. It represents an erosion in values, dignity, spirit, and will—an erosion of the human soul" (p. 17). Skovolt (2001) describes burnout as "a hemorrhaging of the self" (p. 106). According to Maslach and Leiter (1997), factors that lead to a path toward burnout are work overload, lack of control, insufficient reward, breakdown of community, unfairness, and significant value conflicts. Burnout results in personal feelings of depression, loss of morale, feelings of isolation, reduced productivity, and a decreased capacity to cope. Because their well is dry, helpers who are both physically and emotionally depleted have little to give to others.

Skovholt (2001) distinguishes between two kinds of burnout: meaning burnout and caring burnout. If you are experiencing *meaning burnout*, your work in caring for others no longer gives you sufficient meaning and purpose in life. The meaning of your work has been lost and the existential purpose for your work is not apparent. If you are experiencing *caring burnout,* your professional attachments are draining your energy. Like a battery that gets drained, eventually there is no spark left. Caring burnout is the result of a cumulative depletion of your energy to the extent that you are left without a spark. The problem of burnout is particularly critical for people working in systems or in community agencies and experiencing the stresses associated with this work. With the emphasis in this kind of work on giving to others, there is often not enough focus on giving to oneself.

Burnout, whether it be meaning or caring burnout, manifests itself in many ways. Those who experience this syndrome typically find that they are emotionally drained, exhausted, and without energy or enthusiasm. Other symptoms include a cynical attitude toward work and a loss of idealism, trust, concern, and spirit. Helpers talk of feeling pulled by their many projects, most of which seem to have lost their meaning. They feel that what they do have to offer is either not wanted or not received; they feel unappreciated, unrecognized, and unimportant. Feeling ineffective leads to a sense of inadequacy. Helpers go about their jobs in a mechanical and routine way and tend not to see any concrete results or fruits from their efforts. There is a negative shift in responses to others that is characterized by depersonalization, negative attitudes toward clients, a decline of idealism, and general irritability. Often they feel oppressed by the "system" and by institutional demands, which, they contend, stifle any sense of personal initiative. A real danger is that the burnout syndrome can feed off itself, leaving practitioners feeling more and more isolated. They may fail to reach out to one another or to develop a support system. Because burnout can rob us of the vitality we need personally and professionally, it is important to look at some of its causes, possible remedies, and ways of preventing it.

Burnout is not something that happens to you suddenly. Rather, it is an ongoing process with developmental stages. It might be helpful to think of burnout on a continuum rather than in either/or terms. In the beginning of a helping career, the worker might have the motivation to "set the world afire." As you experience the inevitable frustrations and stresses of being a professional helper, this flame may be dampened, and your initial ideals may give way to a cynical and hard view of the world.

Kottler (1993) observes that therapists who experience burnout have probably ignored the signs of their condition for months and even years. He lists a number of key symptoms of burnout: (1) when clients call to cancel, the therapist celebrates with a bit too much enthusiasm; (2) daydreaming and escapist fantasies are common; (3) there is a tendency to cope with prolonged stress by abusing drugs; (4) therapy sessions lose their excitement and spontaneity; (5) the therapist gets behind in paperwork and billings; (6) the therapist's social life suffers; and (7) there is a reluctance to explore the causes and cures of one's condition.

Professional helpers need to see that what they do is worthwhile; yet the nature of their profession is such that they often don't see immediate or concrete results. This lack of reinforcement can have a debilitating effect as counselors begin to wonder whether anything they do makes a difference to anyone. The danger of burnout is greater if helpers practice in isolation, have little interchange with fellow professionals, have demanding or disturbed clients, have few vital interests outside of work, or fail to seek an explanation of their feelings of deadness.

Professionals who limit their work to one type of activity are particularly susceptible to burnout. Many therapists who work alone in their own practice report that they often get caught in the routine of seeing client after client. They find it increasingly difficult to be fully present for their clients, especially when it seems that they are dealing with the same kind of problem over and over. After a while they may well find themselves responding almost mechanically. It may be difficult to rectify this situation if one's livelihood seems to depend on maintaining one's own private practice. Nevertheless, therapists need to question whether sticking to one kind of practice is worth the price they often pay in lack of excitement.

Some Causes of Burnout

There is no single cause of burnout; rather, it is a condition that results from a combination of stressful factors. Burnout is best understood by considering the individual, interpersonal, and organizational factors that contribute to it. Recognizing the causes of burnout can be the first step toward dealing with it. These situations often lead to burnout:

- Doing the same type of work with little variation
- Giving a great deal personally and not getting back much in the way of appreciation or other positive responses
- Lacking a sense of accomplishment and meaning in your work
- Being under constant and strong pressure to produce, perform, and meet deadlines—many of which may be unrealistic
- Working with a difficult population, such as highly resistant clients, involuntary clients, or those who show very little progress or change
- Continuing conflict and tension among staff; an absence of support from colleagues and an abundance of criticism
- Lacking trusting relationships between supervisors and mental health workers, creating conflict rather than teamwork toward commonly valued goals
- Lacking opportunities for personal expression or for taking initiative in trying new approaches; a situation in which experimentation, change, and innovations not only are not rewarded but are actively discouraged
- Continuing dissatisfaction with agency goals and few opportunities to create new goals
- Providing substandard services to clients
- Having unrealistic demands on your time and energy
- Having personally and professionally taxing work without much opportunity for supervision, continuing education, or other forms of in-service training
- Experiencing unresolved personal conflicts beyond the job situation, such as marital tensions or chronic health or financial problems

A number of writers have identified major sources of stress that frequently result in burnout. Kramen-Kahn and Hansen (1998) identify business aspects, economic uncertainty, professional conflicts, time pressures, sense of enormous responsibility, excessive workload, and caseload uncertainties as the most frequently endorsed occupational hazards of psychotherapists. According to Brown and O'Brien (1998), sources of stress that often lead to burnout for crisis intervention and other frontline mental health workers include a lack of full involvement in the decision-making process related to work; feelings that their abilities are not being fully utilized on the job; being taxed by regulations, procedures, and paperwork; and being exposed to discomfort and dangers in their work setting. Sapienza and Bugental (2000) believe one of the main causes of burnout is the pressure of assuming the responsibility of curing the client. Lazarus (2000) views avarice and greed as the major stressors in a therapist's life. Striving to make more and more money often increases work-related pressures and emotional strain. Lazarus emphasizes how essential it is for professionals to replenish themselves. The challenge is to create a style of life that enables professionals to nourish themselves so that they can prevent distress and burnout.

Rather than looking at burnout as something that may afflict you, consider the role you may play in increasing your risk of burnout. Certain personality traits and characteristics can increase your risk factor. Some individual factors such as a compelling need for approval, feeling unappreciated, and striving for unrealistically high goals can increase your risk for burnout. Interpersonal and organizational factors are also causes of burnout.

Individual Factors

Helpers play a role in creating their own burnout. The chances for burnout rise if the person is younger, less self-confident, impulsive, impatient, and dependent on others for approval and affection and has goals and aspirations that are out of tune with reality (Maslach, 1982).

Feeling needed.   In Chapter 1 we talked about the helper's need to be needed. This need can work for or against you. There is a considerable expenditure of energy in thinking about and taking care of those who need you. If this need is great, you may find yourself a prisoner of the demands you have created for yourself based on your own needs. As you are starting out and building a practice, you may be flattered by those who are seeking your help. Indeed, it feels psychologically affirming to be sought after and needed. You may also become impressed with the economic rewards associated with helping people. The temptation is there to not turn away people, for both emotional and financial reasons. Some helpers have a difficult time taking a vacation, especially when they calculate the lost income. Soon these helpers forget that they, too, have needs, which are probably not being met because of their overinvolvement with others and their overcommitments. There are limits to how much you can take on without paying a price in terms of your physical, mental, and emotional health.

Feeling unappreciated.   A major theme heard by those who are suffering from burnout is that they do not feel recognized for who they are or what they do, that they receive little positive feedback, and that they do not feel that their dedication is appreciated. In such a setting helpers are bound to lose their striving for excellence eventually. This lack of recognition is compounded by the fact that you may have entered the helping professions because of your need for recognition and appreciation. You may be sincerely devoted to helping others, yet your efforts may seem meager at times. You will hear more often about what you are failing to do and about your deficiencies than about what you have done well. If appreciation is lacking on the job, it is difficult over a period of time to know whether what you are doing really makes a difference to anyone. This process tends to erode both your ideals and your enthusiasm, which leads to demoralization.

The real challenge is to learn ways of working for your own appreciation and self-worth. Unless you want to depend on clients or colleagues to give you positive feedback and confirmation, it is imperative that you give yourself the appreciation that you might be seeking from others.

Feeling uninspired.   An important factor in burnout is whether your ideals are working for you or against you. In our experience, those who set high goals for themselves seem to have a high need for recognition. They also tend to have high expectations of others. As long as helpers feel satisfied by their efforts, their energy level remains high. But when these helpers get stuck in routine patterns and do not see the fruits of their efforts, they are likely to experience a sense of restlessness.

Most mental health professionals were initially attracted to their careers in large part because of their hope of making a significant difference in the lives of others. One sign of burnout is the dulling of these ideals and the loss of caring about others. The idealism embodied in the desire to help everyone can sometimes be transformed into feelings of cynicism. The ideals that you hold when you begin your career can be a positive force, and this idealism can also be a direct path toward burnout. Your idealism can result in brainstorming ideas that are translated into new projects. Yet if you are not careful, you can get carried away with your enthusiasm and immerse yourself in your work and projects. If your total worth as a person hinges on your projects' bearing fruit, you may experience personal devastation when they cease being rewarding.

The problem of tarnished idealism increases as you come into contact with cynical colleagues who are threatened by your enthusiasm. A seasoned staff member may tear down your ideals and try to convince you that you, too, will harden yourself to painful reality. Your co-workers may tell you of all the things that simply won't work. It is difficult to stay creative and excited in a job environment where those around you are continually chipping away at your efforts to make a difference. If you constantly hear that your proposals for change won't work and if you are without real support for your ideas, you are likely to face psychological erosion, and you might eventually join the ranks of your soured peers. Faced with this onslaught of negative input, many beginners start to doubt themselves and their competence. If you are beginning as a helper, you probably already have many self-doubts. If these doubts are reinforced, you may soon feel disillusioned.

A young man we know recently graduated with a bachelor's degree in psychology and worked briefly in a residential home for adolescents. Paul was greatly disillusioned when he encountered deeply entrenched cynicism in this facility. He quickly learned that both the residents and the staff were committed to the status quo. The apathy he saw in the staff discouraged him and led him to wonder if he wanted to pursue this field.

If you work in an environment where you receive negative bombardment, you would do well to actively seek some source of support either in your job setting or away from it. It would be a mistake to wait for the agency to create this support for you, so ask colleagues to join you in making the time for regular meetings. Learning the fine balance between idealism and realism is essential if you hope to survive as a helping professional.

Interpersonal and Organizational Factors

Maslach and Leiter (1997) tend to focus on the organizational factors, or the social environment, as the prime cause of burnout, rather than placing the blame or responsibility on the individual. The hallmark of the burnout syndrome is a shift in the way professionals view the people they are helping. They change from feeling positive and caring to feeling negative and uncaring. Continuous contact with clients who are unappreciative, upset, and depressed often leads helpers to view all recipients in helping relationships in negative terms. Practitioners may care less, begin to make derogatory comments about their clients, ignore them, and want to move away from them. Dehumanized responses are a core ingredient of burnout. According to Maslach and Leiter, organizations have the power and the resources to do a great deal to prevent burnout

One counselor in an agency notices that she is on the path toward burnout when she becomes too involved with her clients' struggles:

> Sometimes I'm unable to escape personal issues that arise when my clients' problems trigger issues similar to my own. This affects me in a positive way in that it holds me accountable within my own life and keeps me moving toward the best person I can become. Sometimes it affects me negatively when I become overly self-critical.

A vicious circle is operating here. If you get an abundance of negative reactions from others, you will tend to become self-critical and wonder if you are making any difference to those you are supposedly helping. Being critical of and unkind to yourself usually leads to being critical of and unkind to others.

The impact that people around you have should not be overlooked. If you are part of an institutional setting, the quality of your contacts with co-workers and supervisors is extremely important. Co-workers can be helpful in providing support for you, but if there is no climate of trust and openness in the work setting, you become more vulnerable to burnout. If these relationships are strained and the atmosphere is hostile and unsupportive, the chances of burnout are increased.

When we consulted at a state mental hospital, we found that many workers were suffering from burnout. They claimed to have difficult clients, a difficult administration, and difficult colleagues. If you find yourself in a similar situation with this combination of factors, you are in trouble. To help these workers at the state facility, we taught them to seek out others with whom they could talk.

The Experience of Burnout

Burnout is not a simple phenomenon. Helpers are affected in many ways by the strains of constant interaction with people in need of help. As an example, let's consider the case of a counselor named Daniel, who is suffering from many of the symptoms of burnout.

Physically, Daniel is fatigued most of the time. He has accepted an increased caseload and works long hours. He exercises very little because of a lack of time, does not have time to eat regularly or properly, and is so wrapped up in his work that he does not sleep well. He finds it a real chore to get up in the morning. He suffers from headaches that just will not go away as well as a range of other health problems that stem from his stressful lifestyle.

Intellectually, Daniel has lost his curiosity and desire to question or learn. Although when he was in graduate school he enjoyed sharing and discussing ideas about human behavior and counseling, now he cannot be bothered by argumentation, discussion, and revision of his ideas. With all the pressures at work, he finds no time to read or take courses to keep abreast of developments in the field. Instead, he hopes to find quick remedies to deal with the crisis situations that he faces in his daily work.

Emotionally, Daniel has spent so much time focusing on the emotional needs of others that he has failed to recognize his own needs. At one time he was able to provide nurturance for others, yet by chronically neglecting his need for expression he has become indifferent in his professional life and withdrawn from those he loves in his personal life. He is isolated and unable to feel either pain or joy. He feels very alone at work, and he tends to blame himself for not doing well. Because he is not feeling a sense of personal accomplishment, his view of his own worth is also declining. He experiences an increasing sense of wanting to get away from demands and pressures.

Interpersonally, Daniel has lost interest in being with others. He feels "peopled out" and is relieved when clients cancel. He sometimes "forgets" his appointments with clients and fails to show up for staff meetings. When he began his career, Daniel had high hopes of making an impact on the lives of others. Now his ideals are tarnished, and his motivation is low. His job performance is deteriorating, and much of the time he is indifferent. His family is also suffering from his burnout, for he shrinks away from involvement with his wife and children. He just wants everybody to leave him alone and make no more demands on him. He feels emotionally dry and has little energy to listen to what they might want from him. Even minor requests are heard as demands that only burden him more.

Daniel has paid a steep price for ignoring the stressful circumstances that resulted in his indifference. Not only has he become an impaired professional, but he is suffering in his personal life as well. By withdrawing from his friends, family, and co-workers, he has cut off all sources of possible nourishment.

The Impaired Professional

Burnout often contributes to the making of an impaired practitioner. Guy (1987) defines impairment as the "diminution or deterioration of therapeutic skills and abilities due to factors which have sufficiently impacted the personality of the therapist to result in potential incompetence" (p. 199). Impairment can also be viewed as the presence of an illness or severe psychological depletion that is likely to block a professional from being able to deliver effective services, which results in consistently functioning below acceptable practice standards. A number of factors can negatively influence a professional's effectiveness, both personally and professionally, including substance abuse, physical illness, and burnout. Impaired professionals are unable to effectively cope with stressful events, and they are also unable to adequately carry out their professional duties. Those practitioners whose inner conflicts are consistently activated by client material may respond by trying to stabilize themselves rather than facilitating the growth of their clients.

Impaired practitioners clearly contribute to the suffering of their clients rather than alleviating it. For example, sexually exploitive behavior by counselors is often a manifestation of impairment (Emerson & Markos, 1996). Counselors who become sexually involved with clients show personality patterns similar to those of impaired counselors. These shared characteristics include:

- Fragile self-esteem
- Difficulty establishing intimacy in one's personal life
- Professional isolation
- A need to rescue clients
- A need for reassurance about one's attractiveness
- Substance abuse

Because a common characteristic of impairment is denial, professional colleagues may need to confront the irresponsible behavior of an impaired counselor. Herlihy (1996) suggests confronting the impaired counselor with sensitivity, respect, and preparedness.

What are the mental health professions doing to address the difficulties of impaired helping professionals? Barnett and Hillard (2001) conducted a survey of all 59 state and provincial psychological associations (SPPAs). The findings of their survey showed that between 1998 and 1999, 69% of these associations (41 out of 59) reported that a colleague assistance program did not exist for distressed or impaired psychologists. Of these 41 SPPAs, 24% reported that a formal colleague assistance program had been available in the past. Some of the most common reasons given for discontinuing such a program included lack of use (70%), risk of liability too great (10%), and lack of volunteer support (10%). Furthermore, 61% of these 41 SPPAs reported that there were no plans to develop a program in the future, and 54% stated that a need for such recourses was not perceived by the SPPA leadership. The authors of this survey indicate that the profession has been slow to address issues of helper impairment. They suggest that the profession of psychology might emulate the lead of other healing professions that have effective means of preventing, identifying, and treating professional impairment.

Certainly, the lack of leadership from the profession needs to be addressed, but it is ethically imperative that impaired professionals recognize and deal with their impairment regardless of this lack. It is our view that licensing boards could require personal therapy in cases where counselor impairment becomes obvious. Of course, we hope that practitioners themselves will realize that they need therapy for themselves and welcome the opportunity to deal with problems that are keeping them stuck in dysfunctional patterns.

Although we emphasize the personal responsibility of helpers in learning to cope with stress and in preventing burnout, we agree with one of the doctoral students who reviewed our book, who addressed the role of professional organizations and agencies in taking steps to address problems that often lead to burnout:

> I believe that many of our mental health delivery systems are in need of reform, not only for the sake of clients but also for the sake of practitioners. I would like to

see our professional organizations challenged to take a greater role in protecting practitioners as well as clients. We know that many systems are inefficient at best. At their worst, some of them can be harmful to direct service personnel they employ. Personal responsibility on the part of the frontline worker is paramount, indeed. Nevertheless, our professional organizations need to evolve beyond the guild mentality, whose primary purpose is self-protection. Real and meaningful activism and pressure on agencies may be required to reform the trend of hanging the helper out to dry, not to mention the client, in the service of keeping the agency afloat. (Jamie Bludworth, personal communication, April 8, 2001)

Stress can lead to burnout and impairment, but this is not an incurable disease. Rather, it may be helpful to view it in much the same way as you would a virus that infects you because of a weakening of your immune system. You need not be helpless. Just as you are able to cure a disease resulting from a virus, you are also able to cope with the outcome of burnout. In the final chapter we discuss how you can manage stress, prevent burnout, take care of yourself, and retain your vitality as a person and as a professional.

By Way of Review

- One of the hazards of the helping professions is that helpers are typically not very good at asking for help for themselves.

- It is wise to sensitize yourself to both the external and internal factors that contribute to your experience of stress.

- One of the major environmental sources of job stress is the friction that arises out of working in an organization.

- There is a heavy price to pay for being a professional caregiver. No one is immune from the cost of caring for others.

- Being a professional helper often reopens your own psychological wounds. If you are not willing to work on your unfinished business, you might reconsider whether you want to accompany clients on their journey of dealing with their past wounds.

- Most helpers enter their profession with a high degree of idealism. Later, these ideals are sometimes tempered with realism. The danger is that idealism can be transformed into cynicism, which is a step away from burnout.

- There is no single cause of burnout; rather, a combination of individual, interpersonal, and organizational factors lead to burnout. Understanding these factors can help you learn how to prevent or cope with burnout.

- Burnout is often the result of the many demands placed on you by an agency. It is important to learn specific ways of surviving with dignity in an agency setting.

• The impaired professional is an issue that the helping professions seriously need to address. Impairment is frequently the result of long-standing patterns of being burned out and not dealing with the condition.

• Coping with stress effectively is a way to lessen the chances of becoming an impaired helper.

What Will You Do Now?

1. Make a list of some of the environmental factors that are most stressful in your life. Once you have identified external stressors, write in your journal about how you might deal with them differently. What can you do now to minimize at least some of these sources of stress? Develop a plan of action, and try it out for at least a week. Consider making a contract with someone so that you will be accountable for acting to reduce stress in your life.

2. We encourage you to look at the factors in you that are most likely to cause burnout. A common denominator in many cases of burnout is the question of *responsibility*. Helpers may feel fully responsible for what their clients do or don't do; they may assume too much responsibility for the direction of therapy; or they may have extremely high expectations of themselves. How does this description apply to you? In what ways could your assumption of an inordinate degree of responsibility contribute to your burnout?

3. Identify a few of the warning signs that you are not taking care of yourself or that you are close to burnout. For example, you might not be getting adequate sleep, you might be ignoring exercise, or you might be experiencing a variety of physical symptoms. Are you willing to assume responsibility for eliminating something that you are doing that is contributing to your level of fatigue?

4. Arrange an interview with a practicing professional, and ask this person these questions: "What are some of the major stresses you face in your work?" "What are some ways you deal with these stresses?" "What are your thoughts on preventing burnout?"

5. Reflect on the patterns of stress you experience in your life. Think about your responses to the sources-of-stress checklist and the other information presented in this chapter. How do you think stress affects all areas of your life? What are you likely to do to cope with these sources of stress? In your journal, keep track of some stressful activities for a few weeks. Think about practical ways to minimize your stress in a few situations, especially by changing your reactions to them. Try out these new ideas, and write down your observations.

6. For the full bibliographic entry for each of the sources listed here, consult the References and Reading List at the back of the book. One of the best single

sources that deals with burnout and self-care strategies is Skovholt's (2001) book, *The Resilient Practitioner*. Another excellent resource is Maslach and Leiter (1997), *The Truth about Burnout,* which deals with how organizations cause personal stress and what they can do about preventing it. For a discussion of how stress affects your health, see Rice (1999) and G. Corey and Corey (2002). See Kottler (1993) and Guy (1987) for discussions of how stress affects the personal and professional lives of helpers. Kottler's (1997) edited book, *Finding Your Way as a Counselor,* contains a number of excellent articles on topics pertaining to the special demands of those in the helping professions.

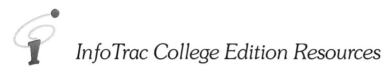

InfoTrac College Edition Resources

For additional readings, explore InfoTrac College Edition, our online library. Go to http://www.infotrac.college.com/wadsworth and select these key word searches:

    counselor W1 stress
    therap* impairment
    impaired W1 therapist
    mental AND health AND burnout

Key words are listed in a format that enables the search engine to locate a wider range of articles in the online university library. Key words should be entered exactly as shown, including asterisks, "W1," "W2," "AND," and other search engine tools.

CHAPTER *15*

Take Care of Yourself

Focus Questions

1. What are some specific ways in which you cope with the stresses you experience? How effective is your stress management?

2. Helpers sometimes engage in a self-defeating internal dialogue. For instance, they may expect that they will be perfect and may burden themselves with fears of making mistakes. What are some examples of your own internal dialogue that may not serve you well? How good are you at challenging self-defeating attitudes and beliefs?

3. It has been said that either you control stress or stress controls you. How would you apply this maxim to yourself at this time in your life?

4. How well do you utilize your time? What are some ways to better organize your time to achieve your priorities?

5. What are some specific ways to lessen the chances of burnout? How can you remain alive both as a person and as a helper?

Aim of the Chapter

In the previous chapter we examined how stress affects you in both your personal and your professional life and how chronically stressful patterns put you on a path toward burnout. This chapter deals with the challenge you face as a helper in retaining your vitality. We will focus on specific strategies for coping with stress effectively but, even more, on developing attitudes, thought patterns, and specific action plans geared to changing your lifestyle so you will be oriented toward health. Staying alive as a person and as a professional is not something that happens automatically; it is the result of a commitment to acquiring habits of thinking and action that promote soundness of mind and body.

It is unrealistic to think that you can eliminate stress from either your personal life or your professional life, but you do not have to be the victim of stress. You can recognize how you are being affected by stress and make decisions about how to think, feel, and behave in stressful situations. You can become aware of your destructive reactions to stress and learn constructive ways of coping with it. In short, you can learn to manage and control stress rather than being controlled by it.

As you saw in Chapter 14, it is important to become aware of both external and internal factors that contribute to negative physical and psychological reactions. Probably the best way to approach stress management is to develop a multipronged strategy tailored to your individual personality and unique situation. Good training programs do not promote a simple formula or a "cookbook" approach for coping with stress. An effective program should be future-oriented, preparing you to adapt particular strategies to various stressful life situations as they arise. You also need to be prepared for inevitable setbacks. Your program should help you identify sources of possible failure and prepare for them. It is essential to stick with your program if you hope to see long-term positive results.

Taking a course on stress management would be an ideal way to learn and apply specific coping skills. If you are interested in learning more about the details of preventive and combative approaches to managing stress, you can carefully select some self-help books, of which there are an increasing number. As with many other endeavors, merely reading about stress management is not enough to combat some of the stresses you face. It is essential that you regularly practice the stress management techniques that you read about, and we encourage you to develop your own strategies for managing stressful experiences. Now, let's take a look at some strategies you might consider.

Cognitive Approaches to Stress Management

Our beliefs largely determine how we interpret events. Therefore, events are not the cause of our stress; it is the meaning we give to these events that regulates our stress level. Albert Ellis, the founder of rational emotive behavior therapy (REBT) and a precursor of cognitive therapy, cites the Stoic philosopher Epictetus: "Men are disturbed not by things, but by the views that they take of them." Cognitive therapists have developed approaches to help people become aware of their cognitions—the dialogue that goes on inside of them—and how their thinking affects how they feel and act. The cognitive approaches offer specific strategies to clients for challenging and changing self-defeating cognitions and for developing sound thinking that leads to less stressful living. In this section we draw heavily from the writings of Ellis and other cognitive therapists, especially Aaron Beck, in presenting the strategies cognitive therapists use that can help you manage stress.

All of us engage in self-defeating thinking and ineffective self-talk from time to time. If you can recognize the nature of your irrational beliefs and understand how they lead to problems, you can begin to convert self-defeating cognitions into self-enhancing ones. In much of the rest of this chapter we discuss cognitive approaches that shed light on how you create much of your own stress by the beliefs you hold and the statements you make to yourself. Because you have this capacity to create stress, you also have the means to lessen its impact. Cognitive strategies can be employed to retain your vitality on both the personal and professional levels, and we describe several approaches to this work. Our examples will be geared primarily to situations that you are likely to encounter in your work as a helping professional.

The A-B-C Theory

Ellis has developed what he calls his A-B-C theory of irrational thinking (Ellis, 1999, 2001b). This theory explains the relationship among events, beliefs, and feelings. According to Ellis, your interpretations of events are frequently more important than what occurs in reality. He calls A an Activating event, B one's Belief system, and C the emotional Consequence. Consider the situation of applying for a new job in an agency and going through an interview. Let's imagine the worst scene. The director of the agency who interviewed you kindly tells you that she does not think you would fit well in the agency. She is not really impressed with your training and experience. You do not get this job, which you badly wanted. The activating event (A) in this case is the situation of being rejected. The (C) is the emotional consequences you experience. If you feel depressed, hurt, let down, and even devastated, the chances are that you hold what Ellis would term "irrational beliefs" about not having been accepted. For example, your beliefs (B) about this rejection might be some combination of the following thoughts: "It is absolutely horrible that I didn't get this job, and it surely proves that I'm incompetent." "I should have gotten this job, and this rejection is unbearable." "I must succeed at every important endeavor, or I'm really worthless." "I failed in this interview; it's a sure sign that I will fail in any other interview I might have." "This rejection means I'm a total failure."

Rational emotive and other cognitive-behavioral therapies are grounded on the premise that emotional and behavioral disturbances are originally learned by the inculcation of irrational beliefs from significant others during our childhood, as well as by our creative inventing of irrational dogmas and superstitions. However, we actively reinstill false beliefs by the processes of autosuggestion and self-repetition (Ellis, 1999, 2001b). It is largely our own repetition of these early-indoctrinated irrational thoughts, rather than a parent's repetition, that keeps dysfunctional attitudes alive within us. Therefore, we mainly have ourselves to hold accountable when we feel and act miserably over our performance as helpers.

To complete the A-B-C model of Ellis (1999, 2001b), we look briefly at D, which is the process of actively and forcefully Disputing irrational beliefs that lead to negative emotional reactions, many of which are stressful. If you are successful in this process of disputing and in substituting constructive thinking for destructive thinking, then you have a basis for thinking, feeling, and acting differently. Thus, instead of feeling depressed about a loss, you can put it in a new perspective and feel appropriately disappointed. Instead of feeling devastated by the lack of universal approval, you can feel appropriately hurt if a significant person rejects you. By changing your beliefs, you also change your feelings, which is a useful way of learning to reduce stress.

Ellis (1999, 2001b) contends that we have the power to control our emotional destiny. He suggests that when we are upset it is well to look to our hidden dogmatic "musts" and absolutistic "shoulds." For Ellis, practically all human misery and serious emotional turmoil is unnecessary. As thinking human beings, we have the ability to observe our beliefs to see how our absolutistic demands and musts largely *create* our destructive feelings and behaviors. Our challenge is to change these demands into strong *preferences* instead of grandiose, unrealistic commands. Because we have the capacity for self-awareness, we can observe and evaluate our goals and purposes and, thus, can change them (Ellis, 1988, 1999, 2001a, 2001b; Ellis & Dryden, 1997; Ellis & Harper, 1997; Ellis & MacClaren, 1998).

Identifying Self-Defeating Internal Dialogue

Those of us who are human services providers often incorporate a wide range of dysfunctional beliefs that impair our capacity to function as effectively as we might with those who seek our assistance. For example, at times we may distort the processing of information, which can easily lead to faulty assumptions and misconceptions. As a helper, you can complicate your life through the process of telling yourself that you must be all-knowing, superhuman, totally congruent, and perfect. If you feel depressed, agitated, or otherwise miserable about the job you are doing, it is essential that you examine your basic assumptions and beliefs to determine how they are influencing what you are doing and how you are feeling. As you become attuned to identifying your faulty thinking, you are in a position to change such patterns (Beck, 1976, 1987; Corey, 2001c; Ellis & Dryden, 1997). Here are a few statements that we often hear helping professionals utter: "I am fully responsible for my clients' outcomes." "I must be successful with every client." "If a client discontinues, it is always my fault." "I should be able to help my clients more." "I must always be available for anyone who needs me." "If a client is in pain, I should take it away." "I should know everything." "If I make a mistake, that means I'm a failure." "Referring a client means that I am inadequate." "If a couple divorces, I was not helpful enough." "I depend on my clients to love and appreciate me to feel worthwhile."

Statements such as these are repeated endlessly by helpers, and as you can see, most of them refer to feelings of inadequacy, a nagging belief that one should be more, and a chronic sense of self-doubt. By assuming the giant share of responsibility for your clients, you are relieving them of the responsibility to direct their own lives, in addition to creating stress for yourself. Read these irrational belief statements again, and underline those statements that you hear yourself making. Do you tend to make any other related statements, especially with regard to your role in assuming responsibility for being the "perfect" helper? What are some examples of other things you say to yourself that often get you into trouble? What are some other beliefs you hold that tend to create stress for you?

Changing Distorted and Self-Defeating Thinking

Aaron Beck developed an approach known as cognitive therapy, which has a number of similarities to rational emotive behavior therapy. Beck (1976, 1987) contends that people with emotional difficulties tend to commit characteristic "logical errors" that tilt objective reality in the direction of self-deprecation. Cognitive therapy perceives psychological problems as stemming from commonplace processes such as faulty thinking, making incorrect inferences on the basis of inadequate or incorrect information, and failing to distinguish between fantasy and reality. A number of systematic errors in reasoning may lead to such faulty assumptions and misconceptions, which are termed *cognitive distortions* (Beck & Weishaar, 2000; Dattilio & Freeman, 1992). Let's examine a few of these errors.

• *Arbitrary inferences* refer to making conclusions without supporting and relevant evidence. This includes "catastrophizing," or thinking of the absolute worst scenario and outcomes for most situations. You might begin your first job as a counselor with the conviction that you will not be liked or valued by either your colleagues or your clients. You are convinced that you fooled your professors and somehow just managed to get your degree, but now people will certainly see through you!

• *Selective abstraction* consists of forming conclusions based on an isolated detail of an event. In this process other information is ignored, and the significance of the total context is missed. The assumption is that the events that matter are those dealing with failure and deprivation. As a counselor, you might measure your worth by your errors and weaknesses, not by your successes.

• *Overgeneralization* is a process of holding extreme beliefs on the basis of a single incident and applying them inappropriately to dissimilar events or settings. If you have difficulty working with one adolescent, for example, you might conclude that you will not be effective in counseling any adolescents. You might also conclude that you will not be effective in working with *any* clients!

• *Magnification and minimization* consist of perceiving a case or situation in a greater or lesser light than it truly deserves. You might make this cognitive error by assuming that even minor mistakes you make in counseling a client could easily create a crisis for the individual and might even result in psychological damage.

• *Personalization* is a tendency for individuals to relate external events to themselves, even when there is no basis for making this connection. If a client does not return for a second counseling session, you might be absolutely convinced that this absence is due to your terrible performance during the initial session. You might tell yourself, "I really let that client down, and now she may never seek help again!"

• *Labeling and mislabeling* involve portraying one's identity on the basis of imperfections and mistakes made in the past and allowing them to define one's true identity. Thus, if you are not able to live up to all of a client's expectations, you might say to yourself, "I'm totally worthless and should turn my degree in right away!"

• *Polarized thinking* involves thinking and interpreting in all-or-nothing terms, or categorizing experiences in either/or extremes. With such dichotomous thinking, events are labeled in black or white terms. You might give yourself no latitude for being an imperfect person and imperfect counselor. You might view yourself as either being the perfectly competent helper (which means you always succeed with all clients) or as a total flop if you are not fully competent (which means there is no room for any mistakes).

• *Language errors and negative thoughts* often produce stress. By becoming aware of the quality of your language, you can get some idea of how your self-talk influences you. Here are some examples of negative thinking:

- I *must* act competently in all situations, and I *must* win people's approval.
- I *can't stand* making mistakes. They prove I'm a total failure.
- I *must* be brilliant, and I *must* perform well at all times. If I'm ever less than brilliant, this is *horrible.*
- I *should* always put the interests of other people before my own. My mission is to help others, and I *shouldn't* be selfish.
- I *ought* to be available when anybody needs me. If I'm not, this shows that I'm not a caring person and that I've probably chosen the wrong profession.

The most direct way to change dysfunctional emotions and behaviors is to modify inaccurate and dysfunctional thinking (Beck, 1976). The cognitive therapist teaches clients how to identify these distorted and dysfunctional cognitions through a process of evaluation. Through a collaborative effort, clients learn to discriminate between their own thoughts and events that occur in reality. They learn the influence that cognition has on their feelings and behaviors and even on environmental events. Clients are taught to recognize, observe, and monitor their own thoughts and assumptions, especially their negative automatic thoughts.

Learning how to answer and to dispute your self-defeating thinking entails identifying your core negative thoughts. Review the common cognitive distortions we have discussed, and think about statements you might be inclined to make that contain these errors. How often do you create stress in yourself with such thoughts? After you have identified a few core self-defeating beliefs, begin to answer them. Answering faulty beliefs is best done by vigorous disputation. One method for disputing unfounded beliefs is illustrated in these examples wherein we provide a dysfunctional belief, a disputation, and a constructive belief.

SELF-STATEMENT: I should always be available for anyone who needs me. If I'm not, this shows that I'm not a caring person.

DISPUTATION: Why must I always be available? Where is it written that if I am not always there when a client wants me I am not a caring person?

CONSTRUCTIVE BELIEF: Although I want to be responsible, there are limits. Sometimes clients may have exaggerated needs. There are times when I may not be emotionally available for all clients.

SELF-STATEMENT: I should be able to do everything well, which means being perfect. Either I'm the perfect helper, or I am worthless.

DISPUTATION: Where did I pick up this belief? Does it make any sense that I should do everything well the first time? Can I do some things less than perfectly and still be outstanding in other areas?

CONSTRUCTIVE BELIEF: Although I like doing well, I can accept imperfection in myself. I can tolerate mistakes. I do not have to be perfect to be capable. Since perfection is an unrealistic ideal, I will be "perfectly satisfied" with being a fallible human.

SELF-STATEMENT: I should always put the interests of other people before my own.

DISPUTATION: Who told me this? Is it really wrong to be concerned about myself? Can't I have self-interests and still be interested in others?

CONSTRUCTIVE BELIEF: I can't show more interest in others than I have for myself. If I don't take care of myself, the chances are slim that I'll be able to be concerned about the interests of others.

Awareness is the first step in self-change, followed by learning how to dispute self-defeating thinking. However, merely identifying faulty beliefs and learning to make functional statements will not alone ensure change. For change to occur, it is essential that you take *action*. You need to test reality and act on your new thoughts and beliefs. For example, assume that you have convinced yourself that your failure to get a certain job does not mean that you are a failure as a person. You can act on this belief by taking the risk of applying for another job that interests you. If you are afraid of people's disapproval, you can put yourself in situations where approval will not always be forthcoming. If you have convinced yourself that making a mistake as a helper is not horrible, you can allow yourself to make a mistake and not feel devastated. Rather than avoiding doing new things that you have wanted to do, you might seek out some of these new ventures and take the chance of being less than perfect.

At times you will have to force yourself to act in new ways that are not comfortable for you if you hope to challenge self-limiting assumptions. For instance, if you have been avoiding giving talks to community groups because you are afraid that you will look like a fool, it might be important to challenge yourself by giving some of these speeches in spite of your fears. The point is that your new beliefs need to be put into action, and this is the hard part in making these changes.

If you hope to prevent stress from controlling you, you need to take an active stance in recognizing how your stresses lead to personal depletion and how they eventually lead to burnout. If you give of yourself continually and ignore the signs of stress and the toll it is taking, you will eventually find that your well runs dry. To be able to give to others, it is essential that you take care of yourself. Skovholt (2001) reminds us that sustaining the personal self requires a constant investment so that we do not become stagnant. Self-care means finding ways to replenish the self: "Personal self-care should focus in part on producing feelings of zest, peace, euphoria, excitement, happiness, and pleasure" (p. 147).

We hope you will make some decisions about specific ways you can better manage stress in your life. You can begin by monitoring how you are affected by stress, and you can follow up by applying some of the specific preventive and combative strategies for stress management that we have discussed. Perhaps one of the major challenges you will face is to retain your vitality and a sense of personal power in the organization where you work. The multiple demands from the agency and your clients can make it difficult to retain a spirit of believing that you are making a difference.

Time Management as a Strategy for Coping With Stress

We often hear students complaining that there are simply not enough hours in the day and night to do everything they want to do. Ask yourself the degree to which you are satisfied with how you are balancing your needs for work and for leisure. How well do you manage to meet your responsibilities at school, at work, and at home? Are you able to keep up with your studies and still maintain a social life? Is life only work, or do you make any time for play? Is life only play, and do you put off work lest it get in the way of your fun? Time is one thing we have in common, for we all have the same amount of time: 24 hours a day, 168 hours a week, and 8,736 hours a year. How you manage this time to your best advantage is a very individual matter, and it is also a good indicator of what you value. We offer some suggestions for ways of keeping better track of what you are doing, what you want to be doing, and what you might do differently.

Before you continue reading, spend a few minutes taking this time management inventory. It will help you assess the danger signals of poor allocation of time. Read each statement, decide whether it is more true or more false as it applies to you, and rate it accordingly with a "T" or an "F."

_____ 1. I often feel confused and unsure of where I am going.
_____ 2. At the end of most days I am amazed at how little I have accomplished.
_____ 3. I have a hard time getting to important tasks and sticking with them.
_____ 4. I often find myself taking on tasks because I am the only one who can do them.
_____ 5. I often feel overwhelmed because I try to do too much in too little time.
_____ 6. No matter how much I do, I feel that I am always behind and never quite caught up.
_____ 7. I find that I am working longer and longer and sometimes wonder if I am accomplishing much.

____ 8. I frequently miss deadlines.

____ 9. I simply have too many irons in the fire.

____ 10. It is very easy for me to put off until tomorrow what I know needs to be done today.

____ 11. I am bothered by many unscheduled interruptions when I am trying to do important work.

____ 12. I am aware of hurrying much of the time and often feel hassled.

____ 13. I just don't have time to attend to important things, because I get lost in dealing with one crisis after another.

____ 14. I tend to be a perfectionist, and this leaves me never feeling satisfied with what I am accomplishing.

____ 15. I feel guilty about leaving work behind me.

If you are interested in making better use of your time, the best place to begin is by monitoring how you are spending time. See whether there are any patterns in the way you are using your time. Are you able to identify particular ways in which you are wasting time? What most gets in the way of effectively using the time you have? If at the end of a day you often find yourself wondering where your time went, you can probably benefit by doing a time study. Several times a day, stop to record what you have done in each half-hour period and how much time it took. At the end of each week simply look for patterns. Ask yourself questions such as "Where is most of my time going?" "Am I enjoying most of the things I do?" "Is there a way that I could cut out some of the things I'm doing, especially if they're not meaningful?" Identifying patterns is an important first step in finding the areas in which you need to improve your time management. You will then be able to make conscious choices of where you want to allocate your limited time.

Once you have made this inventory of how you use your time, the next step is to find some positive way to stop wasting time and to put your time to best use. Here are a few suggestions for effective time management:

- *Identify your long-range goals.* Specify what personal changes you want to make, what kind of interpersonal relationships you would like to develop and maintain, what activities you would like to engage in, and what projects you would like to accomplish. Set goals and reevaluate them periodically.
- *Establish subgoals.* Break down your long-range goals into subgoals that can be accomplished in a shorter period of time. It might be helpful to prioritize your goals, from most important to least important. Develop a plan of action for reaching your subgoals.
- *Prioritize your activities.* Realize that if you plan well today you are likely to be more relaxed tomorrow. Allocate your time according to your priorities. Build recreation time into your schedule.
- *Thin out your schedule.* Realize that you probably won't be able to do all that you need or want to do in any given week. Therefore, focus on what you see as most essential, and prune those activities that are cluttering your life.
- *Evaluate potential new commitments.* Reflect when others ask you to take on new projects. Before you say "yes," make sure that you really want to accept the project—and that you have time in your schedule to spend on it.

- *Avoid procrastination.* Keeping a schedule of what you have to do and when it must be done can give you some sense of pacing yourself. If you know that waiting until the very end causes you stress and makes you function poorly, experiment with completing certain assignments or tasks before the last minute.
- *Identify time wasters.* If you become aware of activities that distract you from doing the important things in your life, write down these time wasters and ways to avoid them. Then, before you engage in these activities again, pause to ask yourself if you are willing to use your time in such a manner.
- *Learn to delegate.* Rather than convincing yourself that you are the only one who can do certain tasks, learn to ask for help and to assign specific tasks to others. Even if some tasks do not get done as well as they might if you had done them yourself, ask yourself if this isn't a better arrangement.
- *Try to do a task only once.* Rather than dealing with paperwork several times, make a quick decision the first time a document comes your way. If you can throw it away rather than filing it, do so.
- *Focus your attention.* You increase your stress level if you attempt to do too many things at once. Concentrate on doing one thing at a time and doing it as well as you can.
- *Strive to live in the present moment.* Experience each moment fully, and avoid ruminating about what you could have done. If you focus on the past or the future, it may be difficult to fully appreciate what you are experiencing now.

Effective use of time is not something that simply happens to you. Instead, it is a skill that you acquire and refine. It is essential to write down your goals and then plan how to spend the time you have. You might organize your schedule by creating a "to-do list" that ranks activities from high priority to low. At the end of each week and each month, review your activities in light of your long-range and short-range goals to determine whether you are putting your time to best use. If you practice a systematic approach to time management, you will probably find that you have more time to use in ways that are meaningful to you.

Here are a few suggestions for developing a systematic approach to managing your time:

- Schedule fixed responsibilities first—classes, work hours, and so forth—then work your study times and other activities around the fixed commitments.
- Figure out your peak-performance, high-energy times and schedule difficult and high-priority tasks then. Adjust your schedule around the times when you get the most done and when you will have the fewest interruptions.
- Leave some unscheduled time for yourself and for unexpected tasks and opportunities.
- Try out your plan for a couple of weeks to see how well it works for you, but be open to revising it. Plans are designed to help you manage your life, not to control you. Realize that it takes time to break old habits and to establish new and more functional ones.

- Create a long-term to-do list that includes all major projects and other critical dates for the term. Put all the due dates on a semester calendar or schedule.
- Make time in your schedule for fun, exercise, meditation, socializing, and down time. Including yourself in your schedule is one important step in preventing burnout.

Monitor Yourself to Prevent Burnout

Because professional burnout is an internal phenomenon that becomes obvious to others only in its advanced stages, you should take special care to recognize your own limits. How you approach your tasks and what you get from doing them are more important than how much you are doing. Ultimately, whether you experience burnout depends on how well you monitor the effects that the stresses of your work have on you and on the quality of your helping.

As you saw in Chapter 14, many sources contribute to the process of burnout, so it stands to reason that many paths can be taken to combat it. You can do much personally to lessen the chances of burning out or to restore yourself. Individual strategies alone, however, are not enough. You need to make effective use of others as a source of support, which requires that you learn certain interpersonal skills. There is also the organizational level to consider. Maslach and Leiter (1997) identify the steep costs of burnout in terms of reduced productivity and the decline in overall quality of life. When burnout reaches the stage of a full-blown problem, treatment is difficult and an organization is faced with major damage control. From Maslach and Leiter's perspective, preventive measures by an organization are wise and prudent investments in the future of that organization. By making this investment in the present, the costs and losses of burnout in the future are forestalled.

You Have Control Over Yourself

We have suggested that to a large extent you create your own stress by the interpretation you give to events. Although you cannot always control these events, you can control how you respond to them and the stance you take toward your life. If you are responsible for contributing to your physical and emotional exhaustion, you can also take action to change this condition. If you fail to recognize your limitations, you ought to be prepared for the price you will pay. Become attuned to the danger signals that you are being depleted, and take seriously your own need for nurturing and for recognition. What follows are some thoughts on what you can do to lessen the chances that you will get stuck in the rut of disillusionment. We encourage you to develop your own strategy for keeping yourself alive personally and professionally.

- Examine your behavior to determine if it is working for you. Ask yourself: "Is what I am doing what I really want to be doing? If not, why am I continuing in this direction?" "What are some things I want to be doing professionally that I am not doing? Who or what is stopping me?" "Am I accepting projects that I really want to reject? If so, why is it so difficult for me to say no?" Once you have answered some of these questions for yourself in an honest way, decide what action to take. For example, if you often say yes when you really want to firmly say no, you can begin to change this behavior.

• Look at your expectations to determine whether they are realistic. Although you may have initially become a helper because you wanted to create a better world, it is essential to temper your ideals with reality if you are to avoid continual frustration. You may expect that you can be all things to all people, and you may think that it is your mission in life always to be available for anyone who needs you. These self-expectations will eventually wear you down. Even though it is hard to accept, there are clients whom you will not be able to help. Regardless of how much you have to offer others, there is a limit to what you can give.

• Recognize that you can be an active agent in your life. If you allow yourself to get into a rut of hopelessness and helplessness, you will feel that your destiny is out of your control. Find other sources of meaning besides your work. These activities and interests can help you at least temporarily escape from job stresses and keep a balance in your life.

• There may be some unpleasant aspects of your job that are difficult to change, but you can approach your work differently. You can rearrange your schedule to reduce your stress. If you have some exceptionally difficult clients, for example, avoid seeing them one after the other. You can also look for new ways to bring your talents and interests to your work—for example, exchange jobs with a colleague for a time. If you stop blaming the institution for your problems and start assuming more control of your own destiny, this shift alone can make a key difference.

• It is easy to become overwhelmed by thinking about all the things that you feel powerless to change. Instead, focus on the aspects of your work that you have the power to change. Creativity grinds to a halt when most of your time is spent thinking of all that you cannot do rather than thinking about what you are able to do, within the limits that are imposed on you.

• Learn your own limits and strive to avoid overextending yourself. Others might not make this easy, so it will take considerable self-discipline to maintain your limits. This means that you will have to struggle with clients who demand things from you that you are not willing to give. The same is true for those who employ you. If you have not been setting limits, it may be extremely difficult to change this pattern, but it is not impossible.

• Look to colleagues and friends. Don't try to internalize all of your concerns and deal with them alone. Colleagues who face the same realities as you on the job can provide you with new information, insights, and perspectives. In the helping professions, the companionship of colleagues can be your greatest asset.

- Create a support group. If you wait for the system to organize a formal support group for you and your co-workers, you may have a long and frustrating wait. You can take the initiative to organize your colleagues to listen to one another and provide help. You can gain strength and hope by forming meaningful alliances with colleagues. Helpers know how to take care of their clients, so they also have the resources to take care of themselves and their fellow workers. Do make your support group a caring and productive one, and avoid getting caught in the trap of using the group as mere gripe sessions. Instead, focus on finding alternative ways of approaching problems.

Don't wait until you are hit with a chronic case of burnout—recognize the early signs and take remedial action quickly. It is best to direct your energies toward preventing this condition.

The real challenge is to learn ways to structure your life so that you can prevent burnout. Prevention is much easier than trying to cure a condition of severe physical and psychological depletion. An important prevention measure to lessen the chance of burnout is to seek diversity in your personal life and in your professional work. This diversity is based on engaging in multiple forms of therapy, engaging in multiple kinds of professional activities, working with multiple types of clients and problems, and balancing professional responsibilities with personal needs (Norcross, 2000). By engaging in a diversity of professional activities, you can often bring vitality to your work.

Several people in the helping professions told us of their personal strategies to prevent burnout:

- "To prevent burnout, I try to exercise daily, take personal time out with friends, go to personal therapy, and talk with co-workers and supervisors."
- "I plan my schedule carefully and make sure not to overextend myself. I take time off for vacations."
- "I take time out for myself to have fun. I do things like reading junk novels, shopping, spending time with my family, and going on vacations, and I always pat myself on the back for all my accomplishments."
- "I learn to say no and set limitations for myself. I try to allow as much time for play as I do for work, and I always try to leave my job at work."
- "I try to manage my time well. I reward myself with little presents. I take time off to go for a bike ride, go out for dinner, or take a bubble bath."
- "I don't bring work home with me. I try to leave my paperwork at school. I also take days off to relax when I need them."
- "I prevent burnout by doing a variety of things such as teaching, taking personal time out, writing, spending time with colleagues doing workshops, and spending lazy time off by being nonproductive."
- "I do my best to focus on those work activities where I can see results. Since I can do only so much with the time I have, I look for ways to get involved in projects that seem personally meaningful."
- "One strategy for coping with the resistance of administrators and colleagues is to deal with it much as I deal with the resistance of my clients. It helps me keep my perspective if I don't take the resistance I encounter personally."

A couple, both social workers, remind themselves continually not to become overwhelmed by the myriad of demands, not to lose sight of why they are in the agency, and not to get lost by being a cog in the production line. They have managed to temper their idealism by accepting that they cannot do everything they wanted to do. They are continuing to learn to cut down rather than taking on more and more. To prevent getting caught in a comfortable rut, they are creative in finding ways to vary their activities. They work with children and adults, co-lead groups, supervise interns, teach, and give in-service presentations. They attempt to develop a tolerant perspective when the agency acts in a petty way, which they do partly by keeping a sense of humor. They both assess their priorities and maintain limits. To be sure, this is not a simple matter; it involves a commitment to self-assessment and an openness to change.

Ways of Staying Alive Personally and Professionally

What can you do to promote your wellness from a holistic perspective? Perhaps the most basic way to retain your vitality as a person and as a professional is to realize that you are not a bottomless pit and cannot give and give without replenishing your reserve. But simply recognizing that you cannot be a universal giver is not enough to keep you alive as a person and a professional. You need an action plan and the commitment to carry out this plan.

Rather than thinking in terms of avoiding burnout and impairment, it is better to strive for wellness. In their study of the characteristics of well-functioning mental health professionals, Coster and Schwebel (1997) surveyed experienced professional psychologists who identified factors that contributed to their ability to function well. The dimensions that were most often mentioned included self-awareness and monitoring; support from peers, spouses, friends, mentors, and colleagues; values; and a balanced life that allowed time for family and friends. Well people are committed to creating a lifestyle that contributes to taking care of their physical selves, challenging themselves intellectually, expressing the full range of their emotions, finding rewarding interpersonal relationships, and searching for a meaning that will give direction to their lives. This holistic approach to well-being requires that we pay attention to the specific aspects of our lifestyle, including how we work and play, how we relax, how and what we eat, how we think and feel, how we keep physically fit, our relationships with others, our values and beliefs, and our spiritual needs. To the degree that we ignore or neglect one or more of these areas, we pay a price in terms of optimal functioning.

One model of wellness that can be applied to practitioners in the helping professions is provided by Myers, Sweeney, and Witmer (2000), who define wellness as "a way of life oriented toward optimal health and well-being in which body, mind, and spirit are integrated by the individual to live more fully within the human and natural community" (p. 252). In their model of the wheel of wellness, Myers and colleagues borrow from the Adlerian perspective and identify five life tasks that are a basic part of healthy functioning: spirituality, self-direction, work and leisure, friendship, and love. We briefly describe each of these components and raise some questions for you to apply to yourself.

- *Spirituality* is an awareness of a being or force that goes beyond the material dimension and gives a deep sense of wholeness or connectedness to the universe. What does spirituality mean to you? How do you get your spiritual needs met?
- *Self-direction* involves a sense of mindfulness and intentionality in meeting the major life tasks. Meyers and colleagues list a sense of worth, healthy sense of control, realistic beliefs, emotional awareness and coping, problem solving and creativity, sense of humor, nutrition, exercise, self-care, gender identity, and cultural identity as components of self-direction. What value do you place on each of these life tasks? To what degree is self-direction important to you? In what ways do you feel in control of your life both personally and professionally?
- *Work and leisure* provide a sense of accomplishment. If you were to analyze your weekly activities, what kind of balance would you find between work and leisure?
- *Friendship* incorporates all of one's social relationships that involve a connection with others. Do you have the kind of friends that you want? Are your friendships nourishing to you?
- *Love* involves long-term, intimate, trusting, compassionate, and mutually committed relationships. Do you have a love relationship in your life? To what degree does that relationship keep you alive emotionally?

We hope you realize that self-care is not a luxury but a necessity if you are to function optimally and effectively as a helping professional. How can you give your client your best if you are not nourished yourself? Is it possible for you to genuinely give to your clients if you are depleted physically and emotionally? Skovholt (2001) notes that those in the helping professions are experts at one-way caring. He warns of the dangers involved if one-way caring relationships are characteristic of helpers' personal lives, and he encourages helpers to learn to nurture the personal self.

Learning to cope with personal and professional sources of stress generally involves making some fundamental changes in your lifestyle. We think it is essential to create an action plan and then make a commitment to carry out this plan. At this point, take some time to ask yourself what basic changes, if any, you are willing to make in your behavior to promote your own wellness. Remember, this is routinely the question you ask your clients. What is your personal strategy for taking care of yourself?

Your personal strategy. Here is a list of suggestions for preventing burnout. You need to find your own way of remaining vital as a professional, but this list may stimulate you to think of some additional methods of preventing or treating burnout. After you think about each suggestion, rate each one using the following code:

A = This approach would be *very meaningful* to me.
B = This approach would have *some value* for me.
C = This approach would have *little value* for me.

_____ 1. Pursue paths to self-care such as meditation, deep relaxation, yoga, and therapeutic massage.

_____ 2. Become involved in peer group meetings where a support system is available.

_____ 3. Find other interests besides my work.

_____ 4. Attend to my health, and take care of my body by exercising and eating well.

_____ 5. Determine whether what I am doing is meaningful or draining.

_____ 6. Do some of the things now that I plan to do when I retire.

_____ 7. Take time for myself to do some of the things that I enjoy doing.

_____ 8. Avoid assuming an inordinate amount of responsibility.

_____ 9. Attend a personal-growth group or some type of personal therapy experience to work on my level of vitality.

_____ 10. Travel or seek new experiences.

_____ 11. Read stimulating books, and do some personal writing.

_____ 12. Exchange jobs for a time with a colleague.

_____ 13. Find nourishment with family and friends.

_____ 14. Work at modifying repetitively stressful situations.

_____ 15. Find a person who will confront and challenge me and who will encourage me to look at what I am doing.

_____ 16. Take short focusing and relaxing breaks during the day.

_____ 17. Seek diversity in my professional activities.

_____ 18. Learn how to work for my own affirmation of my worth rather than looking for external validation.

_____ 19. Make time for my spiritual development.

_____ 20. Rearrange my schedule to reduce stress.

_____ 21. Learn my limits, and learn to set my limits with others.

_____ 22. Pursue some hobbies or do things I truly enjoy.

_____ 23. Get enough rest and sleep.

_____ 24. Take the initiative to begin new projects that have meaning to me.

_____ 25. Become active in a professional organization.

Keep in mind that burnout is not always acute; rather, it is a cumulative process. You can handle only so much stress, and eventually you must pay the price in terms of your physical and psychological health. Recognizing the signs that you are on a path toward impairment demands a high level of honesty. You need to be alert to the subtle indications and then be willing to take action to remedy a situation that will inevitably result in burnout. Reflect on ways in which you can take care of yourself as well as being a helper to others.

Our personal experiences with preventing burnout.   We would like to share with you our own struggles with burnout and the measures we take to keep ourselves fresh. First of all, even though we are aware of the dangers of burnout, we are not immune to it. At different times throughout our professional lives we have wondered about the meaning of our work. We have come to realize that the answer does not lie merely in cutting out activities that we don't enjoy. Much of what we do professionally we like very much, and we have to remind ourselves that we cannot accept all the attractive projects that we may be interested in. The psychological and financial rewards, however high and tempting, do not always compensate for the emotional and physical depletion that results from an over-scheduled professional life. At one time, for example, we scheduled as many as six weeklong residential groups a year. Although these groups were profession-ally rewarding, it took a great deal of energy to lead them, and it necessitated re-arranging our personal life. We eventually began to limit ourselves to two of these weeklong groups a year. In another instance we became aware that too many of our "vacations" were coupled with professional commitments such as giving a workshop or attending a convention. Although we see this mixture as a good bal-ance, we nevertheless realized that we missed real vacations that were separate from any professional commitments.

Another way in which we attempt to prevent burnout is to pay attention to the early signals that we are overextending ourselves, and we involve ourselves in diverse projects. We engage in a variety of professional tasks, such as teaching, consulting, doing groups and workshops, and writing books. Besides offering our services to others, we recognize our need for input from others in the field, and we attend workshops for our own personal and professional development. Being aware of the demands that our profession puts on us, we are highly con-scious of living a healthy lifestyle. Therefore, we pay attention to our nutritional habits, and no matter how busy we are, we make the time that we need for ad-equate rest and regular exercise. As part of our lifestyle, we made the decision to live in a remote mountain community. But this remoteness and our busy sched-ules kept us, at times, from seeing our friends and colleagues. We had to realize that we could easily separate ourselves too much from relationships that were much needed and a source of joy and support for us. Thus, we made extra efforts to schedule blocks of time with our friends and to maintain and to nourish these valued relationships.

By Way of Review

- Because it is next to impossible to eliminate stress from your life, the crucial question is "Does stress control you, or do you control stress?"

- You do not have to be the victim of stress, for you have the capacity to rec-ognize situations that lead to stress, and you can make decisions about how you will think, feel, and behave in response to these situations.

- There are both preventive and combative strategies for coping with stress. Self-monitoring is the first step in developing an effective stress management program.

- Some of the most useful ways of managing stress are the cognitive ap-proaches. These include changing your distorted self-talk, learning time manage-ment skills, and applying them to daily life in a systematic fashion.

- Learning to recognize and cope with the reality of professional burnout is essential for your survival as a helper. Intense involvement with people over a period of time can lead to physical and psychological exhaustion.

- Because burnout is not something that suddenly happens to you, recognizing the early signs is an important step toward prevention.

- If you work in an agency, it is a challenge to retain your integrity, sense of direction, enthusiasm, and vitality. It is important to learn specific ways of surviving with dignity in an organization.

- If you work in an environment where there is a great deal of negativity, it is good to seek sources of positive support, both on your job and at home.

- Just as there are many sources of burnout, there are multiple ways to prevent and combat it. Individual, interpersonal, and organizational strategies can be devised.

What Will You Do Now?

1. If you have trouble doing everything that you want with the time you have available, consider trying the time management strategies that we described. Keep a written record of what you do in the coming week. At the end of the week, add up the hours you are spending on personal, social, job, and academic activities. Review your activities, and ask yourself if you are spending the time you have in the ways you want.

2. List three to five things you can do to better cope with stress (relaxation exercises, meditation, exercise). Put this list where you can see it easily, and use it as a reminder that you are in charge of creatively reducing stress.

3. Find a person in the helping professions who is willing to be interviewed about burnout. Focus your discussion with this person on what he or she does to keep alive personally and professionally. Questions to consider include "What do you find to be the major source of burnout?" and "What do you do to prevent burnout?"

4. Think about how you are when you are at work and when you are on vacation. Ask someone who knows you in both situations to describe you in these situations. Does this person see you as the same in both contexts, or different? Use this exercise as a way of thinking about how your work affects your personal life.

5. Self-care and self-renewal involve a balanced attention to our physical, emotional, mental, social, and spiritual dimensions. Identify some specific ways you can achieve greater balance in your life to continue your self-renewal process. In your journal write down some ideas about patterns that you may want to

change to enhance the balance in your life. Then make an action plan that will assist you in coping with stress by using some of the preventive and combative strategies discussed in this chapter.

6. For the full bibliographic entry for each of the sources listed here, consult the References and Reading List at the back of the book. For a useful book on self-care, see Skovholt (2001). See Kottler (1997) for various articles describing how individuals address the challenges they have faced in retaining their vitality in the helping professions. See George (1998) for a practical guidebook for coping with stress. See G. Corey and Corey (2002) for ideas on self-renewal and retaining your vitality. See Ellis (1999, 2000, 2001a, 2001b) for cognitive techniques in learning ways of disputing dysfunctional beliefs that often lead to stress. For specific time management strategies, we recommend George (1998) and Rice (1999).

Concluding Comments

You can get into a powerless stance if you become overly ambitious and try to fill the bill of an "ideal helper." Remember that the challenges we have presented throughout these chapters do not have to be addressed immediately or all at once. You may want to accomplish more than there is time for, so identify clear priorities of what you most want to accomplish. Setting priorities is essential if you want to maintain a sense of stability. At this point, we encourage you to dream and allow yourself to envision the helper you want to become. You can begin now to reach your visions by becoming an active and questioning student and by putting yourself fully into your fieldwork activities. We hope you will become excited by your journey of self-exploration as you learn about the helping professions.

The process of becoming a helper is intrinsically related to the process of becoming a person. In this book we have emphasized the importance of looking at your life and of understanding your motivations. Although it is not essential for you to be problem-free, we have stressed the importance of being a model for your clients. Reflect on whether what you do in your own life is what you encourage for your clients. If you urge your clients to take the risks that growth entails, it is essential that you do this in your own life.

This is a good time to reflect on the personal meaning this book has held for you. Do you still think the helping professions are for you? What do you think you can bring to your work? How might your work affect your personal life? What are the greatest challenges you expect to face? Do you now have a different perspective on the concerns that were addressed in this book? At this point, what do you see as your major strengths and some of your limitations? What steps could you take to work on your limitations? How can you build on your strengths?

Now that you have completed the book, return to Chapter 1 and once again complete the Self-Assessment: An Inventory of Your Attitudes and Beliefs about Professional Helping. You took this inventory as a pretest at the beginning of the course, and now, as the course is ending, you can use this self-inventory to determine the degree to which any of your attitudes and beliefs about helping may have changed. Additionally, read the Focus Questions at the beginning of each chapter again. Can you answer all of these questions now? Have your answers to some of these questions changed as you have acquired new knowledge from the book and in your course? We highly recommend that you also look at the key points at the end of each chapter in the By Way of Review section as a way to consolidate your key learnings. Finally, from the What Will You Do Now? section at the end of each chapter, choose one activity that is meaningful to you and that you are willing to pursue. Challenge yourself to extend your learning experience by taking the initiative to complete these projects on your own. If you have been keeping a journal, continue to write about the experiences you are having in your training program as a way to extend the self-reflection process.

We dedicated this book to you, our readers, who are most likely preparing for a career in one of the helping professions. We hope that you see more clearly how the kind of person you are is so vitally linked to the kind of helping professional that you can become. Best of luck in your continuing journey!

InfoTrac College Edition Resources

For additional readings, explore InfoTrac College Edition, our online library. Go to http://www.infotrac.college.com/wadsworth and select these key word searches:

cognitive W1 therapy
stress W1 management AND cognitive
time W1 management AND stress
prevention W2 burnout

Key words are listed in a form that enables the search engine to locate a wider range of articles in the online university library. Key words should be entered exactly as shown, including asterisks, "W1," "W2," "AND," and other search engine tools.

References
and Reading List

Acuff, C., Bennett, B. E., Bricklin, P. M., Canter, M. B., Knapp, S. J., Moldawsky, S., & Phelps, R. (1999). Considerations for ethical practice of managed care. *Professional Psychology: Research and Practice, 30*(6), 563–575.

Albom, M. (1997). *Tuesdays with Morrie.* New York: Doubleday.

Alle-Corliss, L., & Alle-Corliss, R. (1998). *Human service agencies: An orientation to fieldwork.* Pacific Grove, CA: Brooks/Cole.

Alle-Corliss, L., & Alle-Corliss, R. (1999). *Advanced practice in human service agencies: Issues, trends, and treatment perspectives.* Pacific Grove, CA: Brooks/Cole.

American Association for Marriage and Family Therapy. (2001). *AAMFT code of ethics.* Washington, DC: Author.

American Counseling Association. (1995). *Code of ethics and standards of practice.* Alexandria, VA: Author.

American Psychiatric Association. (1994). *Diagnostic and statistical manual of mental disorders* (4th ed.). Washington, DC: Author.

American Psychological Association. (1992). *Ethical principles of psychologists and code of conduct.* Washington, DC: Author.

American Psychological Association, Division 44. (2000). Guidelines for psychotherapy with lesbian, gay, and bisexual clients. *American Psychologist, 55*(12), 1440–1451.

American School Counseling Association. (1998). *Ethical standards for school counselors.* Alexandria, VA: Author.

Anderson, M. J., & Ellis, R. (1988). On the reservation. In N. A. Vacc, J. Wittmer, & S. B. DeVaney (Eds.), *Experiencing and counseling multicultural and diverse populations* (2nd ed., pp. 107–126). Muncie, IN: Accelerated Development.

Anderson, S. K., & Kitchener, K. S. (1996). Nonromantic, nonsexual posttherapy relationships between psychologists and former clients: An exploratory study of critical incidents. *Professional Psychology: Research and Practice, 27*(1), 59–66.

Arredondo, P., Toporek, R., Brown, S., Jones, J., Locke, D., Sanchez, J., & Stadler, H. (1996). Operationalization of multicultural counseling competencies. *Journal of Multicultural Counseling and Development, 24*(1), 42–78.

Association for Counselor Education and Supervision. (1993, Summer). Ethical guidelines for counseling supervisors. *Spectrum, 53*(4), 3–8.

Association for Specialists in Group Work. (1998). Best practice guidelines. *Journal for Specialists in Group Work, 23*(3), 237–244.

Association for Specialists in Group Work. (1999). Principles for diversity-competent group workers. *Journal for Specialists in Group Work, 24*(1), 7–14.

Association for Specialists in Group Work. (2000). Professional standards for the training of group workers. *Journal for Specialists in Group Work, 25*(4), 327–342.

Atkinson, D. R., Morten, G., & Sue, D. W. (Eds.). (1998). *Counseling American minorities: A cross-cultural perspective* (5th ed.). Boston, MA: McGraw-Hill.

Atkinson, D. R., Thompson, C. E., & Grant, S. K. (1993). A three-dimensional model for counseling racial/ethnic minorities. *The Counseling Psychologist, 21*(2), 257–277.

Austin, K. M., Moline, M. M., & Williams, G. T. (1990). *Confronting malpractice: Legal and ethical dilemmas in psychotherapy.* Newbury Park, CA: Sage.

Axelson, J. A. (1999). *Counseling and development in a multicultural society* (3rd ed.). Pacific Grove, CA: Brooks/Cole.

Baird, B. N. (1996). *The internship, practicum, and field placement handbook: A guide for the help-*

ing professions. Upper Saddle River, NJ: Prentice-Hall.

Barnett, J. E., & Hillard, D. (2001). Psychological distress and impairment: The availability, nature, and use of colleague assistance programs for psychologists. *Professional Psychology: Research and Practice, 32*(2), 205–210.

Beck, A. T. (1976). *Cognitive therapy and the emotional disorders.* New York: New American Library.

Beck, A. T. (1987). Cognitive therapy. In J. K. Zeig (Ed.), *The evolution of psychotherapy* (pp. 149–178). New York: Brunner/Mazel.

Beck, A. T., & Weishaar, M. E. (2000). Cognitive therapy. In R. J. Corsini & D. Wedding (Eds.), *Current psychotherapies* (6th ed., pp. 241–272). Itasca, IL: F. E. Peacock.

Becvar, D. S., & Becvar, R. J. (2000). *Family therapy: A systemic integration* (4th ed.). Needham Heights, MA: Allyn & Bacon.

Bednar, R. L., Bednar, S. C., Lambert, M. J., & Waite, D. R. (1991). *Psychotherapy with high-risk clients: Legal and professional standards.* Pacific Grove, CA: Brooks/Cole.

Bergin, A. E. (1991). Values and religious issues in psychotherapy and mental health. *American Psychology, 46*(4), 393–403.

Bernard, J. M., & Goodyear, R. K. (1998). *Fundamentals of clinical supervision* (2nd ed.). Needham Heights, MA: Allyn & Bacon.

Bersoff, D. N. (1999). *Ethical conflicts in psychology* (2nd ed.). Washington, DC: American Psychological Association.

Bitter, J. R. (1987). Communication and meaning. Satir in Adlerian context. In R. Sherman & D. Dinkmeyer (Eds.), *Systems of family therapy: An Adlerian integration* (pp. 109–142). New York: Brunner/Mazel.

Bitter, J. R. (1988). Family mapping and family constellation: Satir in Adlerian context. *Individual Psychology: The Journal of Adlerian Theory, Research, and Practice, 44*(1), 106–111.

Brammer, L. M. (1993). *The helping relationship: Process and skills* (5th ed.). Boston: Allyn & Bacon.

Brems, C. (2001). *Basic skills in psychotherapy and counseling.* Pacific Grove, CA: Brooks/Cole.

Brockett, D. R., & Gleckman, A. D. (1991). Countertransference with the older adult: The importance of mental health counselor awareness and strategies for effective management. *Journal of Mental Health Counseling, 13*(3), 343–355.

Brown, C., & O'Brien, K. M. (1998). Understanding stress and burnout in shelter workers. *Professional Psychology: Research and Practice, 29*(4), 383–385.

Burke, M. T., & Miranti, J. G. (Eds.). (1995). *Counseling: The spiritual dimension.* Alexandria, VA: American Counseling Association.

Calfee, B. E. (1997). Lawsuit prevention techniques. In *The Hatherleigh guide to ethics in therapy.* New York: Hatherleigh Press.

Calhoun, K. S., Moras, K., Pilkonis, P. A., & Rehm, L. P. (1998). Empirically supported treatments: Implications for training. *Journal of Consulting and Clinical Psychology, 66,* 151–162.

Campbell, J. M. (2000). *Becoming an effective supervisor: A workbook for counselors and psychotherapists.* Philadelphia, PA: Accelerated Development (Taylor & Francis).

Canter, M. B., Bennett, B. E., Jones, S. E., & Nagy, T. F. (1994). *Ethics for psychologists: A commentary on the APA ethics code.* Washington, DC: American Psychological Association.

Carlson, J., Sperry, L., & Lewis, J. A. (1997). *Family therapy: Ensuring treatment efficacy.* Pacific Grove, CA: Brooks/Cole.

Cohen, R., & Cohen, J. (2000). *Chiseled in sand: Perspectives on change in human services organizations.* Pacific Grove, CA: Brooks/Cole.

Cooper, C. C., & Gottlieb, M. C. (2000). Ethical issues with managed care: Challenges facing counseling psychology. *The Counseling Psychologist, 28*(2), 179–236.

Corey, G. (2000). *Theory and practice of group counseling* (5th ed.) and *Manual.* Pacific Grove, CA: Brooks/Cole.

Corey, G. (2001a). *The art of integrative counseling.* Pacific Grove, CA: Brooks/Cole.

Corey, G. (2001b). *Case approach to counseling and psychotherapy* (5th ed.). Pacific Grove, CA: Brooks/Cole.

Corey, G. (2001c). *Theory and practice of counseling and psychotherapy* (6th ed.) and *Manual.* Pacific Grove, CA: Brooks/Cole.

Corey, G., Corey, C., & Corey, H. (1997). *Living and learning.* Belmont, CA: Wadsworth.

Corey, G., & Corey, M. (2002). *I never knew I had a choice* (7th ed.). Pacific Grove, CA: Brooks/Cole.

Corey, G., Corey, M., & Callanan, P. (2003). *Issues and ethics in the helping professions* (6th ed.). Pacific Grove, CA: Brooks/Cole.

Corey, G., Corey, M., Callanan, P., & Russell, J. M. (1992). *Group techniques* (2nd ed.). Pacific Grove, CA: Brooks/Cole.

Corey, G., Corey, M., & Haynes, R. (1998). *Ethics in action CD-ROM (student version).* Pacific Grove, CA: Brooks/Cole.

Corey, G., Corey, M., & Haynes, R. (2000). *Evolution of a group Student video and workbook.* Pacific Grove, CA: Brooks/Cole.

Corey, G., & Herlihy, B. (1996). Counselor training and supervision. In B. Herlihy & G. Corey (Eds.), *ACA ethical standards casebook* (5th ed., pp. 275–278). Alexandria, VA: American Counseling Association.

Corey, G., & Herlihy, B. (1997). Dual/multiple relationships: Toward a consensus of thinking. In *The Hatherleigh guide to ethics in therapy* (pp. 193–205). New York: Hatherleigh Press.

Corey, M., & Corey, G. (2002). *Groups: Process and practice* (6th ed.). Pacific Grove, CA: Brooks/Cole.

Cormier, S., & Hackney, H. (1999). *Counseling strategies and interventions* (5th ed.). Boston: Allyn & Bacon.

Coster, J. S., & Schwebel, M. (1997). Well-functioning in professional psychologists. *Professional Psychology: Research and Practice, 28*(1), 5–13.

Cottone, R. R. (2001). A social constructivism model of ethical decision making in counseling. *Journal of Counseling and Development, 79* (1), 39–45.

Cottone, R. R., & Tarvydas, V. M. (1998). *Ethical and professional issues in counseling.* Upper Saddle River, NJ: Merrill/Prentice-Hall.

Crawford, I., Humfleet, G., Ribordy, S. C., Ho, F. C., & Vickers, V. L. (1991). Stigmatization of AIDS patients by mental health professionals. *Professional Psychology: Research and Practice, 22*(5), 357–361.

Crawford, I., McLeod, A., Zamboni, B. D., & Jordan, M. B. (1999). Psychologists' attitudes toward gay and lesbian parenting. *Professional Psychology: Research and Practice, 30*(4), 394–401.

Crawford, R. (1999). Law and ethics: Comparisons and contrasts. In P. Stevens (Ed.), *Ethical casebook for the practice of marriage and family counseling* (pp. 17–39). Alexandria, VA: American Counseling Association.

Crespi, T. D., Fischetti, B. A., & Butler, S. K. (2001, January). Clinical supervision in the schools. *Counseling Today, 7*, 28, & 34.

Cummings, N. A. (1995). Impact of managed care on employment and training: A primer for survival. *Professional Psychology: Research and Practice, 26*(1), 10–15.

Dalton, J. H., Elias, M. J., & Wadersman, A. (2001). *Community psychology: Linking individuals and communities.* Belmont, CA: Wadsworth/Thomson Learning.

Daniels, J. A. (2001). Managed care, ethics, and counseling. *Journal of Counseling and Development, 79*(1), 119–122.

Dattilio, F. M., & Freeman, A. (1992). Introduction to cognitive therapy. In A. Freeman & F. M. Dattilio (Eds.), *Comprehensive casebook of cognitive therapy* (pp. 3–11). New York: Plenum.

Davis, S. R., & Meier, S. T. (2001). *The elements of managed care: A guide for helping professionals.* Pacific Grove, CA: Brooks/Cole.

Diller, J. V. (1999). *Cultural diversity: A primer for the human services.* Pacific Grove, CA: Brooks/Cole.

Dilley, J. W., & Marks, R. (Eds.) (1998). *The UCSF AIDS health project guide to counseling: Perspectives on psychotherapy, prevention, and therapeutic practice.* San Francisco, CA: Jossey-Bass.

Dilley, J. W., Pies, C., & Helquist, M. (Eds.) (1993). *Face to face: A guide to AIDS counseling.* San Francisco, CA: UCSF AIDS Health Project.

Doyle, R. E. (1998). *Essential skills and strategies in the helping process* (2nd ed.). Pacific Grove, CA: Brooks/Cole.

Dworkin, S. H., & Gutierrez, F. J. (1992). *Counseling gay men and lesbians: Journey to the end of the rainbow.* Alexandria, VA: American Association for Counseling and Development.

Edlin, G., Golanty, E., & Brown, K. (2000). *Essentials for health and wellness* (2nd ed.). Sudbury, MA: Jones & Bartlett.

Egan, G. (2002). *The skilled helper: A problem-management approach to helping* (7th ed.). Pacific Grove, CA: Brooks/Cole.

Ekbom, C. (2000). Interview with Dr. Gerald Corey. *The Wisconsin Counselor, 19*(1), 15–21.

Elkins, D. N. (1994, August). *Toward a soulful psychology: Introduction and overview.* Paper presented at the meeting of the American Psychological Association, Los Angeles.

Ellis, A. (1988). *How to stubbornly refuse to make yourself miserable about anything—yes, anything!* Secaucus, NJ: Lyle Stuart.

Ellis, A. (1999). *How to make yourself happy and remarkably less disturbable.* San Luis Obispo, CA: Impact.

Ellis, A. (2000). *How to control your anxiety before it controls you.* New York: Citadel.

Ellis, A. (2001a). *Feeling better, getting better, and staying better.* Atascadero, CA: Impact.

Ellis, A. (2001b). *Overcoming destructive thoughts, feelings, and behaviors.* Amherst, New York: Prometheus Books.

Ellis, A. (2002). *Overcoming resistance: Rational-emotive therapy with difficult clients* (rev. ed.). New York: Springer.

Ellis, A., & Crawford, T. (2001). *Making intimate connections: Seven guidelines for great relationships and better communication.* Atascadero, CA: Impact.

Ellis, A., & Dryden, W. (1997). *The practice of rational-emotive therapy* (rev. ed.). New York: Springer.

Ellis, A., & Harper, R. A. (1997). *A new guide to rational living* (3rd ed.). North Hollywood, CA: Wilshire Books.

Ellis, A., & MacClaren, C. (1998). *Rational emotive behavior therapy: A therapist's guide*. Atascadero, CA: Impact.

Emerson, S., & Markos, P. A. (1996). Signs and symptoms of the impaired counselor. *Journal of Humanistic Education and Development, 34*, 108–117.

Erikson, E. (1963). *Childhood and society* (2nd ed.). New York: Norton.

Erikson, E. (1982). *The life cycle completed*. New York: Norton.

Ezell, M. (2001). *Advocacy in the human services*. Pacific Grove, CA: Brooks/Cole.

Faiver, C. M., Eisengart, S., & Colonna, R. (2000). *The counselor intern's handbook* (2nd ed.) Pacific Grove, CA: Brooks/Cole.

Faiver, C. M., Ingersoll, R. E., O'Brien, E., & McNally, C. (2001). *Explorations in counseling and spirituality: Philosophical, practical, and personal reflections*. Pacific Grove, CA: Brooks/Cole.

Faiver, C. M., & O'Brien, E. M. (1993). Assessment of religious beliefs form. *Counseling and Values, 37*(3), 176–178.

Farber, B. A. (1983). Psychotherapists' perceptions of stressful patient behavior. *Professional Psychology: Research and Practice, 14*(5), 697–705.

Fontana, D. (1999). *Learn to meditate: A practical guide to self-discovery and fulfillment*. San Francisco: Chronicle Books.

Foos, J. A., Ottens, A. J., & Hill, L. K. (1991). Managed mental health: A primer for counselors. *Journal of Counseling and Development, 69*(4), 332–336.

Frame, M. W. (1999). The impaired counselor. In P. Stevens (Ed.), *Ethical casebook for the practice of marriage and family counseling* (pp. 103–121). Alexandria, VA: American Counseling Association.

Fujimura, L. E., Weis, D. M., & Cochran, J. R. (1985). Suicide: Dynamics and implications for counseling. *Journal of Counseling and Development, 63*(10), 612–615.

Gabbard, G. (April, 1995). What are boundaries in psychotherapy? *The Menninger Letter,* Vol. 3, No. 4, pp. 1–2.

George, M. (1998). *Learn to relax: A practical guide to easing tension and conquering stress*. San Francisco: Chronicle Books.

Getz, J. G., & Protinsky, H. O. (1994). Training marriage and family counselors: A family-of-origin approach. *Counselor Education and Supervision, 33*(3), 183–200.

Gill-Wigal, J., & Heaton, J. A. (1996). Managing sexual attraction in the therapeutic relationship. *Directions in Mental Health Counseling, 6*(8), 4–15.

Glosoff, H. L., Corey, G., & Herlihy, B. (1996). Dual relationships. In B. Herlihy & G. Corey (Eds.), *ACA ethical standards casebook* (5th ed., pp. 251–257). Alexandria, VA: American Counseling Association.

Glosoff, H. L., Garcia, J., Herlihy, B., & Remley, T. P. (1999). Managed care: Ethical considerations for counselors. *Counseling and Values, 44*(1), 8–16.

Goldenberg, I., & Goldenberg, H. (2000a). *Family therapy: An overview* (5th ed.). Pacific Grove, CA: Brooks/Cole.

Goldenberg, I., & Goldenberg, H. (2000b). *A workbook for family therapy: An overview* (5th ed.). Pacific Grove, CA: Brooks/Cole.

Goleman, D. (1995). *Emotional intelligence*. New York: Bantam Books.

Goodman, R. W., & Carpenter-White, A. (1996). The family autobiography assignment: Some ethical considerations. *Counselor Education and Supervision, 35*(3), 230–238.

Guy, J. D. (1987). *The personal life of the psychotherapist*. New York: Wiley.

Guy, J. D. (2000). Holding the holding environment together: Self-psychology and psychotherapist care. *Professional Psychology: Research and Practice, 31*(3), 351–352.

Haas, L. J., & Cummings, N. A. (1991). Managed outpatient mental health plans: Clinical, ethical, and practical guidelines for participation. *Professional Psychology: Research and Practice, 22*(1), 45–51.

Hamilton, J. C., & Spruill, J. (1999). Identifying and reducing risk factors related to trainee-client sexual misconduct. *Professional Psychology: Research and Practice, 30*(3), 318–327.

Hanna, S. M., & Brown, J. H. (1999). *The practice of family therapy: Key elements across models* (2nd ed.). Pacific Grove, CA: Brooks/Cole.

Hanson, C. E., Skager, R., & Mitchell, R. R. (1991). Counselors in at-risk prevention services: An innovative program. *Journal of Mental Health Counseling, 13*(2), 253–263.

Hatherleigh guide to ethics in therapy. (1997). New York: Hatherleigh Press.

Hering, N. (2000). Managed care: Notes from the underground. *The California Therapist, 12*(4), 36–38.

Herlihy, B. (1996). When a colleague is impaired: The individual counselor's response. *Journal of Humanistic Education and Development, 34*, 118–127.

Herlihy, B., & Corey, G. (1996a). *ACA ethical standards casebook* (5th ed.). Alexandria, VA: American Counseling Association.

Herlihy, B., & Corey, G. (1996b). Confidentiality. In B. Herlihy & G. Corey (Eds.), *ACA ethical standards casebook* (5th ed., pp. 205–209). Alexandria, VA: American Counseling Association.

Herlihy, B., & Corey, G. (1997a). *Boundary issues in counseling: Multiple roles and responsibilities.* Alexandria, VA: American Counseling Association.

Herlihy, B., & Corey, G. (1997b). Codes of ethics as catalysts for improving practice. In *The Hatherleigh guide to ethics in therapy* (pp. 39–59). New York: Hatherleigh Press.

Herr, E. L. (1991). Challenges to mental health counselors in a dynamic society: Macrostrategies in the profession. *Journal of Mental Health Counseling, 13*(1), 6–10.

Hersch, L. (1995). Adapting to health care reform and managed care: Three strategies for survival and growth. *Professional Psychology: Research and Practice, 26*(1), 16–26.

Ho, D. Y. F. (1985). Cultural values and professional issues in clinical psychology: Implications from the Hong Kong experience. *American Psychologist, 40*(11), 1212–1218.

Hoffman, M. A. (1991a). Counseling the HIV-infected client: A psychosocial model for assessment and intervention. *The Counseling Psychologist, 19*(4), 467–542.

Hoffman, M. A. (1991b). Training mental health counselors for the AIDS crisis. *Journal of Mental Health Counseling, 13*(2), 264–269.

Hogan-Garcia, M. (1999). *The four skills of cultural diversity competence: A process for understanding and practice.* Pacific Grove, CA: Brooks/Cole.

Hogan-Garcia, M., & Scheinberg, C. (2000). Culturally competent practice principles for planned intervention in organizations and communities. *Practicing Anthropology, 22*(2), 27–29.

Homan, M. (1999). *Promoting community change: Making it happen in the real world* (2nd ed.). Pacific Grove, CA: Brooks/Cole.

Housman, L. M., & Stake, J. E. (1999). The current state of sexual ethics training in clinical psychology: Issues of quantity, quality, and effectiveness. *Professional Psychology: Research and Practice, 30*(3), 302–311.

Hutchins, D. E., & Cole Vaught, C. G. (1997). *Helping relationships and strategies* (3rd ed.). Pacific Grove, CA: Brooks/Cole.

Hwang, P. O. (2000). *Other-esteem: Meaningful life in a multicultural society.* Philadelphia, PA: Accelerated Development (Taylor & Francis)

Ivey, A. E., & Ivey, M. B. (1998). Reframing DSM-IV: Positive strategies from developmental counseling and therapy. *Journal of Counseling and Development, 76*(3), 334–350.

Ivey, A. E., & Ivey, M. B. (1999). *Intentional interviewing and counseling: Facilitating client development in a multicultural society* (4th ed.). Pacific Grove, CA: Brooks/Cole.

Ivey, A. E., D'Andrea, M., Ivey, M. B., & Simek-Morgan, L. (2002). *Theories of counseling and psychotherapy: A multicultural perspective* (5th ed.). Boston: Allyn & Bacon.

Ivey, A. E., Pedersen, P. B., & Ivey, M. B. (2001). *Intentional group counseling: A microskills approach.* Pacific Grove, CA: Brooks/Cole.

Jaffe, D. T. (1986). The inner strains of healing work: Therapy and self-renewal for health professionals. In C. D. Scott & J. Hawk (Eds.), *Heal thyself: The health of health care professionals.* New York: Brunner/Mazel.

James, R. K., & Gilliland, B. E. (2001). *Crisis intervention strategies* (4th ed.). Pacific Grove, CA: Brooks/Cole.

Jensen, J. P., & Bergin, A. E. (1988). Mental health values of professional therapists: A national interdisciplinary survey. *Professional Psychology: Research and Practice, 19*(3), 290–297.

Jones, C. L., & Higuchi, A. (1996). Landmark New Jersey lawsuit challenges "no cause" termination. *Practitioner Focus, 9*(2), 1 & 13.

Jones, L. (1996). *HIV/AIDS: What to do about it.* Pacific Grove, CA: Brooks/Cole.

Kain, C. D. (1996). *Positive HIV affirmative counseling.* Alexandria, VA: American Counseling Association.

Kanel, K. (1999). *A guide to crisis intervention.* Pacific Grove, CA: Brooks/Cole.

Karon, B. P. (1995). Provision of psychotherapy under managed health care: A growing crisis and national nightmare. *Professional Psychology: Research and Practice, 26*(1), 5–9.

Kelly, E. W. (1995a). Counselor values: A national survey. *Journal of Counseling and Development, 73*(6), 648–653.

Kelly, E. W. (1995b). *Spirituality and religion in counseling and psychotherapy.* Alexandria, VA: American Counseling Association.

Kiser, P. M. (2000). *Getting the most from your human service internship: Learning from experience.* Pacific Grove, CA: Brooks/Cole.

Kottler, J. A. (1992). *Compassionate therapy: Working with difficult clients.* San Francisco, CA: Jossey-Bass.

Kottler, J. A. (1993). *On being a therapist* (rev. ed.). San Francisco, CA: Jossey-Bass.

Kottler, J. A. (Ed.). (1997). *Finding your way as a counselor.* Alexandria, VA: American Counseling Association.

Kottler, J. A. (2000). *Nuts and bolts of helping.* Boston: Allyn & Bacon.

Kottler, J. A., & Blau, D. S. (1989). *The imperfect therapist: Learning from failure in therapeutic practice.* San Francisco, CA: Jossey-Bass.

Kottler, J. A., & Brown, R. W. (2000). *Introduction to therapeutic counseling: Voices from the field* (4th ed.). Pacific Grove, CA: Brooks/Cole.

Kramen-Kahn, B., & Hansen, N. D. (1998). Rafting the rapids: Occupational hazards, rewards, and coping strategies of psychotherapists. *Professional Psychology: Research and Practice, 29*(2), 130–134.

Kramer, S. A. (1990). *Positive endings in psychotherapy: Bringing meaningful closure to therapeutic relationships.* San Francisco, CA: Jossey-Bass.

Lawson, D. M., & Gaushell, H. (1988). Family autobiography: A useful method for enhancing counselors' personal development. *Counselor Education and Supervision, 28*(2), 162–167.

Lawson, D. M., & Gaushell, H. (1991). Intergenerational family characteristics of counselor trainees. *Counselor Education and Supervision, 30*(4), 309–321.

Lazarus, A. A. (1994). How certain boundaries and ethics diminish therapeutic effectiveness. *Ethics and Behavior, 4*(3), 255–261.

Lazarus, A. A. (1998). How do you like these boundaries? *The Clinical Psychologist, 51*(1), 22–25.

Lazarus, A. A. (2000). Multimodal replenishment. *Professional Psychology: Research and Practice, 31*(1), 93–94.

Lazarus, A. A. (2001). Not all "dual relationships" are taboo: Some tend to enhance treatment outcomes. *The National Psychologist, 10*(1), 16.

Lee, C. C. (1997a). *Multicultural issues in counseling: New approaches to diversity* (2nd ed.). Alexandria, VA: American Counseling Association.

Lee, C. C. (1997b). The problems and pitfalls of multicultural counseling. In C. C. Lee (Ed.), *Multicultural issues in counseling: New approaches to diversity* (pp. 3–13). Alexandria, VA: American Counseling Association.

Lee, C. C. (1997c). New approaches to diversity: Implications for multicultural counselor training and research. In C. C. Lee (Ed.), *Multicultural issues in counseling: New approaches to diversity* (pp. 353–360). Alexandria, VA: American Counseling Association.

Lee, W. M. L. (1999). *An introduction to multicultural counseling.* Philadelphia, PA: Accelerated Development (Taylor & Francis).

Lewis, J. A., Lewis, M. D., Daniels, J. A., & D'Andrea, M. J. (1998). *Community counseling: Empowerment strategies for a diverse society* (2nd ed.). Pacific Grove, CA: Brooks/Cole.

Loar, L. (1995). Brief therapy with difficult clients. *Directions in Mental Health Counseling, 5*(12), 3–11.

Loeschen, S. (1998). *Systematic training in the skills of Virginia Satir.* Pacific Grove, CA: Brooks/Cole.

Lum, D. (1999). *Culturally competent practice: A framework for growth and change.* Pacific Grove, CA: Brooks/Cole.

Lum, D. (2000). *Social work practice and people of color: A process-stage approach* (4th ed.). Pacific Grove, CA: Brooks/Cole.

MacCluskie, K. C., & Ingersoll, R. E. (2001). *Becoming a 21st century agency counselor: Personal and professional explorations.* Pacific Grove, CA: Brooks/Cole.

Mackelprang, R. W., & Salsgiver, R. O. (1999). *Disability: A diversity model approach in human service practice.* Pacific Grove, CA: Brooks/Cole.

Margolin, G. (1982). Ethical and legal considerations in marital and family therapy. *American Psychologist, 37*(3), 788–801.

Marino, T. W. (1996). The challenging task of making counseling services relevant to more populations. *Counseling Today,* 1 & 6.

Martin, S. (1999). Revision of ethics code calls for stronger former client sex rule. *APA Monitor, 30*(7), 44.

Maslach, C. (1982). *Burnout: The cost of caring.* Englewood Cliffs, NJ: Prentice-Hall (Spectrum).

Maslach, C., & Leiter, M P. (1997). *The truth about burnout.* San Francisco: Jossey-Bass.

McCarthy, P., Sugden, S., Koker, M., Lamendola, F., Maurer, S., & Renninger, S. (1995). A practical guide to informed consent in clinical supervision. *Counselor Education and Supervision, 35*(2), 130–138.

McGoldrick, M., & Carter, B. (1999). Self in context: The individual life cycle in systemic perspective. In B. Carter & M. McGoldrick (Eds.) *The expanded family life cycle: Individual, family, and social perspectives* (3rd ed., pp. 27–46). Boston: Allyn & Bacon.

McGoldrick, M., Gerson, R., & Shellenberger, S. (1999). *Genograms: Assessment and intervention* (2nd ed.). New York: Norton.

Meier, S. T., & Davis, S. R. (2001). *The elements of counseling* (4th ed.). Pacific Grove, CA: Brooks/Cole.

Miller, W. R. (Ed.). (1999). *Integrating spirituality into treatment: Resources for practitioners.* Washington, DC: American Psychological Association.

Miller, W. R., & Thoresen, C. E. (1999). Spirituality and health. In W. R. Miller (Ed.), *Integrating spirituality into treatment: Resources for practitioners* (pp. 3–18). Washington, DC: American Psychological Association.

Miranti, J., & Burke, M. T. (1995). Spirituality: An integral component of the counseling process. In M. T. Burke & J. G. Miranti (Eds.), *Counseling: The spiritual dimension* (pp. 1–3). Alexandria, VA: American Counseling Association.

Modrak, R. (1992). Mass shootings and airplane crashes: Counselors respond to the changing face of community crisis. *Guidepost: AACD Newsletter, 34*(8), 4.

Mosak, H., & Shulman, B. (1988). *Life style inventory.* Muncie, IN: Accelerated Development.

Murphy, B. C., & Dillon, C. (1998). *Interviewing in action: Process and practice.* Pacific Grove, CA: Brooks/Cole.

Myer, R. A. (2001). *Assessment for crisis intervention: A triage assessment model.* Pacific Grove, CA: Brooks/Cole.

Myers, J. E. (1990). Aging: An overview for mental health counselors. *Journal of Mental Health Counseling, 12*(3), 245–259.

Myers, J. E., Sweeney, T. J., & Witmer, J. M. (2000). The wheel of wellness counseling for wellness: A holistic model. *Journal of Counseling and Development, 78*(3), 251–266.

National Association for the Education of Young Children. (1998). *Code of ethical conduct and statement of commitment.* Washington, DC: Author.

National Association of Social Workers. (1999). *Code of ethics.* Washington, DC: Author.

National Board for Certified Counselors. (1997). *Code of ethics.* Alexandria, VA: Author.

National Council on Family Relations. (1997). *NCFR Ethical principles and guidelines.* Minneapolis, MN: Author.

National Organization of Human Service Education. (2000). Ethical standards of human service professionals. *Human Service Education, 20*(1), 61–68.

Neimeyer, R. A. (2000). Suicide and hastened death: Toward a training agenda for counseling psychology. *The Counseling Psychologist, 28*(4), 551–560.

Nelson-Jones, R. (1993). *Lifeskills helping: Helping others through a systematic people-centered approach.* Pacific Grove, CA: Brooks/Cole.

Nessman, A., & Herndon, P. (2000, December). New Jersey settlement offers strong protections for psychologists. *Monitor on Psychology, 31*(11), 20–21.

Neukrug, E. S. (1999). *The world of the counselor: An introduction to the counseling profession.* Pacific Grove, CA: Brooks/Cole.

Neukrug, E. S. (2000). *Theory, practice, and trends in human services: An overview of an emerging profession* (2nd ed.). Pacific Grove, CA: Brooks/Cole.

Newman, R. (1996). Supreme Court affirms privilege. *APA Monitor, 27*(8), 44.

Newman, R., & Bricklin, P. M. (1991). Parameters of managed mental health care: Legal, ethical, and professional guidelines. *Professional Psychology: Research and Practice, 22*(1), 26–35.

Nichols, M. P., & Schwartz, R. C. (2001). *Family therapy: Concepts and methods* (5th ed.). Boston: Allyn & Bacon.

Norcross, J. C. (2000). Psychotherapist self-care: Practitioner-tested, research-informed strategies. *Professional Psychology: Research and Practice, 31*(6), 710–713.

Nystul, M. (1999). Interview with Dr. Gerald Corey. *Individual Psychology, 55*(1), 15–25.

Okun, B. F. (2002). *Effective helping: Interviewing and counseling techniques* (6th ed.). Pacific Grove, CA: Brooks/Cole.

Okun, B. F., Fried, J., & Okun, M. L. (1999). *Understanding diversity: A learning-as-practice primer.* Pacific Grove, CA: Brooks/Cole.

Olarte, S. W. (1997). Sexual boundary violations. In *The Hatherleigh guide to ethics in therapy* New York: Hatherleigh Press.

Patterson, C. H. (1989). Values in counseling and psychotherapy. *Counseling and Values, 33,* 164–176.

Patterson, C. H. (1996). Multicultural counseling: From diversity to universality. *Journal of Counseling and Development, 74*(3), 227–231.

Patterson, L. E., & Welfel, E. R. (2000). *The counseling process* (5th ed.). Pacific Grove, CA: Brooks/Cole.

Pedersen, P. (2000). *A handbook for developing multicultural awareness* (3rd ed.). Alexandria, VA: American Counseling Association.

Perkinson, R. R. (1997). *Chemical dependency counseling: A practical guide.* Thousand Oaks, CA: Sage.

Plante, T. G. (1999). A collaborative relationship between professional psychology and the Roman Catholic church: A case example and suggested principles for success. *Professional Psychology: Research and Practice, 30*(6), 541–546.

Ponterotto, J. G., Casas, J. M., Suzuki, L. A., & Alexander, C. M. (1995). *Handbook of multicultural counseling.* Thousand Oaks, CA: Sage.

Pope, K. S., Keith-Spiegel, P., & Tabachnick, B. G. (1986). Sexual attraction to clients: The human therapist and the (sometimes) inhuman training system. *American Psychologist, 41*(2), 147–158.

Pope, K. S., Sonne, J. L., & Holroyd, J. (1993). *Sexual feelings in psychotherapy: Explorations for therapists and therapists-in-training.* Washington, DC: American Psychological Association.

Pope, K. S., & Vasquez, M. J. T. (1998). *Ethics in psychotherapy and counseling: A practical guide for psychologists* (2nd ed.). San Francisco, CA: Jossey-Bass.

Powers, R. L., & Griffith, J. (1986). *The individual psychology client workbook.* Chicago: The Americas Institute of Adlerian Studies.

Powers, R. L., & Griffith, J. (1987). *Understanding life-style: The psycho-clarity process.* Chicago: The Americas Institute of Adlerian Studies.

Prieto, L. R. (1996). Group supervision: Still widely practiced but poorly understood. *Counselor Education and Supervision, 35*(4), 295–307.

Purkey, W. W., & Schmidt, J. J. (1996). *Invitational counseling: A self-concept approach to professional practice.* Pacific Grove, CA: Brooks/Cole.

Radeke, J. T., & Mahoney, M. J. (2000). Comparing the personal lives of psychotherapists and research psychologists. *Professional Psychology: Research and Practice, 31*(1), 82–84.

Ray, D., & Altekruse, M. (2000). Effectiveness of group supervision versus combined group and individual supervision. *Counselor Education and Supervision, 40*(1), 19–30.

Remley, T. P. (1996). The relationship between law and ethics. In B. Herlihy & G. Corey, (Eds.), *ACA ethical standards casebook* (5th ed., pp. 285–292). Alexandria, VA: American Counseling Association.

Remley, T. P., & Herlihy, B. (2001). *Ethical, legal, and professional issues in counseling.* Upper Saddle River, NJ: Merrill/Prentice-Hall.

Remley, T. P., Herlihy, B., & Herlihy, S. B. (1997). The U.S. Supreme Court decision in *Jaffee v. Redmond:* Implications for counselors. *Journal of Counseling and Development, 75*(3), 213–218.

Remley, T. P., & Sparkman, L. B. (1993). Student suicides: The counselor's limited legal liability. *The School Counselor, 40,* 164–169.

Rice, P. L. (1999). *Stress and health* (3rd ed.). Pacific Grove, CA: Brooks/Cole.

Richards, P. S., & Bergin, A. E. (1997). *A spiritual strategy for counseling and psychotherapy.* Washington, DC: American Psychological Association.

Richards, P. S., & Bergin, A. E. (Eds.). (2000). *Handbook of psychotherapy and religious diversity.* Washington, DC: American Psychological Association.

Richards, P. S., Rector, J. M., & Tjeltveit, A. C. (1999). Values, spirituality, and psychotherapy. In W. R. Miller (Ed.), *Integrating spirituality into treatment: Resources for practitioners* (pp. 133–160). Washington, DC: American Psychological Association.

Ridley, C. R. (1995). *Overcoming unintentional racism in counseling and therapy: A practitioner's guide to intentional intervention.* Thousand Oaks, CA: Sage.

Rowe, J. W., & Kahn, R. L. (1998). *Successful aging.* New York: Pantheon.

Salisbury, W. A., & Kinnier, R. T. (1996). Posttermination friendship between counselors and clients. *Journal of Counseling and Development, 74*(5), 495–500.

Sampson, E. E. (2000). Reinterpreting individualism and collectivism: Their religious roots and monologic versus dialogic person-other relationships. *American Psychologist, 55*(12), 1425–1432.

Sapienza, B. G., & Bugental, J. F. T. (2000). Keeping our instruments finely tuned: An existential-humanistic perspective. *Professional Psychology: Research and Practice, 31*(4), 458–460.

Satir, V. (1983). *Conjoint family therapy* (3rd ed.). Palo Alto, CA: Science and Behavior Books.

Satir, V. (1989). *The new peoplemaking.* Palo Alto, CA: Science and Behavior Books.

Satir, V., & Baldwin, M. (1983). *Satir: Step by step.* Palo Alto, CA: Science and Behavior Books.

Satir, V., Bitter, J. R., & Krestensen, K. K. (1988). Family reconstruction: The family within— a group experience. *Journal for Specialists in Group Work, 13*(4), 200–208.

Schank, J. A., & Skovholt, T. M. (1997). Dual-relationship dilemmas of rural and small-community psychologists. *Professional Psychology: Research and Practice, 28*(1), 44–49.

Schultz, D., & Schultz, S. E. (2001). *Theories of personality* (7th ed.). Pacific Grove, CA: Brooks/Cole.

Seppa, N. (1996, August). Supreme Court protects patient-therapist privilege. *APA Monitor, 27*(8), 39.

Sheehy, G. (1992). *The silent passage.* New York: Random House.

Sheehy, G. (1995). *New passages: Mapping your life across time.* New York: Random House.

Sherman, M. D., & Thelen, M. H. (1998). Distress and professional impairment among psychologists in clinical practice. *Professional Psychology: Research and Practice, 29*(1), 79–85.

Shulman, B., & Mosak, H. (1988). *Manual for life style assessment.* Muncie, IN: Accelerated Development.

Shuman, D. W., & Foote, W. (1999). *Jaffee v. Redmond's* impact: Life after the Supreme Court's recognition of a psychotherapist-patient privilege. *Professional Psychology: Research and Practice, 30*(5), 479–487.

Silven, D., & Caldarola, T. J. (1993). The HIV-positive client. In J. W. Dilley, C. Pies, & M. Helquist (Eds.), *Face to face: A guide to AIDS counseling* (pp. 15–25). San Francisco, CA: UCSF AIDS Health Project.

Silverman, M. M. (2000). Rational suicide, hastened death, and self-destructive behaviors. *The Counseling Psychologist, 28*(4), 540–550.

Skovholt, T. M. (2001). *The resilient practitioner: Burnout prevention and self-care strategies for counselors, therapists, teachers, and health professionals.* Boston: Allyn & Bacon.

Slaikeu, K. A. (1990). *Crisis intervention: A handbook for practice and research.* Boston: Allyn & Bacon.

Sleek, S. (1994, December). Ethical dilemmas plague rural practice. *APA Monitor, 25*(12), 26–27.

Sleek, S. (1995, July). Group therapy: Tapping the power of teamwork. *APA Monitor, 26*(7), 1, 38–39.

Smith, D., & Fitzpatrick, M. (1995). Patient-therapist boundary issues: An integrative review of theory and research. *Professional Psychology: Research and Practice, 26*(5), 499–506.

Sonne, J. L., & Pope, K. S. (1991). Treating victims of therapist-patient sexual involvement. *Psychotherapy, 28,* 174–187.

Steinman, S. O., Richardson, N. F., & McEnroe, T. (1998). *The ethical decision-making manual for helping professionals.* Pacific Grove, CA: Brooks/Cole.

Sue, D. (1997). Counseling strategies for Chinese Americans. In C. C. Lee (Ed.), *Multicultural issues in counseling: New approaches to diversity* (2nd ed., pp. 173–187). Alexandria, VA: American Association for Counseling and Development.

Sue, D. W. (1992). The challenge of multiculturalism: The road less traveled. *American Counselor, 1*(1), 6–14.

Sue, D. W. (1996). Ethical issues in multicultural counseling. In B. Herlihy & G. Corey (Eds.), *ACA ethical standards casebook* (5th ed., pp. 193–200). Alexandria, VA: American Counseling Association.

Sue, D. W., Arredondo, P., & McDavis, R. J. (1992). Multicultural counseling competencies and standards: A call to the profession. *Journal of Counseling and Development, 70*(4), 477–486.

Sue, D. W., Bernier, Y., Durran, A., Feinberg, L., Pedersen, P. B., Smith, E. J., & Vasquez-Nuttal, E. (1982). Position paper: Cross-cultural counseling competencies. *The Counseling Psychologist, 10*(2), 45–52.

Sue, D. W., Carter, R. T., and colleagues. (1998). *Multicultural counseling competencies: Individual and organizational development.* Thousand Oaks, CA: Sage.

Sue, D. W., Ivey, A., & Pedersen, P. (1996). *A theory of multicultural counseling and therapy.* Pacific Grove, CA: Brooks/Cole.

Sue, D. W., & Sue, D. (1999). *Counseling the culturally different: Theory and practice* (3rd ed.). New York: Wiley.

Sumerel, M. B., & Borders, L. D. (1996). Addressing personal issues in supervision: Impact of counselors' experience level on various aspects of the supervisory relationship. *Counselor Education and Supervision, 35*(4), 268–286.

Sweitzer, H. F., & King, M. A. (1999). *The successful internship: Transformation and empowerment.* Pacific Grove, CA: Brooks/Cole.

Szasz, T. (1986). The case against suicide prevention. *American Psychologist, 41*(7), 806–812.

Tan, S. Y. (1997). The role of the psychologist in paraprofessional helping. *Professional Psychology: Research and Practice, 28*(4), 368–372.

Teyber, E. (2000). *Interpersonal process in psychotherapy: A relational approach* (4th ed.). Pacific Grove, CA: Brooks/Cole.

Thomlison, B. (2002). *The family assessment workbook: A beginner's practice guide to family assessment and intervention.* Pacific Grove, CA: Brooks/Cole.

Tice, C., & Perkins, K. (1996). *Mental health issues and aging: Building on the strengths of older persons.* Pacific Grove, CA: Brooks/Cole.

Tjeltveit, A. C. (2000). There is more to ethics than codes of professional ethics: Social ethics, theoretical ethics, and managed care. *The Counseling Psychologist, 28*(2), 242–252.

Trull, T. J., & Phares, E. J. (2001). *Clinical psychology: Concepts, methods, and profession* (6th ed.). Belmont, CA: Wadsworth/Thomson Learning.

Vacc, N. A., & Clifford, K. F. (1988). Individuals with a physical disability. In N. A. Vacc, J. Wittmer, & S. B. DeVaney (Eds.), *Experiencing and counseling multicultural and diverse populations* (2nd ed., pp. 169–188). Muncie, IN: Accelerated Development.

Watts, R. E., Trusty, J., Canada, R., & Harvill, R. L. (1995). Perceived early childhood family influence and counselor effectiveness: An exploratory study. *Counselor Education and Supervision, 35,* 104–110.

Wehrly, B. (1995). *Pathways to multicultural counseling competence: A developmental journey.* Pacific Grove, CA: Brooks/Cole.

Weihemayer, E. (2001). *Touch the top of the world.* New York: Dutton.

Weikel, W. J. (1990). A multimodal approach in dealing with older adults. *Journal of Mental Health Counseling, 12*(3), 314–320.

Weinrach, S. G., & Thomas, K. R. (1998). Diversity-sensitive counseling today: A postmodern clash of values. *Journal of Counseling and Development, 76*(2), 115–122.

Welfel, E. R. (2002). *Ethics in counseling and psychotherapy: Standards, research, and emerging issues* (2nd ed.). Pacific Grove, CA: Brooks/Cole.

Werth, J. L. (1996). *Rational suicide? Implications for mental health professionals.* Washington, DC: Taylor & Francis.

Werth, J. L., & Holdwick, D. J. (2000). A primer on rational suicide and other forms of hastened death. *The Counseling Psychologist, 28*(4), 511–539.

Westefeld, J. S., Range, L. M., Rogers, J. R., Maples, M. R., Bromley, J. L., & Alcorn, J. (2000). Suicide: An overview. *The Counseling Psychologist, 28*(4), 445–510.

Whiston, S. C., & Emerson, S. (1989). Ethical implications for supervisors in counseling of trainees. *Counselor Education and Supervision, 28*(4), 318–325.

White, J. L., & Parham, T. A. (1990). *The psychology of blacks: An African-American perspective* (2nd ed.). Englewood Cliffs, NJ: Prentice-Hall.

Wilcoxon, S. A., Walker, M. R., & Hovestadt, A. J. (1989). Counselor effectiveness and family-of-origin experiences: A significant relationship? *Counseling and Values, 33*(3), 225–229.

Wiederman, M. W., & Sansone, R. A. (1999). Sexuality training for professional psychologists: A national survey of training directors of doctoral programs and predoctoral internships. *Professional Psychology: Research and Practice, 30*(3), 312–317.

Woodside, M., & McClam, T. (2002). *An introduction to human services* (4th ed.). Pacific Grove, CA: Brooks/Cole.

Woody, R. H. (1998). Bartering for psychological services. *Professional Psychology: Research and Practice, 29*(2), 174–178.

Woody, R. H., & Woody, J. D. (2001). *Ethics in marriage and family therapy: Understanding the 2001 Ethics Code from the American Association for Marriage and Family Therapy.* Washington, DC: American Association for Marriage and Family Therapy.

Wrenn, C. G. (1962). The culturally encapsulated counselor. *Harvard Educational Review, 32,* 444–449.

Wrenn, C. G. (1985). Afterword: The culturally encapsulated counselor revisited. In P. Pedersen (Ed.), *Handbook of cross-cultural counseling and therapy* (pp. 323–329). Westport, CT: Greenwood Press.

Wubbolding, R. E. (1988). *Using reality therapy.* New York: Harper & Row (Perennial Library).

Wubbolding, R. E. (1996). Working with suicidal clients. In B. Herlihy & G. Corey (Eds.), *ACA ethical standards casebook* (5th ed., pp. 267–274). Alexandria, VA: American Counseling Association.

Wubbolding, R. E. (2000). *Reality therapy for the 21st century.* Philadelphia, PA: Brunner-Routledge (Taylor & Francis).

Yalom, I. D. (1995). *The theory and practice of group psychotherapy* (4th ed.). New York: Basic Books.

Yarhouse, M. A., & VanOrman, B. T. (1999). When psychologists work with religious clients: Applications of the general principles of ethical conduct. *Professional Psychology: Research and Practice, 30*(6), 557–562.

Zinnbauer, B. J., & Pargament, K. I. (2000). Working with the sacred: Four approaches to religious and spiritual issues in counseling. *Journal of Counseling and Development, 78*(2), 162–171.

Zur, O. (1999). The demonization of dual relationship: How prohibition on non-sexual dual relationships compromises effective therapy and keeps incompetent therapists in business. *Critical thinking about psychology series, monograph #2.* Oakland, CA: Independent Thinking Review.

Zur, O. (2000a). Going too far in the right direction: Reflections on the mythic ban of dual relationships. *The California Psychologist, 33*(4), 14–16.

Zur, O. (2000b). In celebration of dual relationships. *The Independent Practitioner, 20,* 97–100.

Name Index

Subject Index